Vertigo Rehabilitation Protocols

Dario Carlo Alpini • Antonio Cesarani
Guido Brugnoni

Vertigo Rehabilitation Protocols

Springer

Dario Carlo Alpini
"Don Carlo Gnocchi" Foundation
Milano
Italy

Guido Brugnoni
Istituto Auxologico Italiano
Milano
Italy

Antonio Cesarani
UOC Audiologia Dip. Scienze Cliniche e Comunità
Università degli Studi di Milano
Milano
Italy

ISBN 978-3-319-05481-0 ISBN 978-3-319-05482-7 (eBook)
DOI 10.1007/978-3-319-05482-7
Springer Cham Heidelberg New York Dordrecht London

Library of Congress Control Number: 2014940284

Printed on acid-free paper

Springer is part of Springer Science+Business Media (www.springer.com)

Foreword

In the last years, rehabilitation gained more and more interest in the medical field at least in the industrialized world. On one hand, clinical and epidemiological evidences highlight the importance of rehabilitation as a complimentary, but indispensable, part of the therapeutic pathway, on the other hand rehabilitation per se is the main therapeutic approach to chronic diseases.

Although drugs and surgery are first directed toward the resolution of a lesion or a dysfunction, they themselves may become source of lesion or dysfunction. Rehabilitation is not able to solve a lesion but it is always directed to restore a dysfunction and avoid a handicap.

Rehabilitation, per se or as a part of a wider therapeutic project, is aimed to return a patient to her/his own living and working environment. In other words, rehabilitation is mainly aimed to reduce the social impact, and thus at the end the social costs of a disease, an accident, a trauma, etc.

At the beginning, the goal of rehabilitation was the recovery of the motor functions but, progressively, it became a more and more complex medical discipline directed to restore every function of the human being, motor, psychological or cognitive.

Due to the complexity of the action field of rehabilitation and its "social" ultimate goal, sometimes rehabilitation resembles more a restoration art than a medical science. (About this argument see "don Carlo Gnocchi's *Restoration of the Human Person*, Milan, 1946.)

Furthermore, some diseases or disturbances may be not healed but only managed. Rehabilitation is frequently the most complete and less expensive approach to management of chronic disorders.

Equilibrium disturbances are becoming more and more frequent in the western industrialized countries, maybe due to particular aspects of the modern life with substantial changes in the life rhythm and feeding, or the modification of the epidemiology or the increase of degenerative diseases and viral infections, and last but not least, the increase in the average age of life.

Rarely equilibrium disturbances are dangerous to life but always they are annoying and expensive, both due to various investigations frequently employed to formulate a diagnosis and the loss of working days due to the resolution of the problem.

The authors of these book dedicated their last 25 years to study the vestibular system and to refine their approach to patient in order to optimize both the diagnostic pathway and, especially, the therapeutic approach. In their experience, the functional diagnosis and rehabilitation are the cornerstones of a daily cost-effective work.

The functional approach to equilibrium disturbances falls in the field of the so-called neuro-otology, a sort of super specialty which starts from otolaryngology to reach neurology passing through general medicine, ophthalmology, orthopedics, endocrinology, virology and physical medicine.

A valid rehabilitation is effective and efficient, that is to say that it is able to obtain the best and lasting functional result in the most time- and cost-saving way.

Along the chapters of this book the authors lead the reader to the management of the most frequent equilibrium disturbances, from the acute viral vestibular neuritis to elderly unsteadiness, through cervicogenic vertigo, quite a distinctive vertigo of the PC and tablet age, always keeping in mind the rehab key words, *effectiveness* and *efficiency*: simple life style advices and complex exercises are blended to obtain the best and lasting therapeutic result.

We can state that the authors approach vertigo dizziness and unsteadiness more along the pathway of the fuzzy logic than the evidence based guidelines, but always leaning on solid neurophysiological basis.

We are grateful to the authors that decided to share their experience, due to successes and failures, including tradition and innovation, guidelines and common sense, always directed to *restore* the unbalanced human being.

Prof. Pasquale Ferrante
Ordinary Professor of Microbiology
and Clinical Microbiology,
University of Milan,
Milan, Italy

Adjunct Visiting Professor,
Department of Neuroscience,
Temple University,
Philadelphia, PA, USA

Scientific Director Clinical Institute
"Città Studi" Milan,
Milan, Italy

Preface

Vertigo is one of the most frequently experienced physical disturbances and is probably also the most interdisciplinary symptom. As Thomas Brandt highlighted in his book "*Vertigo. Its Multisensory Syndromes*" [1], understanding vertigo may be approached through taking into account how vision, hearing, and proprioception interact with vestibular cues and result in the distinct dynamic balance of human beings. As detailed in chapter 1, human balance is unique along the evolutionary scale. Human bipedalism-based balance is a continuous challenge against gravity. Life, in general, is a challenge for every kind of living being. However, bipedalism-based balance presents both a challenge and opportunities for humans to change their habitat, their interaction with the environment, and their interaction with other humans. Humans have the possibility of changing the rules of gravity, changing the rules of life; they are able to walk, run, jump, and swim, and they may also become able to skate, fly, and more. Modern life demonstrates how humans are able to change the rules of the game of life, combining challenges and opportunities. The problem of vertigo arises from how the vestibular system adapts to the opportunities of modern life.

Inner ear vestibular organs and the subcortical vestibular system developed to control the balance of the dinosaurs approximately 400 million years ago. With similar vestibular systems, *Homo sapiens* had a span of only 150,000 years to adapt to managing the balance of a complex multisegmental body that was continuously moving and continuously close to falling. In only the past 100 years, modern *Homo sapiens*, who often live in a high-velocity world, have had to adapt to managing the balancing required by modern life while still using the same vestibular system. Vertigo reminds *Homo sapiens* that gravity exists, that the body has structural limits, and that sometimes we overwhelm the rules of life, exceeding the rules of our biology and overpowering our natural limits. It seems that vertigo says to us, "Hey, you are on the Earth, you can't fly, you can't live so fast, you need rest, you can't change more quickly than your vestibular system can adapt to your lifestyle!"

Thus, vertigo is a part of the experience of modern human life for the majority of our lives. Children enjoy playing in vertigo-provoking manners, such as playing ring-around-the-rosy or on the seesaw; many adults enjoy carousels and rollercoasters and many adults enjoy challenging gravity, experiencing an exciting adrenergic vertigo. Vertigo as pleasure or vertigo as suffering is always with us, reminding us that we are dino-sapiens, living here and now. Because of this role, vertigo may deeply impact a patient's life. Vertigo patients deeply suffer because they have become a restricted *Homo sapiens*, frequently no longer *erectus* and sometimes a bit less *sapiens*.

The purpose of vestibular rehabilitation is to restore an adequate relationship between the patient and the Earth, even if it is through a damaged vestibular system. Since the 1940s, when Cawthorne and Cooksey first proposed vestibular rehabilitation, the recommended physical exercises have not changed significantly, whereas the scientific approach to vertigo has changed and is a "work in progress." For this reason, the foreword is devoted to a virologist and the first chapter to the adaptation of the vestibular system to bipedalism-based human balance, the subsequent chapters on vestibular disorders begin with considering the patient as a complex biomechanical and biological system interacting with a specific disease, and each rehabilitation protocol ends with specific suggestions regarding the mutual impact of disease and lifestyle.

Reference

1. Brandt T. Vertigo: its multisensory syndromes. Springer, London (1991 first edition, 1999, second edition)

Milan, Italy — Dario Carlo Alpini
Milan, Italy — Antonio Cesarani
Milan, Italy — Guido Brugnoni
February 2014

Contents

Part I

Human Balance and Rehab

From Bipedalism to the Vestibulo-vertebral Unit

1

1.1 Introduction

Vertigo and dizziness are symptoms very common in the population. The self-reported prevalence among the working population is 20 % [1] and increases with age [2, 3]. The symptoms are often reported to be severe enough to constitute a handicap for daily activities [1, 2, 4, 5]. Moreover, with a frequency of close to 2 %, dizziness ranges among the most common reasons for consulting a primary care physician. Nearly 45 % of outpatients with dizziness are seen and treated by general practitioners or family physicians [6].

Dizziness as a nonspecific symptom can be caused by a variety of disorders. These include peripheral vestibular disorders (e.g. benign paroxysmal positional vertigo, BPPV), central vestibular disorders (e.g. Wallenberg's syndrome), cardiovascular disorders (e.g. orthostatic arterial hypotension), ocular disorders (e.g. double vision due to ocular motor nerve palsy), somatosensory disorders (e.g. polyneuropathy) and others [7].

Vertigo and dizziness are also frequently associated with other common diseases and conditions, such as migraine [8], motion sickness [9], faints [10] and anxiety [11, 12].

In epidemiologic studies, vertigo and dizziness have a prevalence ranging from 5 to 10 %; according to different age classes, they are particularly common over 40 years of age; they are the first reason for a medical visit in patients over 65 years [13].

In women, the symptoms are more frequent than in men in most age groups except for ≥70 years. The prevalence is similar across the various age groups except that in women, acute vertigo is lower for the age group 40–49 years [14].

Although there are some specific drugs for the treatment of these symptoms and specific treatment for the major part of the causes of vertigo and dizziness, rehabilitation seems to be the most effective tool for the therapy of vertigo and dizziness. The so-called vestibular rehabilitation (VR) is a special rehabilitation of motion intolerance and imbalance problem based on the head, body and coordinated eye exercises.

D.C. Alpini et al., *Vertigo Rehabilitation Protocols*,
DOI 10.1007/978-3-319-05482-7_1,

In the mid-1940s, an English otolaryngologist, Sir Terence Cawthorne, observed that some patients who experienced dizziness did better or recovered sooner when performing rapid head movements. In cooperation with a physiotherapist, Mr. Cooksey, he developed a regimen of exercises which, with some modifications, are nowadays still used. The Cawthorne–Cooksey protocol is based on the concepts of habituation and sensory substitution. These concepts are not sufficient to explain the therapeutic effects of vestibular rehabilitation.

Vertigo and dizziness are conscious symptoms, and the disturbances are not disequilibrium or nystagmus but the *consciousness* of disequilibrium and nystagmus. Thus, rehabilitation must not only be pointed to the resolution of objective disorder, but it must be aimed to the resolution of subjective consciousness of the disorder itself, too.

Such a particular kind of treatment needs a particular theoretical basis. This is the reason why we structured our method of rehabilitation on a particular model of the vestibular system.

The first consideration that moved us to propose a personal model was the need of thinking about a clear and satisfactory definition of equilibrium.

According to Massion [15], equilibrium control is correlated to postural control. Postural control is a behaviour that involves "the maintenance of the alignment of body posture and the adoption of an appropriate vertical relationship between body segments to counteract the forces of gravity and allows the maintenance of upright stance". According to Norrè [16], balance function "consists of a sensorimotor complex. The goal of this function is: stabilization of the visual field and maintenance of the erect standing position".

Both these two important concepts don't explain, in our opinion, the ultimate goal of this sensorimotor complex. Why is stabilization of the visual field or maintenance of the upright stance necessary? Why does balance "work in a subconscious way, and in normal conditions why is 'well-feeling' present rather than a detailed perception of every change"?

The sensorimotor complex that controls balance that we can name equilibrium system is aimed to allow the animal man to be a *man*, that is to say, interacting into the environment, communicating with the environment and learning from the environment itself. *Into, with and from* are the keys to understand the reason why the human vestibular system is so complicated and equilibrium is so important for animals, in general, and for man, in particular. *Into, with and from* are the practical keys of the exercises we will propose in this book.

During evolution human beings conquered an upright posture that allowed, progressively, the *Homo erectus* to become *habilis* and then *sapiens*. The conquering of the upright stance represents a specific step into evolution, and the upright stance is the base of bipedalism. Anthropological studies [17, 18] identified bipedalism as the specific sign of evolution from primates to *Homo* which required both anatomical adaptations, specifically the atlo-occipital junction and the lumbosacral joint, and neurophysiological adaptations, specifically the head-to-trunk dynamic stabilization during movement. In this condition the vestibular system had to evolve to satisfy the needs of *Homo erectus* and, according to Skoyles [17], is the vestibular evolution that allowed specific cognitive evolution of mankind.

Humans are in fact biologically novel in several respects including language, dexterity and complex culture. One trait which tends to get overlooked is bipedality. This is perhaps because two legged locomotion is biologically common. However, the manner in which humans stand, walk and run only occurs in our own species.

The human body is arranged vertically such that the head, trunk, legs and feet and their links in the neck, spine, pelvis, knees and ankles dynamically balance together to form an upright "antigravity pole". Since these segments and their points of articulation are not fixed, and the downward force of gravity never stops, the erect body exists always an inch or two away from falling. There is no locomotive use of holds, as with other primates. That the body is constantly upright is due to the unending skeletal–muscular adjustment of posture (in the manner of a Segway scooter or iBOT wheelchair). The habitual stance of no other animal has this total dependence upon the maintenance of vertical balance.

Bipedalism, as a descriptive term for the use of two legs for standing and locomotion, can be applied to a variety of animals. These include, as an occasional method of locomotion, primates (such as macaques, chimpanzees, bonobos, gorillas), birds (in general and as a specialization in flightless ones such as penguins, ostriches and emus) and extinct reptiles (*Tyrannosaurus rex*).

Humans are habitual and obligate bipeds that engage in a wide and diverse variety of erect locomotion (walking, running, skipping, jumping and dancing) and, apart from a brief period in infancy, normally (unlike all other primates) do not engage in any form of quadrupedalism. Other obligate bipedal mammals such as kangaroos exist, but they hop rather than walk or run. Humans use their upper limbs exclusively for non-locomotion such as manipulation, clubbing, carrying, throwing and arm gestures. In contrast, the upper and lower limbs of nonhuman primates engage regularly both in locomotion and non-locomotion.

Given the central role of the balance faculty in human biped standing and locomotion, it might be expected that it could be impaired during development. The impairment of this faculty would, however, not underlie all individuals with balance problems since balance can also be affected by dysfunction to sensory input or the motor coordination needed to make balance adjustments. Only one developmental condition exists that can be directly attributed to the central impairment of the balance abilities needed for bipedalism: the very rare autosomal recessive balance disorder of disequilibrium syndrome [19].

As noted above, there is a close link between cerebral cortical processing abilities including those in the frontal cortex and balance. Between *australopithecine species* and *H. erectus*, there was a marked increase in brain size particularly of the cerebral cortex. Such an increase would have provided increased numbers of cortical circuits with which to model the anticipation needed to control erect balance. Only with *H. erectus* did balance become sufficiently competent to allow for endurance running [20]. Together this argues that a radical enhancement of erect balance competences occurred between the *australopithecine* and *Homo species*.

On the basis of the over-mentioned considerations, it is clear that the importance of the interaction of the vestibular system with the vertebral apparatus is to allow

Homo to become *erectus*, to explore the environment, to interact *with* the environment and to learn *from* the environment. For this reason, we think it is important to begin our book showing the so-called vestibulo-vertebral unit.

1.2 The Vestibulo-vertebral Unit

The importance of the head as reference in dynamic control of balance is supported by evidence that the head itself supports three types of sensors: the vestibular system, which is sensitive to both gravity forces and the head, itself, accelerations; vision which is able to stabilize the head and the body with respect to the external space; and the neck muscle proprioceptive input which conveys the position of the head with respect to the trunk providing an "error signal" to the central vestibular system in order to optimize vestibulospinal control.

The head stabilized in space serves as a reference frame for the postural organization of the rest the body. In fact, while vertical alignment and centre of pressure displacement control during quiet standing are strictly important in postural control, head stability is important for balance in dynamic conditions like walking [21]. Static and dynamic head stabilization is obtained through proper tonic and phasic contraction of the cervical muscles. Due to spine biomechanics, also dorsal and paravertebral muscles contribute to head stabilization in space.

In this way, it is possible to define the cooperation between vestibular cues and vertebral muscle activity as a functional unity, that is to say, the vestibulo-vertebral unit.

Because head stabilization occurs during different tasks and conditions, some investigators speculate that motor system utilizes a top–down control schema. The top–down schema corrects head displacements preventing upward transmission of movements from the trunk so that the head remains stable in the space providing an inertial guidance system [22]. The stabilization of the head is thought to improve the interpretation of vestibular input for balance. In fact, head stabilization reduces the inertial acceleration on the otolithic membrane and semicircular canals, improving the estimation of gravitational acceleration and providing a stable gravitational reference. Head stabilization also decreases the retinal slip of the image of the world, and, specifically, the decrease of retinal slip allows a more accurate visual control of the environment. Head control is not directly influenced by input from sensorial systems; rather the complex high order of sensory mechanisms combines inputs forming frames of reference; so each sensory cue has a value of reference against which the changes of signal are interpreted. Finally frames of reference of each cue are used to create body schema that is defined as "a combined standard against which all subsequent changes of posture are measured".

The internal representation of body schema allows the CNS to represent body geometry, body kinetics and the attitude of the body with respect to gravity.

The importance of different body parts in the definitions of body schema relies on the specific characteristic of each segment itself. For example, the feet inform the position and attitude of support surface and the forces that are exerted by the support surface on the body; the importance of the trunk in the representation of body schema is justified by the fact that the trunk is the segment with bigger mass; a primary role of the head in body schema is justified by the fact that visual and labyrinthine systems are located in the head and inform on the position of the line of gravity and the horizontal; moreover inputs from neck proprioceptors control the relationship between the trunk and head.

This process leads to a better evaluation of the movement of the body segments with respect to the segment of reference and the position of the subjects with respect to the external world.

Vestibular function depends also on the blood supply and venous drainage. The vascular inner ear system is regulated by the sympathetic and parasympathetic cervical system. In this way, the so-called vestibulo-vertebral functional unit of the vascular and autonomic cervico-cephalic systems has to be taken into account.

1.3 Head Stabilization Control

1.3.1 Vestibular Reflexes

During each movement of the head and/or body, it is necessary that the image of the perceived surrounding has to remain on the same place on the retina [23]. Thus, the image of the perceived part of the environment must change in a very quick way. During head movement, the eye has to make movements relative to the skull in such a way as to guarantee immobilization of the image projection on the retina. If there is a "retinal sip", the vision is blurred; the surrounding is perceived as moving around. As a result, during head movement the required eye movement has to be "compensatory", in order to cancel the effect of the head movement. Such eye movement is executed in a reflexive manner, without conscious intervention, and it is called vestibulo-ocular reflex (VOR).

The achievement of correct erect standing position, both in static and in dynamic conditions, requires continuous adaptation of counterreaction of the antigravity muscles to the gravity force, in order to stabilize head position and to maintain the erect position itself. Maintaining upright position of the body is acquired via a continual to-and-fro movement of the centre of gravity (CoG) around the point of mass equilibrium. This movement is called "postural sway". It is achieved in a reflexive manner by means of the so-called vestibulospinal reflexes (VSR). The control of correct head position is possible through the activation of the neck muscles by means of a part of the VSR (the so-called vestibulo-collic reflex, VCR) and the cervical reflexes.

1.3.2 Cervical Proprioception

The receptors of the cervical region play a separate and particular role and constitute what can be considered as a "secondary labyrinth" [23]. In a clinical context, attention has been devoted to the neck with respect to a possible origin of vertigo, the so-called cervical vertigo. Furthermore its role in the posture of the head and the body seems undeniable. The cervical region with its structures intervenes in the elaboration of balance reflexes. Neck–body reflexes as well as cervical influences upon eye position have been described. The task of neck proprioceptors is to inform the centres about movement or change of position of the head, as this concerns a differential movement between the head and trunk. This is the fundamental difference from the vestibular system which is sensitive to head movements relative to space. Both sensory systems provide specific and proper information, thus complementing one another.

Peripheral proprioceptors of the muscles and the joints have a feedback control on the vestibular nuclei through spino-vestibular pathways. Neuromuscular spindles and Golgi receptors are dynamometers, and they are particularly sensitive to variations in muscle length and tension. Joint receptors, Ruffini and Golgi bodies, give information regarding the position of a joint and its movement. The portion of the neck including the first three vertebrae is particularly involved during the major part of everyday head movements. The paravertebral muscles of this region are very rich in proprioceptors. They are especially concentrated in the splenius capitis, the rectus capitis major, the longissimus capitis and the semispinalis capitis. These muscles compose the deep plane of the nuchal muscles. The splenius is just more superficial. They act in the extension homolateral bending and rotation of the head. During head movements they discharge to the vestibular nuclei.

The direct projection from the first three cervical roots to the inferior vestibular nucleus has been described and the convergence of the cervical and labyrinth inputs on vestibular nuclei has been showed. Convergence regards especially inputs from the horizontal semicircular canal: the electrical stimulation of the vestibular nerve induces action potentials in the contralateral abducens nerve. This response is increased when also neck roots are simultaneously stimulated. Thus, facilitatory convergences of proprioceptive inputs from C2–C3 receptors on the medial vestibular nucleus of the opposite side and an inhibition on the ipsilateral muscles have been demonstrated. The latency between electrical stimulation of the dorsal cervical roots and vestibular nucleus response is only 2 ms; thus direct projections from neck to vestibular nuclei have been hypothesized. Proprioceptive nuchal afferents on the Schwalbe nucleus have been demonstrated, and it has been shown that neurons in the dorso-caudal portion of the Deiters nucleus receive tonic cervical inputs, while the neurons in the rostro-ventralis portion receive especially otolithic inputs. Roller nucleus and the accessory group Y receive ipsilateral projections from the cervical muscles, and cerebellar projections on the nodulus and the flocculus have been demonstrated, and projections on the cerebellar anterior lobus have been described.

Proprioceptive convergences in 80 % of the neurons in the suprasylvian parietal cortical vestibular area have been demonstrated and sensitive inputs run through IA and IIA fibres that rise along the spinal cord and through the spino-reticular and spino-cerebellar fasciculus that seem to send direct projections to the vestibular nuclei.

From cervical proprioceptors arise the cervicospinal reflexes (CSR): bending the neck and turning the head relative to the body evoke reflexes in the limb muscles either in decerebrate cats or in human beings.

These reflexes interact with the vestibulo-collic reflex (VCR) which is a part of the vestibulospinal reflexes (VSR).

Vestibulo-collic reflex moves the head and interferes with the VOR for stabilizing the visual field. The VCR rotates the head in the plane of the canal. Natural canal stimulation results in contraction of neck muscles to counter the applied angular acceleration and thus results in stabilization of the head. VCR augments the VOR for image stabilization during head movement. Cervico-ocular reflex and cervico-collic reflex act to generate compensatory shifts of gaze which oppose those produced by rotation of the head. While the gain of COR is too small to make a significant contribution to gaze stability, the CCR is capable of generating large changes in neck muscle activity, which influences gaze and head position. In controlling gaze the VCR and CCR damp oscillations of the head and produce counter-rotations that partially compensate for the rotation of the body, while the VOR compensates for residual rotation of the head with respect to space. In animals with vestibular lesions, COR and CCR increase to compensate partially. Head stabilization contributes to gaze stabilization [24].

1.4 Autonomic Cervico-cephalic System

1.4.1 Sympathetic Supply to the Head and Neck

The preganglionic fibres, which supply the head and neck, arise from the spinal segments *T1–T2*. They enter the sympathetic trunk and travel upward to synapse in one of the three ganglia in the neck:

1. The *superior cervical ganglion* (located anterior to vertebrae C1, C2)
2. The *middle cervical ganglion* (small, often absent, lying anterior to C6)
3. The *inferior cervical ganglion* which is usually fused with the first thoracic ganglion to form the *cervicothoracic* (or *stellate*) *ganglion* (located anterior to C7 and the neck of the first rib)

Each of these ganglia gives rise to:

1. Cardiac branches.
2. Branches to blood vessels, sweat glands and hair follicles in the neck and head. The superior ganglion sends branches to spinal nerves C1–C4, the middle ganglion to spinal nerves C5–C6 and the cervicothoracic ganglion to spinal nerves C7 and C8–T1.
3. Vascular branches which pass to the vertebral, common, internal and external carotid arteries. Some of these branches "hitchhike" along the arteries and their branches to reach their targets in the head and neck. The superior ganglion sends branches along the internal and external carotid arteries to reach structures in the orbit, face, nasal and oral cavities and pharynx. The middle ganglion sends branches along the inferior thyroid artery to reach the larynx, trachea and upper oesophagus. The inferior ganglion sends branches to the subclavian and vertebral arteries.

1.4.2 Parasympathetic Supply to the Head and Neck

There are four ganglia in the head: ciliary, pterygopalatine, otic and submandibular.

The parasympathetic fibres of the oculomotor nerve enter the orbit with the inferior division of the nerve and synapse in the *ciliary ganglion*, which is located just lateral to the optic nerve. The postganglionic fibres with the short ciliary nerves enter the eye to supply the sphincter pupillae (that constricts the pupil) and ciliary muscles. Parasympathetic fibres also travel along the superior branch of the oculomotor nerve to supply the smooth muscle component of the levator palpebrae superioris.

The parasympathetic fibres of the facial nerve supply the lacrimal gland, the mucous glands of the nose and palate and the submandibular and sublingual salivary glands. The fibres which supply the lacrimal, nasal and palatine glands leave the facial nerve (at its genu inside the petrous bone as the greater petrosal nerve), pass through the pterygoid canal (at the root of the pterygoid process as the nerve of the pterygoid canal) and terminate in the *pterygopalatine ganglion* (located in the pterygopalatine fossa). The postganglionic fibres travel in the branches of the ganglion or the maxillary nerve to reach the nasal and palatine glands. Other preganglionic fibres leave the facial nerve in its *chorda tympani* branch. This nerve passes over the internal surface of the tympanic membrane before emerging from the skull through a small fissure, the petrotympanic fissure, in the temporal bone. It joins the lingual nerve (a branch of the mandibular nerve) to travel to, and synapse in, the *submandibular ganglion*, which is suspended from the lingual nerve. The postganglionic fibres either pass into the submandibular gland or rejoin the lingual nerve to reach the sublingual gland.

The parasympathetic fibres of the glossopharyngeal nerve supply the parotid gland. The preganglionic fibres travel with the tympanic branch into the tympanic plexus in the middle ear. The fibres emerge from this plexus as the *lesser petrosal nerve*, which synapses in the *otic ganglion* (located medial to the mandibular nerve, just below the foramen ovale). The postganglionic fibres then hitchhike the auriculotemporal nerve (a branch of the mandibular nerve) to reach the parotid gland.

1.5 The Cervico-oto-ocular Interaction

Interspecies and human neuroanatomy provide the most important advances on the influence of some tracts and cortical areas on others and how they may be felt as secondary sensorineural otic symptoms.

The protagonism of constant deep pain, trigemino-vascular auditive control, somatosensorial-auditory multimodal integration, cortical and subcortical sound broadband interpretation, corticofugal modulation and limbic behavioural interferences as CNS phenomena has been demonstrated in referred otic symptom pathophysiology.

In 2005 and 2007, Franz et al. [25, 26] widely investigated the neurophysiological connections between the inner ear and intrinsic ocular function, connections mediated via trigeminal nerve and cervical sympathetic system.

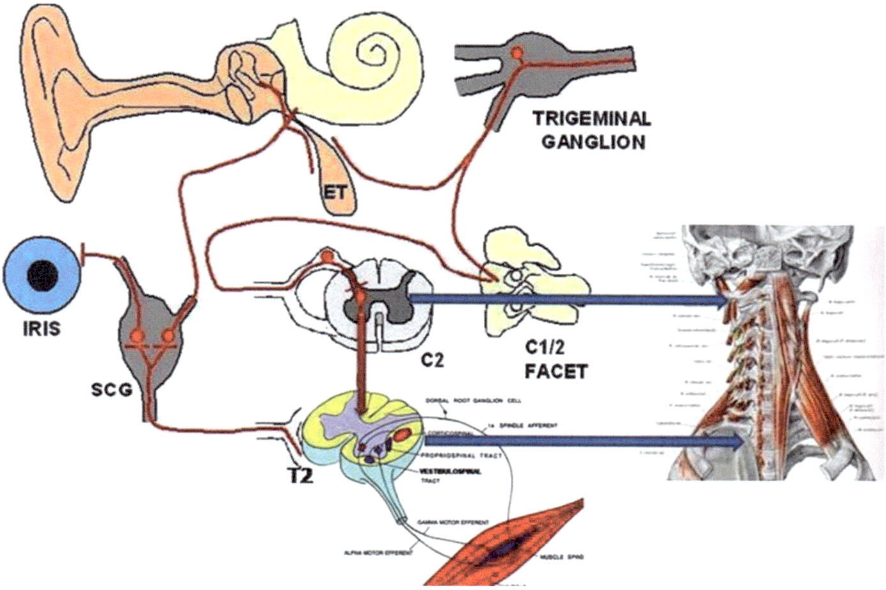

Fig. 1.1 Shows pathway that links first cervical joints and the autonomic nervous system influencing Eustachian tube function. In this hypothetical reflex pathway, irritation of facet joints can first lead to an activated anterior cervical sympathetic system via an independent pathway in the mediolateral cell column. Trigeminal nerve, in which its afferents come from the temporomandibular joint (TMJ), contributes to modulate both middle (Eustachian tube) and inner ear functions (blood flow regulation and thus endolymph production) and intrinsic oculomotricity (Original figure by Prof. Burkhard Franz, Melbourne (Australia). Modified and reproduced with permission)

They focused their attention to Ménière's disease. Ménière's disease not only includes the symptom complex consisting of attacks of vertigo, low-frequency hearing loss and tinnitus but comprises symptoms related to the Eustachian tube, the upper cervical spine, the temporomandibular joints and the autonomic nervous system. Particularly these authors observed some patients presenting normal hearing levels, a mild Eustachian tube dysfunction, mydriasis on the side of the affected ear and a functional disorder of the upper cervical spine. These patients were given a diagnosis of cervicogenic oto-ocular (COO) syndrome.

The authors described the hypothetical reflex (Fig. 1.1) pathway that links joint injury and the autonomic nervous system, where Eustachian tube function is under their influence and is the critical link. In this hypothetical reflex pathway, irritation of facet joints can first lead to an activated anterior cervical sympathetic system via an independent pathway in the mediolateral cell column; it can simultaneously lead to an axon reflex involving nociceptive neurons, resulting in neurogenic inflammation and the prospect of a Eustachian tube dysfunction. The Eustachian tube dysfunction is responsible for a disturbed middle ear–inner ear pressure relationship. This reflex pathway is supported by recent animal experiments [27]. These experiments highlight also the role of the trigeminal nerve. The temporomandibular joint (TMJ) trigeminal afferents contribute to modulate both middle (Eustachian tube) and inner ear functions (blood flow regulation and thus endolymph production) and intrinsic oculomotricity.

An integral model concerning neurological, anatomical and physiological perspectives offers a wider angle for the multiple auditory innervation pattern involving the *trigeminal* nerve. Vass et al. [28–30] found that the trigeminal vascular system innervation in guinea pigs controls cochlear and vestibular labyrinth function. This plays an important role in regulating and balancing cochlear vascular tone and vestibular labyrinth channel and may be responsible for the symptomatic complexity of some cochlear diseases related to inner ear blood flow. Trigeminal ophthalmic fibre projection to the cochlea through the basilar and anterior inferior cerebellar arteries may play an important role in vascular tone in quick and vasodilatatory responses to intense noise. Inner ear diseases that produce otic symptoms such as sudden hearing loss, vertigo and tinnitus can originate from reduced cochlear blood flow due to the presence of abnormal activity in the trigeminal ganglion.

The link between the TMJ, trigeminal nerve and middle ear has an embryological explanation. TMJ development and other neighbouring structures in humans (such as the pharynx, Eustachian tube and tympanic cavity) are complex. The mandible is formed from the ventral part of Meckel's cartilage, which is the first branchial arch. The ossicles (the malleus, incus and partially stapes) are formed from the dorsal part of Meckel's cartilage and Reichert's cartilage (second branchial arch). The malleus has a double origin in these ossicles; the anterior process originates from the mesenchymal cells (os goniale), through intramembranous ossification, and the rest form from Meckel's cartilage, through endochondral ossification. The malleus is related to the TMJ (condylar and temporal blastemas) by fibrous connections (lateral pterygoid muscle) passing through the petrotympanic fissure, which Rees named the discomalleolar ligament. These lateral pterygoid muscular fibrous connections then form the interarticular disc in Meckel's cartilage by mechanic stimulation of this muscle.

The neurological, vascular and ligamental communication between the TMJ and the middle ear is preserved during TMJ development and continues during adult life because of continuity of Meckel's cartilage through the petrotympanic fissure (causing an incomplete closing in adults). This fissure holds the chorda tympani nerve in its middle ear egress to the TMJ, among other ear–TMJ vestige structures. The medial pterygoid muscle and the tensor tympani muscle develop from the temporal blastema. These structures (along with the tensor veli palatini) are innervated by the trigeminal mandibular branch (V3), in turn innervating the masticatory muscles coming from the first branchial arch mesoderm.

The ossicular chain and middle ear muscles primarily belong to the chewing system (i.e. embryologically) but finally serve the auditory system.

1.6 From the Neck to the Inner Ear (Through the Vertebrobasilar System)

The vertebral artery is a major artery in the neck. It branches from the subclavian artery, where it arises from the postero-superior portion of the subclavian artery. It ascends thought the foramina of the transverse processes of the sixth cervical vertebrae. Then, it winds behind the superior articular process of the atlas. It enters the cranium through the foramen magnum where it unites with the opposite vertebral artery to form the basilar artery (at the lower border of the pons).

The vertebral artery can be divided into four divisions:

- V1, it runs posterocranial between the longus colli and the m. scalenus anterior; it is also called "pre-foraminal division".
- V2, it runs cranial through the foramina in the cervical transverse processes of the cervical vertebrae C2; it is also called foraminal division.
- V3, it is the part that rises from C2, from the latter foramen on the medial side of the rectus capitis lateralis, curving behind the superior articular process of the atlas. Then, it lies in the groove on the upper surface of the posterior arch of the atlas and enters the vertebral canal by passing beneath the posterior atlanto-occipital membrane.
- V4, it pierces the dura mater and inclines medial to the front of the medulla oblongata.

At the junction between the medulla oblongata and the pons, two vertebral arteries join into the *basilar artery*, forming the *so*-called vertebrobasilar system, which supplies blood to the posterior part of the circle of Willis and anastomoses with blood supplied to the anterior part of the circle of Willis from the internal carotid arteries.

The basilary artery ascends in the central gutter (sulcus basilaris) inferior to the pons and divides into the posterior cerebral arteries and the superior cerebellar artery just inferior to the pituitary stalk. From the basilar artery arises the anterior inferior cerebellar artery (supplying the superior and inferior aspects of the cerebellum), as well as smaller branches for the supply of the pons (the pontine branches). In under 15 % of the people, the basilar artery gives rise to the labyrinthine artery; generally, the *labyrinthine artery* (*auditory artery*, *internal auditory artery*), a long slender branch of the anterior inferior cerebellar artery (85–100 % cases) or basilar artery (<15 % cases), arises from near the middle of the artery; it accompanies the vestibulocochlear nerve through the internal acoustic meatus and is distributed to the internal ear.

CNS interaction between the somatosensory system and multilevel vestibular tracts is a fundamental property of the auditory system. Cranial and cervical muscular dysfunction producing hypertonicity and muscular spasm can irritate the nerves and blood vessels by muscular trapping.

The vascular relationship between the TMJ and the middle ear may explain otic symptoms in the presence of a vascular reflex from TMJ disorders. The most medial branches of the posterior group of the tympanic anterior *artery* (behind the TMJ) irrigate the tympanic cavity and the outflow of the inner ear that is completely drained by the vein of the cochlear aqueduct.

1.7 From the Inner Ear to the Spine (Through Venous Drainage)

The veins of the vestibule and semicircular canals accompany the arteries and, receiving those of the cochlea at the base of the modiolus, unite to form the *internal auditory veins* (or *veins of labyrinth*) which end in the posterior part of the superior petrosal sinus or in the transverse sinus [31]. The common modiolar vein enters the bony channel immediately adjacent to the aqueduct to become the vein of the cochlear aqueduct which in turn drains via the inferior petrous sinus into the internal jugular veins (IJVs). Injury or occlusion of this vessel would be particularly significant since it is widely believed to provide virtually the entire venous drainage of the cochlea [32].

The cochlear aqueduct and the internal auditory canal communicate with the subarachnoid space; in the guinea pig model, an occlusion of the veins of the cochlear aqueduct results in an increase of perilymphatic and endolymphatic pressure and a decrease of cochlear blood flow and endolymphatic potential. Furthermore, since many of the venous vessels in the scala tympani have little or no bony covering and are essentially exposed to the perilymphatic space, the venous system is a route of entry for the cells participating in the inner ear inflammatory process.

Another interesting point is that the blood leaves the brain by using the back propulsion of the residual arterial pressure (vis a tergo), complemented by anterograde respiratory mechanisms (vis a fronte). The latter consist of the thoracic pump increased venous outflow during inspiration:

The increase of negative thoracic pressure improves the aspiration of blood toward the right atrium. In addition to vis a tergo and vis a fronte, postural mechanisms play a fundamental role in ensuring a correct cerebral venous return.

The pattern of cerebral venous drainage changes, even under physiological conditions, depending on the body position. In the prone or supine position, the outflow through the IJVs is favoured, whereas passing to the upright position transfers most of the encephalic drainage to the vertebral *veins*.

Corrosion cast study highlights the complexity of the venous network in the cranio-cervical junction.

Schematically, two descending cerebral venous outflow tracks can be distinguished: the internal jugular veins anteriorly and the vertebral venous system posteriorly. The latter is composed of the external and internal vertebral venous plexuses, which are anastomosed by way of the intervertebral and basivertebral veins.

In the cervical region, the vertebral venous system is mainly represented by the anterior internal vertebral venous plexus, the vertebral artery venous plexus and the deep cervical veins.

As far as this posterior outflow track is concerned, the anterior, posterior and lateral condylar veins and the *anterior condylar confluent* (ACC) represent the most important connections between the intracranial cerebral venous circulation and the vertebral venous systems.

The posterior and lateral condylar veins allow for connections with the external vertebral venous system, whereas the anterior condylar veins are predominantly related to the internal vertebral venous plexus. It is noteworthy that even though the diameters of the anterior and lateral condylar veins were important, they were connected to the internal jugular vein by only a small anastomosis between the jugular bulb or internal jugular vein and the ACC.

Venous flow from the jugular bulb through the anterior condylar vein and into the anterior internal vertebral venous plexus occurs efficaciously by way of the ACC regardless of how indirect this pathway might seem.

The ACC appeared as an anatomical constant whose major tributaries, size-wise, were the anterior and lateral condylar veins, inferior petrosal sinus and internal jugular vein. The ACC was also connected to the carotid artery venous plexus by the inferior petrooccipital vein and to the prevertebral venous plexus. The numerous anastomoses of the ACC make it a crossroad between the cavernous sinus, dural venous sinuses of the posterior fossa and posterior cervical outflow tracks. ACC is a "common canal" of the inferior petrosal sinus and the anterior condylar vein of the junction of the inferior petrosal sinus and internal jugular vein sinus posteriorly.

From a physiological point of view, one should also consider that the same postural influences affecting cerebral venous drainage might redirect the circulation of the internal and external vertebral venous systems. For instance, the cranial (as opposed to caudal) connections of the anterior internal vertebral venous plexus with the anterior condylar vein could offer a cranial escape route for thoracic and abdominal venous return when thoracic pressure and abdominal pressure are increased concomitantly. One could even consider venous blood from the anterior internal vertebral venous plexus draining into the superior ophthalmic vein and cavernous sinus through the basilar plexus and inferior petrosal sinuses and thus terminally into the pterygoid plexus and facial veins.

Cervico-cephalic drainage system is complicated: cerebral, neurocranial and cervical venous blood might take different common, but variable, outflow tracks depending on posture, pressure and anatomical variations. Anterior, lateral and posterior condylar veins and occipital and mastoid emissary veins provide connections between the posterior fossa dural sinuses and internal jugular vein system with the cervical vertebral venous system. These emissary veins allow for encephalic blood to drain into the cervical internal and external vertebral venous plexuses, which represent the major outflow tract for encephalic drainage in the upright position.

Conclusions

The human equilibrium system is a very complex system aimed to allow the motor *and* the cognitive evolution of human beings. The vestibular system that subserves this complex sensory–psychomotor function, the human equilibrium, has been adapted to bipedalism. Vertigo and dizziness are the consciousness of inappropriate control of human bipedalism. In this way, vestibular rehabilitation has to be interpreted as a rehabilitation of bipedalism, both as motor and cognitive functions.

References

1. Yardley L, Owen N, Nazareth I, Luxon L (1998) Prevalence and presentation of dizziness in a general practice community sample of working age people. Br J Gen Pract 48:1131–1135
2. Chu Y-T, Cheng L (2007) Vertigo and dizziness. Acta Neurol Taiwan 16:50–60
3. Gopinath B, McMahon CM, Rochtchina E, Mitchell P (2009) Dizziness and vertigo in an older population: the Blue Mountains prospective cross-sectional study. Clin Otolaryngol 34:552–556
4. Mendel B, Bergenius J, Langius A (1999) Dizziness symptom severity and impact on daily living as perceived by patients suffering from peripheral vestibular disorder. Clin Otolaryngol Allied Sci 24:286–293
5. Chawla N, Olshaker JS (2006) Diagnosis and management of dizziness and vertigo. Med Clin North Am 90:291–304
6. Sloane PD (1989) Dizziness in primary care. Results from the national ambulatory medical care survey. J Fam Pract 29:33–38
7. Geser R, Straumann D (2012) Referral and final diagnoses of patients assessed in an academic vertigo center. Front Neurol 3:169. doi:10.3389/fneur.2012.00169
8. Neuhauser H, Leopold M, von Brevern M, Arnold G, Lempert T (2001) The interrelations of migraine, vertigo, and migrainous vertigo. Neurology 56:436–441
9. Dai M, Raphan T, Cohen B (2007) Labyrinthine lesions and motion sickness susceptibility. Exp Brain Res 178:477–487
10. Newman-Toker DE, Dy FJ, Stanton VA, Zee DS, Calkins H, Robinson KA (2008) How often is dizziness from primary cardiovascular disease true vertigo? A systematic review. J Gen Intern Med 23:2087–2094
11. Eckhardt-Henn A, Best C, Bense S, Breuer P, Diener G, Tschan R et al (2008) Psychiatric comorbidity in different organic vertigo syndromes. J Neurol 255:420–428
12. Staab JP, Ruckenstein MJ (2003) Which comes first? Psychogenic dizziness versus otogenic anxiety. Laryngoscope 113:1714–1718
13. Neuhauser HK, von Brevern M, Radtke A, Lezius F, Feldmann M, Ziese T et al (2005) Epidemiology of vestibular vertigo: a neurotologic survey of the general population. Neurology 65:898–904
14. Bisdorff A, Bosser G, Gueguen R, Perrin P (2013) The epidemiology of vertigo, dizziness, and unsteadiness and its links to co-morbidities. Front Neurol 4:29
15. Massion J (1996) Woollacott posture and equilibrium. In: Bronstein AM, Brandt T, Woollacott MH (eds) Clinical disorders of balance. Posture and Gait Arnold Ed, London
16. Norrè ME (1990) Posture in otoneurology. Acta Oto-Rhino-Laryngol Belgica 44(2–3):55–364
17. Skoyles JR (2006) Human balance, the evolution of bipedalism and disequilibrium syndrome. Med Hypotheses 66:1060–1068
18. Spoor F, Wood B, Zonneveld F (1994) Implications of early hominid labyrinthine morphology for evolution of human bipedal locomotion. Nature 369:645–648
19. Humphrey N, Skoyles JR, Keynes R (2005) Human hand-walkers: five siblings who never stood up. CPNSS Discussion Paper 77, London: LSE Research. http://eprints.lse.ac.uk/archive/00000463
20. Bramble DM, Lieberman DE (2004) Endurance running and the evolution of Homo. Nature 432:345–352

21. Nadeau S, Amblard B, Mesure S, Bourbonnais D (2003) Head and trunk stabilization strategies during forward and backward walking in healthy adults. Gait Posture 18(3):134–142
22. Gracovetsky S (2002) Le role des membres superieurs dans le control du pelvis et du cou durant la marche. Revue de Medicine Vertebrale 8:4–8
23. Cesarani A, Alpini D (1999) Vertigo and Dizziness Rehabilitation. Springer, Milan
24. Montfoort I, Willem PA, Kelders A, van der Geest JN, Schipper IB, Louw Feenstra L, de Zeeuw CI, Frens MA (2006) Interaction between ocular stabilization reflexes in patients with whiplash injury. Invest Ophthalmol Vis Sci 47(7):2881–4
25. Franz B, Altidis P, Altidis B, Collis-Brown G (1999) The cervicogenic otoocular syndrome: a suspected forerunner of Ménière's disease. Int Tinnitus J 5(2):125–130
26. Franz B, Anderson C (2007) The potential role of joint injury and eustachian tube dysfunction in the genesis of secondary Ménière's disease. Int Tinnitus J 13(2):132–137
27. Franz B, Anderson CR (2007) The effect of the sympathetic and sensory nervous system on active eustachian tube function in the rat. Acta Otolaryngol 127(3):265–272
28. Vass Z, Dai CF, Steyger PS, Jancsó G, Trune DR, Nuttall AL (2004) Co-localization of the vanilloid capsaicin receptor and substance P in sensory nerve fibers innervating cochlear and vertebro-basilar arteries. Neuroscience 124(4):919–927
29. Dai CF, Steyger PS, Wang ZM, Vass Z, Nuttall AL (2004) Expression of Trk A receptors in the mammalian inner ear. Hear Res 187(1–2):1–11
30. Zheng J, Dai C, Steyger PS, Kim Y, Vass Z, Ren T, Nuttall AL (2039) Vanilloid receptors in hearing: altered cochlear sensitivity by vanilloids and expression of TRPV1 in the organ of corti. J Neurophysiol 90(1):444–455
31. Ciuman RR (2009) Communication routes between intracranial spaces and inner ear: function, pathophysiologic importance and relations with inner ear diseases. Am J Otolaryngol 30: 193–202
32. Ruız DSM, Gailloud P, Rufenacht DA, Delavelle J, Henry F, Fasel JHD (2002) The craniocervical venous system in relation to cerebral venous drainage. AJNR Am J Neuroradiol 23: 1500–1508

Functional Organization of Human Balance Control as Basis for Rehabilitation Planning: The *MCS* Model

2

In 1999, we proposed a model of equilibrium system called *MCS* [1]. *MCS* is the acronym for *mechanic*, *cybernetic* and *synergetic*. It is a model and not a theory. In fact, under an epistemological point of view, *theory* is a complex of logical argumentations that it is as valid as it is *true*. *Model* is a complex of logical argumentations that it is as valid as it is *useful*. In this way, we proposed a model aimed to the treatment of vertigo and dizziness, on the basis of neurophysiology of the vestibular system and movement control and the most recent knowledge about cognitive processing and motor learning.

As we stated in the Introduction, human equilibrium is a complex sensory–psychomotor function [2]: complex sensorial cues are processed into the vestibular nuclei and cerebellum, mainly, and, on the basis of emotional, psychological and volitional condition of the subjects, they provide adequate motor reflexes in order to interact with the environment. The vestibular system can be considered the dedicated neurophysiological system that subserves this complex sensory–psychomotor function.

In other words, vestibular and extra-vestibular *reflexes* interact in order to provide different *functions* that harmonically lead to finalistic and ergonomic *behaviours* that allow human beings to dynamically interact with other subjects and the environment.

Reflexes may be considered the basic elements of the human balance control. Thinking under a *mechanic* (*M*) point of view, balance results by the *sum* of these *reflexes*, the contemporary but distinct activation of some or all of the reflexes, according to the need: gaze, standing and walking. Reflexes involved in balance control can be subdivided into two groups:

- Ocular reflexes: vestibulo-ocular reflex (VOR), optokinetic reflexes (OKR) and cervico-ocular reflexes (COR). These reflexes are aimed to the stabilization of the visual field.
- Spinal reflexes: vestibulospinal reflexes (VSR), vestibulocollic reflexes (VCR), cervico-collic reflexes (CCR), cervicospinal reflexes (CSR) and stretch reflexes (SR). These reflexes are aimed at the maintenance of upright stance and maintenance of postural control during moving (walking, stepping, jumping, etc.).

Reflexes are activated by sensorial stimuli and act on muscles, such as the oculomotor, antigravity and dynamic muscles. The muscles arrange the different body

D.C. Alpini et al., *Vertigo Rehabilitation Protocols*,
DOI 10.1007/978-3-319-05482-7_2, © Springer International Publishing Switzerland 2014

segments or move different body long bones (arms and legs) acting through the joints. Under a *mechanic* point of view, also sensorial cues, muscles and joints have to be considered as basic elements. Thus, vertigo and dizziness rehabilitation has to start restoring basic element activity, that is to say, that the first phase of rehab can be considered a *mechanic* phase: simple vestibular stimulations, joint mobilizations, massages, muscle exercises, etc.

In neurophysiological organization each reflex is not always well distinguishable from others. Frequently peripheral cues, such as visual or labyrinthine inputs, convey on the same vestibular nuclei or the same reticular formation. In fact, Lackner [3] stated that, under natural conditions, during movement, it is not possible to activate only single peripheral input. He remembered [4, 5] that the so-called vestibular nuclei are real multisensorial relays. They are the true *balance* nuclei that act together with the cerebellum and reticular formations and the supratentorial structures until the parieto-temporal cortex (the so-called vestibular cortex). Norrè [6] proposed to distinguish two complex reflexes each controlled from different sensorial inputs but generally elaborated in the vestibular nuclei and cerebellum: the Balance Ocular Reflex (BOR) and the Balance Spinal Reflex (BSR).

BOR and BSR represent a higher level of physiological organization in which different reflexes dynamically interact in order to provide complex *functions*: oculomotor (BOR) and postural (BSR) functions. *Cybernetic* [7] helps in approaching this higher level of complexity. In other words, thinking under a cybernetic point of view means that all the structures, peripheral and central, that contribute to the BOR and BSR constitute a *system*. A system is a network of different structures *interconnected* to reach a common goal. In this case the goal is human balance control.

A system [8] is defined as any collection of components arranged and interconnected in a definite way and any collection of communicating materials and processes which together perform some function.

By this point of view, the labyrinths, eyes, vestibular nuclei, paravertebral receptors, antigravity extensor muscles, plantar receptors, etc. constitute a system controlling static and dynamic balance.

The behaviour of any system is determined by:

- The characteristics of the component or subsystems (e.g. threshold of stimulation of gamma-motoneurons or characteristic of endolymph)
- The communication between components and their feedbacks (e.g. internuclear vestibular connections, cerebello-vestibular inhibitory pathways)
- The input signals or variables to the systems (e.g. vestibular cues, proprioceptive information, etc.)

2.1 The Human Balance Control System

The Human Balance Control System (HBCS), according to cybernetic, is a complex, open, causal, time-varying system. Every complex open system is regulated by the same functional rules. These rules are the basic characteristics of the HBCS, and they regulate the functional rehabilitation of vertigo and dizziness.

Complex systems are arranged according to the following general laws:

- Totality: every component of the system correlates with the other components. In this way a modification of one component has an effect on the other parts and on the whole system, for example, a modification of the proprioceptive inputs may modify the vestibulo-ocular reflex and modification of the centre of gravity may modify the activity of antigravity lower limb muscles.
- Feedback: every open system is a circular system in which the outputs (eye movements, head movements, antigravity contractions, etc.) of the system act as input themselves: muscle activity is itself a proprioceptive input to the system that controls the effectiveness of equilibrium output (the so-called *reafference*).
- Equifinality: in a circular self-regulated system, the same functional effect can be obtained by means of action of different components or different arrangements of system components. This is the basis for compensatory phenomena during the course of a vestibular lesion: Balance is maintained using different sensorimotor strategies in different persons and/or in different conditions. The same balance results are obtained both in normal subjects and in compensated vestibular patients when the interrelations between the different components of the system have been modified.
- Calibration: a system is steady if the components of the system remain within personally defined limits. This is why symptom threshold may be different in different patients. By the cybernetic point of view, we can state that, generally speaking, pharmacotherapy mainly acts in modifying the calibration of the vestibular system.
- Redundance: balance control is based on redundant sensorial inputs (visual, proprioceptive, vestibular, somatoesthesic) and redundant motor programmes (motor redundance). Especially in aged patients, symptoms are often due to a reduction of redundance level both in sensorial and in motor aspects. Treatment has to be aimed to increase redundance teaching on how to use residual sensorial information and how to optimize residual motor skills.
- Preference: although balance control is based on multisensorial cues (vestibular, proprioceptive, visual, somatoesthesic, auditory), every subject is preferentially [9] arranged in a precise and "personal" sensorimotor organization. Each subject maintains her/his antigravity position using preferentially visual or vestibular or proprioceptive or somatoesthesic inputs. During rehabilitative treatment, exercises have to be planned following preferential sensorimotor strategies, if they are again effective for balance maintenance or in order to modify sensorimotor preferential strategies if the "natural" condition, due to diseases, becomes ineffective.

Cybernetic laws regulate static and dynamic balance, stabilization of visual field and dynamic stabilization of the head during movement. The second phase of rehab can be called *cybernetic* phase because exercises are aimed to restore more complex balance reactions, automatic postural adjustments and motor reactions.

Anyway, cybernetic laws don't cover cognitive aspects that, in human beings, underlay motor balance skills, that is to say, the behavioural aspects of balance. In fact, vertigo experience per se, very frequently, has a strong negative impact on daily life activities, more than the functional vestibular impairment. In other words, vestibular lesion provokes functional impairment but behavioural changes lead to disability. The difference between lesion, impairment and disability is well known in general rehabilitation. The same concept has to be adopted in vertigo and dizziness rehab.

Lesion acts on a reflex (e.g. vestibular neuritis) or a vestibular organ (e.g. benign paroxysmal positioning vertigo) or muscles (e.g. antigravity sarcopenia in the elderly), that is to say, lesion represents the *mechanic* phase of a balance disorder.

Impairment regards the effect of the lesion on a function (e.g. oscillopsia or unsteadiness), that is to say, impairment represents the *cybernetic* phase of a balance disorder.

Disability is the consequence of behavioural changes that follows a vestibular impairment. This passage from vestibular impairment to behavioural disability has been clearly described by Brandt and co-workers [10, 11] that identified the phobic postural vertigo (PPV). PPV is a form of balance disorder where behavioural aspects overwhelm functional impairment and sometimes a lesion is not recognizable. PPV may represent the behavioural, cognitive and negative evolution of acute vestibular neuritis, benign paroxysmal positioning vertigo, Ménière disease, etc. [12, 13].

Mechanic and cybernetic models don't take into account the behavioural aspects of human balance control. The brain [14] perceives the continuing serial and intermodal integrated inner and outer stimuli, and it programmes coordinate reactions, physical and/or psychical. Perception ability is the basis of movement learning, and it is sometimes more important than a motor production skill. This is true especially for that particular motor skill named "balance". Human balance control acts in an unconscious, automatic, ergonomic, low-energy-expending, goal-specific way. Symptoms, especially chronic dizziness and unsteadiness, may be interpreted as the consciousness of loss of automatic balance responses, non-ergonomic stance, high-energy-expending gait and so on [15].

According to Haken's [16] *synergetic* model of complex phenomena, biological, social, economic or physical, every observable phenomenon is the macroscopic result of microscopic arrangements of its components that act together to produce the phenomenon itself. By this point of view a system can be subdivided into different levels. Each lower, microscopic, level is directly communicating and interconnected with the upper, macroscopic, level. Furthermore, a stable macroscopic phenomenon is the consequence of harmonic interconnection of variable microscopic phenomena.

Human balance control represents the macroscopic phenomenon, highest level, apparently similar in healthy subjects. It is the result of the interaction of two main, lower level functions: orientation and coordination

In each moment of our life, in every condition of our daily life, we have the continuing but unconscious perception of the geometry, dimension of our body (itself *orientation*) and the relationship of our body with the surrounding world (itself orientation into the environment).

The surrounding world is perceived as stable independently by our movements thanks to the *coordination* between head and body movements and eye movements [17].

Maintaining a quiet sitting position or stance is, generally, perceived as no-effort activities, thanks to the *coordination* between adequate low-spending energy tonic antigravity muscle contraction and gravity force.

Even quiet walking is, generally, perceived as a no-effort activity, thanks to *coordination* of tonic muscle contraction with dynamic phasic muscle contraction in harmony with the gravity force and the destabilizing forces produced during movement itself.

Synergetic rehabilitation means to restore the unconsciousness of body orientation and the automatic coordination between the eyes, head and body and tonic and phasic muscle contractions both in static and dynamic activities. Finally a synergetic approach to vestibular rehab is intended to recover a harmonic interaction between coordination and orientation.

Synergetic rehab phase is the third phase of vertigo and dizziness rehab; it is possible only when basic element activity and functions are sufficiently restored. Synergetic phase is aimed to recover disability [18].

References

1. Cesarani A, Alpini D (1999) Vertigo and dizziness rehabilitation. The MCS method. Springer, Milan/Heidelberg
2. Cullen KE (2012) The vestibular system: multimodal integration and encoding of self-motion for motor control. Trends Neurosci 35:185–196
3. Lackner JR (1992) Multimodal and motor influences on orientation: implications for adapting to weightless and virtual environments. J Vest Res 2:307–322
4. Lackner JR (1988) Some proprioceptive influences on the perceptual representation of body shape and orientation. Brain 111:281–297
5. Lackner JR (1992) Sense of body position in parabolic flight. Ann NY Acad Sci 656: 329–335
6. Norrè ME (1990) Posture in otoneurology. Acta Oto-Rhino-Laryngol (Belgica) 44(2–3):55–364
7. Ashby WR (1956) An introduction to cybernetics. Chapman & Hall Ltd, London
8. Von Bertalanffy L (1962) General system theory – a critical review. In: General system yearbook, vol 7. pp 1–20
9. Watzlawick P, Beavin JH, Jackson DD (1967) Pragmatic of human communication. Norton & Co, New York
10. Brandt T, Huppert D, Dieterich M (1994) Phobic postural vertigo: a first follow-up. J Neurol 241:191–195
11. Brandt T (1996) Phobic postural vertigo. Neurology 46:1515–1519
12. Kapfhammer HP, Mayer C, Hock U, Huppert D, Dieterich M, Brandt T (1997) Course of illness in phobic postural vertigo. Acta Neurol Scand 95:23–28
13. Brandt T, Srupp M (2012) Artificial neural network posturography detects the transition of vestibular neuritis to phobic postural vertigo. J Neurol 259:182–184
14. George FH (1962) The brain as a computer. Pergamon Press, Oxford
15. Bronstein AM, Brandt T, Woollacott MH (eds) (1996) Clinical disorders of balance. Posture and Gait Arnold Ed., London
16. Haken H (2006) Synergetics of brain function. Int J Psychophysiol 60(2):110–124
17. Latash ML (1993) Control of human movement. Human Kinetics Publishers, Champaign
18. Borel L, Lopez C, Péruch P, Lacour M (2008) Vestibular syndrome: a change in internal spatial representation. Neurophysiol Clin 38:375–389

3 The Treatment Diagnosis

3.1 Introduction

This chapter is aimed to provide those who plan rehabilitation (usually a medical doctor) or perform rehabilitation (usually a physiotherapist) the minimal clinical elements necessary to prepare both a customized rehab planning and eventual modifications of the planned treatment. In fact, the protocols we propose in the following chapters are based on some common aspects of the considered diseases, but it is well known that rehab has to be as customized as possible.

Furthermore, it is also possible that the patient is evolved, or involved, during the time between rehabilitation planning and beginning of treatment. Spontaneous or drug-induced evo-involution may be sometimes predictable, sometimes not; thus it is necessary that both the doctor and the physiotherapist have a common clinical approach to the patient in order to ameliorate doctor–patient–physiotherapist communication and, consequently, the treatment of the patient itself.

In the previous chapter, we highlighted the difference between lesion, impairment and disability. Thus, the evaluation of the patient needs to identify the combination of these three aspects in each patient. Clinical tests are used to prepare the so-called treatment diagnosis. This kind of diagnosis is different from etiologic or pathogenetic diagnosis. They have to be formulated before rehab proposal, and this kind of diagnosis is not in the scope of this book, and for them we suggest specific papers [1–4].

Treatment diagnosis is specifically aimed to prepare a pharmaco-rehab plan. Instrumental tests may be useful to refine the *treatment* diagnosis but not strictly necessary. Furthermore, it is a specific choice of the authors to highlight clinical (also called bedside) tests to allow vertigo and dizziness rehab as cost-effective as possible.

D.C. Alpini et al., *Vertigo Rehabilitation Protocols*,
DOI 10.1007/978-3-319-05482-7_3, © Springer International Publishing Switzerland 2014

3.2 Case History

Case history is often the key of a correct medical diagnosis and an effective rehab.

The first diagnostic task is to differentiate between vertigo and dizziness or unsteadiness (VDU), ruling out the many varieties of specific dizziness.

Generally speaking, VDU is the awareness of some dysfunction in the balance mechanisms, that is, a dysfunction in the balance mechanisms becomes a conscious experience. The sensation is characterized by feelings of "spatial disorientation", whereof the illusion of false movement is the most characteristic. According to Bisdorff et al. [5], the following descriptions can be transposed into the corresponding medical terms:

Vertigo: "a feeling that things are spinning or moving around"

Dizziness: "a feeling of being light-headed, 'swimmy'or giddy"

Unsteadiness: "feeling unsteady, about to lose balance"

Vertigo is strictly linked with a spinning sensation around the head. The basic impression is the sensation of loss of stable subjective relationship with the environment. In this way less typical sensations must be included and are called "atypical" vertigo. On the other hand, syncopes, blackout, drop attacks, odd sensations in the head, etc. have to be denied as primary "vertigo" sensations, but they can accompany true vertigo. Vertigo is very similar to what is experienced on a carrousel.

Dizziness may result from disturbances of integrating structures within the central nervous system. Dizziness is sometimes confused with unsteadiness and the term is often used popularly. It includes a multitude of symptoms related to the vestibular system or other aspects of the nervous system. Dizziness may be applied to physical, emotional or intellectual disturbances, which common denominators are the sensation of loss of stability and a disruption of the pattern in which the individual is aware of her/his surrounding and its relationship to her/him, whether these refer to her/his physical orientation in space, her/his emotional equilibrium or intellectual clarity. Dizziness is very similar to what is experienced on a boat or when drunk.

Both vertigo and dizziness may be spontaneous or provoked by movement of the head and/or the body, thus presenting as acute sudden unpredictable attacks.

Unsteadiness is the awareness that movement such as capability to maintain the desired steady gait or high-energy movement is not performed correctly. Unsteadiness is strictly correlated to dynamic interaction with the environment.

While patients may feel vertigo or dizziness even if lying supine or sitting, unsteadiness is perceived when walking, frequently out of one's own home [6].

Spontaneous Vertigo and Dizziness attacks cannot be treated by means of rehab.

In rehab planning, it is important to pay particular attention also to the following aspects:

- Vertigo or dizziness or unsteadiness. It is important to note which is the main symptom or if there is a particular and/or recurrent sequence between vertigo/ dizziness and unsteadiness. For example, after a whiplash injury, dizziness appears when the patient removes the collar performing normal activities, while vertigo appears during rotation or backward and forward movement of the head and unsteadiness accompanies daily life movements. In vestibular neuritis, spontaneous vertigo is the onset symptom but chronic dizziness and unsteadiness lead to functional impairment and/or to disability.

- Onset of the symptoms, e.g. immediately after a whiplash, or the day after, or when collar is removed, or after a cervical physiotherapy session, in the morning rather than in the evening, etc.
- Direction of vertigo rotation or the side of prevalent unsteadiness.
- Remission/provocation with particular position of the head/neck.
- Combination with spine pain and stiffness, with brachial paraesthesias, with neurovegetative symptoms such as nausea and vomiting, with cognitive symptoms such as amnesia and attention disturbances and with auditory symptoms such as hearing loss and tinnitus.
- Loss of consciousness associated with spontaneous or provoked vertigo/dizziness.
- Headache and/or migraine immediately after vertigo attack or in the following days/weeks/months.
- Temporal distance between any first medical visit and symptom onset.
- Temporal onset of each symptom and reciprocal combination.
- Frequency of spontaneous attacks.
- Intensity that can be quantified on a decimal Visual Analogue Scale (VAS).
- Duration: continuing, sub-continuing, transient and recurrent.
- Temporal correlation with hearing disturbances: no hearing disturbances, hearing symptoms before, during, after vertigo attacks, etc.

During anamnesis the modality by which the patient tells her/his own history can suggest to the clinician some other characteristics, such as anxiety, restlessness or depression. Sometimes specific psychometric scales can be used, but they are generally boring and not well accepted by the subject. During anamnesis the examiner can, if necessary, simply evaluate attention disturbances with easy temporal orientation (number of the present day, etc.), cultural (name of the popes, etc.), memory (series of numbers, etc.) and logic reversal ability tasks.

Minimal case history information to be collected
Onset main symptom (vertigo dizziness or unsteadiness)
Main symptom at the moment of the rehab planning and the beginning of rehab
Symptoms to be spontaneous or provoked

3.3 Clinical Examination

In the previous chapter, we showed that human balance control is mainly based on orientation and coordination control:

1.a Body segments orientation
1.b Orientation with respect to the environment
2.a Coordination of the environment exploration (mainly through oculomotion and visual field stabilization)
2.b Coordination of the navigation into the environment

Orientation and coordination are the complex, dynamic, instant-by-instant interaction of:

1. Visual field stabilization, through head-to-trunk stabilization and the so-called Balance Ocular Reflex (BOR)
2. Antigravity static (posture) or dynamic (gait) control through the so-called Balance Spinal Reflex (BSR)

Due to the same lesion, in each specific patient, these aspects of balance control may be differently impaired and leading, or not, to specific disabilities. Thus it is necessary for each patient to collect specific information about these different aspects.

According to the *MCS* model, clinical examination may start evaluating the basic elements (M) of the balance control, then investigating main balance functions (C) and, at least, documenting aspects connected with cognition and behaviour (S).

3.3.1 Eye Movements

In clinical practice, the investigator is in front of the patient. First, the examiner lifts suddenly her/his right thumb in front of the patient (at about 50 cm from his eyes) asking her/him to fixate it without moving her/his head, then the examiner lifts the left then the right and continues lifting alternatively as the patient continues fixating on them producing *saccadic* eye movements. The most important features that can be noted are the latency of the eye movements and their conjugation. Also dysmetrias can be revealed because sometimes patients are not able to fixate the thumb with only one saccade but they require adjustments of the eye movements.

Then the examiner asks to the patient to fixate on his right thumb placed at 50 cm from the patient's eyes, during a slow continuing to-and-fro movement. In this case a *smooth pursuit* can be elicited. The most important feature that can be noted is the regularity of the movement that must be continuous and harmonic.

3.3.2 Vestibulo-ocular Reflex

The connections of the inner ear semicircular canals to the extraocular muscle nuclei permits the vestibulo-ocular reflex (VOR). The semicircular canals comprise three pairs of accelerometers arranged roughly in three orthogonal planes, one set on each side of the head. In humans and other erect primates, the vertical canals are large compared with those in quadrupeds, a point of some relevance in that we have greater ability to assess the horizontal than the vertical canals. Whereas the adequate stimulus is acceleration, because of the nature of the flow of fluids through narrow tubes of large radius of curvature, VIII cranial nerve carries velocity (first integral) information to the vestibular nuclei. Further integration to position occurs at a central level and this information is fed to various motor nuclei in the brainstem and cord as well as to the cerebellum and cerebral cortex.

VOR functions in three cardinal planes. Stimulation or inhibition of complementary pairs of canals results in appropriate movement of the eyes ensuring adequate foveation during head movement. The system has a wide dynamic range sufficient to stabilize a retinal image on the fovea through most movements. This is necessary as the only other oculomotor mechanism available for image stabilization is the pursuit and optokinetic system, which functions poorly above 1 Hz.

Measures of the function of individual semicircular canals are invaluable for diagnosing peripheral vestibular loss, such as superior or inferior vestibular neuritis. At present measurement of semicircular canal function relies on measures of horizontal semicircular canal responses to caloric or rotational stimulation. At the bedside, the eye movement response to brief, unpredictable, passive, horizontal head rotations (called head impulses) is an important clinical indicator of the functional state of the horizontal semicircular canals. According to the so-called Halmagyi test named also head impulse test or head thrust test, HIT or HTT) [7–10], the examiner places one hand on top of the head, the other beneath the chin, and for each impulse, moves the head abruptly through a small angle up or down (about 10–20°) with unpredictable timing, while the person attempts to maintain fixation on the earth-fixed target (usually the nose of the examiner). Changing the direction of the head movement, from horizontal to vertical, is possible to selectively activate vertical canals. Patients with bilateral loss of semicircular canal function show loss of all vertical canal responses, as well as loss of horizontal canal responses. Patients with complete unilateral loss of vestibular function, e.g. after surgery for vestibular schwannoma, show reduced or absent responses for the affected anterior, posterior and horizontal canals, leaving the responses of the healthy vertical and horizontal canals a little affected.

Otolith–ocular reflexes may be investigated by means of a modified Halmagyi test using a brisk but small translational impulse of the head. This procedure is called head heave test (HHT) [11].

One of the cardinal signs of abnormal vestibular function is nystagmus. Nystagmus (ny) is a biphasic involuntary movement of both eyes (generally) and it is constituted by a slow displacement of the eyes in a direction (slow phase of nystagmus) followed by a rapid return of the eyes in the primary position of the gaze. Nystagmus is classified as follows:

Spontaneous nystagmus. It is present without any provocative manoeuvre. Vestibular nystagmus is caused by an imbalance between the paired vestibular structures. The nystagmus is called first degree if present only when gaze is directed toward the fast phase, second degree if present in the primary position or third degree if present when the eyes are deviated in the direction of the slow phase. Removal of fixation typically enhances the nystagmus if the lesion is peripheral and the eyes drift markedly toward the deranged side (fast phase toward the healthy side). This can be seen clinically with Frenzel's glasses that have high dioptre convergence lenses which allow a magnified view of the eyes of the patient, without the patient being able to fixate due to the blur produced by the lenses.

Gaze-evoked nystagmus. It is elicited by eccentric position of the eyes that the patient has to maintain for at least 20 s. When bilateral, it is usually a sign of central disorders due to a deficit of the central gaze neural integrator localized in the medial vestibular nucleus and in the prepositus hypoglossi nucleus.

Positional nystagmus. Nystagmus may readily be induced or, if already present, modified by changes in position of the head. The conventional method is the Hallpike manoeuvre [12]. In this, the patient sits on a couch and the examiner firmly grasps the head which is turned 60° toward one shoulder. The patient is instructed to keep the eyes open and to fixate the examiner's forehead. The patient's head is rapidly lowered below the level of the couch and the eyes observed for any nystagmus. After an interval of 30 s, if nystagmus is not found, or after the nystagmus ceases, the patient is returned to sitting position. Again, any nystagmus is normally noted. The test is repeated if nystagmus is found to see if there is any adaptation. After this, the test is performed with the opposite ear dependent. The variables noted are latency to onset of nystagmus, its duration and adaptation, its direction and, finally, associated symptoms. If any nystagmus is found after the Hallpike manoeuvre, nystagmus has to be investigated in the supine position, in head-hanging position and with brisk turning of the head to one side while the patient is in the supine position, the so-called McClure manoeuvre [13]. Typical benign positional nystagmus indicates a peripheral dysfunction, it presents a latency and it is generally horizontal rotatory, usually geotropic, fatiguable and adaptable. Although it is generally unilateral, occasionally what seems to be bilateral benign positional nystagmus occurs.

Typical central positional nystagmus occurs in a wide variety of lesions, especially those involving the vestibulo-cerebellum. Spontaneous vertical nystagmus, either upward or downward, can often be modified by positional testing using the conventional Hallpike manoeuvre or by placing the subject supine or prone. If the nystagmus is increased in prone position, it is usually decreased lying supine. Nystagmus induced by canal stimulation can also be profoundly modified by alteration in the position of the head, due to otolith/semicircular canal interaction.

Vibration nystagmus. Mastoid or suboccipital stimulation by means of a 100 Hz vibration delivered by a specific vibration apparatus [14] evoked a nystagmus when canals or maculae are unbalanced. In whiplash patients, it is very frequent to observe nystagmus induced only by paravertebral cervical stimulation of one side, generally by the same side of more pronounced cervical muscle tension and pain, probably due to overstimulation of cervical muscle spindles.

Head shaking nystagmus. In some patients, vigorous head shaking may generate a nystagmus that is not clinically apparent. The head shaking test (HST) (20–30 full cycles at around 2 Hz followed by Frenzel's glasses observation) is claimed to be a useful addition to the clinical vestibular examination

Cervical nystagmus. It is due to the activation of the cervico-ocular reflex (COR). It is elicited by the rotation of the subject with the head still. This provokes a stimulation of the neck muscles (stretching reflex), a stimulation of the vestibular nuclei and the elicitation of a nystagmus directed toward the opposite side of body rotation. In normal subjects nystagmus usually don't appear; thus the gain of the COR has been calculated to be very low (about 0.1). In patients cervical nystagmus can be more easily observed especially when the labyrinth is hypofunctional. Cervical nystagmus evocation is difficult to perform as "bedside" test.

Optokinetic nystagmus. Optokinetic nystagmus (OKN) is a nystagmus elicited by the rotation of the environment with respect to the patient. It is a compensatory movement of the eyes to pursue a target displacement with more width than the visual field. It can be assessed as "bedside" test with a small stripped drum rotated in front of the patient. This is basically a pursuit task and not surprisingly correlates well with other pursuit measures.

BOR minimal tests to be performed
Evaluation of saccades and smooth pursuit
HHT and HHT
Gaze ny
Spontaneous (under Frenzel's glasses) ny
Head shaking ny
Hallpike and McClure manoeuvres

3.3.3 Posture

The direct observation of patient behaviour, even during case history collecting, may contribute information that is otherwise overlooked.

The active and passive movements of the head with respect to the neck, the trunk and the pelvis must be estimated. Pain and movement limitations have to be noted and in a certain way quantified (e.g. by means of Maigne's "star scheme" [15]). Normal human movement is based on functionally adequate posture and achieved through the integration of fundamental movement patterns with an adequate balance of mobility and stability to meet the demands of the task at hand.

The human system will migrate toward predictable patterns of movement in response to pain or in the presence of weakness, tightness or structural abnormality. Over time, these pain-attenuated movement patterns lead to protective movement and fear of movement, resulting in clinically observed impairments such as decreased range of movement (RoM), muscle length changes and declines in strength. Functional restoration requires a working knowledge of functional patterns and a map of dysfunctional patterns to gain clinical perspective and design an effective treatment strategy.

Palpations of paravertebral extensory muscles, with special regard to those of the neck and the back, have to be performed in order to appreciate hypo- or hypertonicity of the muscles. Simple muscular force tests for the arm and leg extensory are useful. General muscular tonus can be simply evaluated by asking the patient to resist with his/her thumb and index finger, contacting them in a circle, the opposite force of the examiner.

Trigger and tender points may be routinely searched along all paravertebral muscles, and temporomandibular joint may be inspected in static and dynamic positions of the jaw (opening, protrusion, etc.).

3.3.4 Stance

Most common human activities require the ability to stabilize the human body in upright stance to counteract perturbations and to allow voluntary movements. The standing human is an unstable physical structure. To counteract the effects of gravity and comply with the requirements to stabilize the body during voluntary movements, there is a continuous modulation of motor activity, especially in the so-called antigravity muscles, based on the also continuously changing afferent sensory information. The postural control of the standing human can therefore be considered in part a dynamic feedback control. Furthermore, based on experience and visual information, the standing human may foresee perturbations or changing requirements in advance, thus adding a substantial degree of anticipatory or feed-forward control. To evaluate the significance on postural control of observations or test results, it is necessary to bear in mind the physiological background and ability to maintain upright stance.

Regarding the clinical evaluation of stance, the classical Romberg test [15, 16] (standing with eyes closed) is easily applied even in the office and may yield some information. A patient unable to perform a Romberg test with feet together will probably have prominent difficulties in everyday life [17]. During this test particular attention has to be paid to the direction of the slow phase rather than fast compensation. The Romberg test with feet in tandem position is less appropriate as it requires a better than ordinary postural control and will yield a high degree of false-positive results. A Romberg test with the neck extended, however, may contribute further information. In this position the lateral semicircular canal is brought into line with the gravity vector. A patient with a vestibular lesion causing ataxia and nystagmus falls in the direction of the slow phase of nystagmus, while a patient with a cerebellar cause may fall toward the fast phase or the slow phase depending on the site of the lesion.

Stance control is depending on multisensorial cues: vestibular, visual and proprioceptive. Sensorial interaction may be evaluated by means of Clinical Test of Sensory Interaction on Balance (CTSIB) [18, 19]. It uses combinations of three visual and two support surface conditions. Visual conditions include the use of a blindfold for eliminating visual input and a visual-conflict dome for producing inaccurate input. The dome is constructed from a white, 30 cm diameter paper lantern (with horizontal ribs). An opening for the patient's neck and head was cut into the lantern, leaving about 270° circumference. When properly fitted, the visual-conflict dome moves in phase with the patient's head movement, and the patient's eyes are about 20.3 cm from the front of the dome. Peripheral vision is restricted completely at the top, bottom and sides. The support-surface conditions include the use of any hard, flat surface that ensures accurate orientation information from the somatosensory system and a firm, compliant, 50×50×8 cm section of medium-density foam that reduces the accuracy of the orientation [20]. CTSIB consists of six sensory conditions (1, eyes open and firm surface; 2, eyes closed and firm surface; 3, eyes open, visual conflict and firm surface; 4, eyes open and unstable surface; 5, eyes closed and unstable surface; and 6, eyes open, visual conflict and unstable surface). Static balance is considered to be altered when an individual cannot remain at least 30 s in each of the six conditions [21].

To counteract the destabilizing forces of gravity, the inertia of the body, and external perturbations and the feet exert force against the support surface. In the anteroposterior plane, there are two types of corrective forces: rotational torque, about the ankle joints, and horizontal (front to back) shear force. Each is generated using a different strategy of postural movement [22].

The "ankle strategy" uses torque about the ankle joints to resist gravity and rotate the body as a relatively rigid mass about the ankles. Constant ankle torques can be used to maintain offset centre of gravity (CoG) positions. Active ankle torques move the CoG over relatively large distances to new positions of equilibrium. Because the moment of inertia of the body around the ankles is large, only relatively slow CoG movements can be made using the ankle strategy.

When the CoG is located near the limits of stability, or when the support surface is shorter and the feet are long, normal subjects use the "hip strategy" to perform corrective postural movements. This strategy uses rapid rotational acceleration of the hips to generate transient horizontal shear forces against the support surface. Because the moment of inertia of the trunk is small relative to that of the body around the ankles, the hip strategy can produce rapid forward and backward shifts in CoG position. However the distances over which the CoG can be moved with this strategy are relatively small, compared to that provoked by the ankle strategy.

Clinically they may be investigated observing the reaction of the patient to the examiner's pushes (Fig. 3.1a, b). If the examiner applies to the patient a gentle, prolonged, relatively large amplitude push, the patient has to react through ankle strategy. If the examiner applies to the patient a brisk, fast, relatively small amplitude push, the patient has to react through hip strategy.

Healthy subjects are able to adopt the strategy adequate to the task, ankle or hip, in an automatic and unconscious way. Unsteadiness and/or dizziness sometimes is the consequence of inappropriate use of ankle–hip strategies.

During voluntary movements particular strategies must be planned: anticipatory postural adjustments and compensatory reactions. In fact, voluntary movement perturbs equilibrium for two reasons: the performance of a movement changes the body geometry and thus displaces the centre of gravity position resulting in equilibrium disturbance and the internal muscle forces which are the origin of the movement are accompanied by reaction forces acting on the supporting body segments and will tend to displace them. This will disturb both the position of these segments and equilibrium. Voluntary limb movements are virtually always associated with changes in activity of postural muscles. Some of these changes occur prior to the movement and can be addressed as "anticipatory" [23]. Their assumed role is to minimize perturbations of the vertical posture that would otherwise be induced by the

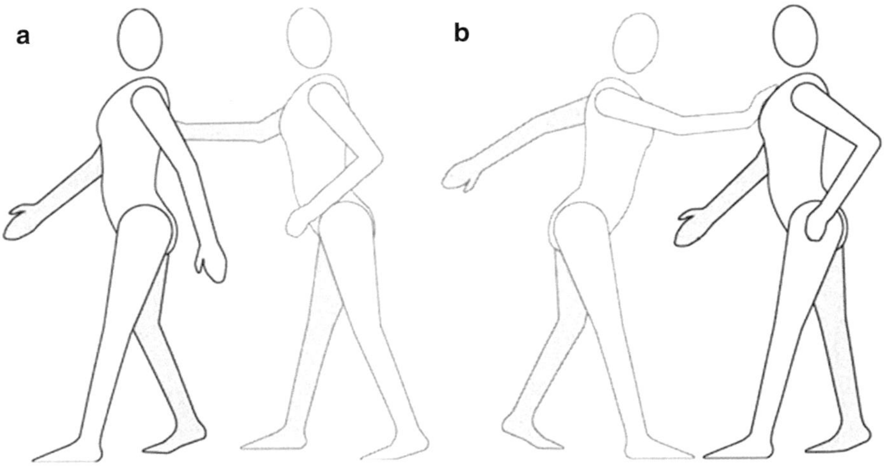

Fig. 3.1 (**a**, **b**) Equilibrium reactions to pushing stimulation by the therapist (Originally published in Cesarani and Alpini [35] published by Springer© 1999)

movement. Anticipatory adjustments are initiated by the subject, and they try to predict postural perturbations associated with a planned movement and minimize them. Anticipatory postural adjustments serve altogether to control balance and to stabilize posture.

Another group of reactions in postural muscles occur later. This group can be considered "compensatory reactions" to balance perturbations induced by the intended movements. They are initiated by sensory feedback triggering signals as other postural corrections to perturbations. They deal with actual perturbations of balance that occur due to a suboptimal efficiency of the anticipatory components.

Both anticipatory adjustments and compensatory reactions are assumed to be preprogrammed and differ in their relative timing with respect to the limb movement and method of triggering and present their own central organization, and they are under the control of cortical areas.

In VDU rehab perspective, anticipatory adjustments and compensatory reactions to flexo-extension of the head and to passage from bipedal or monopodalic stance have to be noted:

1. Asking the patient to bend backward or forward, his/her head and pelvis have to move in the opposite way.
2. Asking the patient to stand on one leg, first she/he has to shift the weight on the standing leg and then lift the other.

Sometimes dizziness and/or unsteadiness is the consequence of inappropriate anticipatory adjustments and compensatory reactions.

To investigate dynamic influence of vestibular impairment on static and dynamic postural control, according to Magnusson [24] the combination of the clinical head-shake test with Romberg and/or stepping test may be performed. The patient does headshakes for 10 s, standing with his back against a wall, then rapidly takes four steps forward. If there is an evident deviation or fall toward the side of the fast phase of nystagmus induced by a previous headshake test, this may be taken as suggesting a posterior fossa lesion. Patients with compensated peripheral vestibular lesions seem to deviate only slightly.

3.4 Cervico-cephalic Interaction

In natural condition, eye movements are coupled with head and/or body movements. Maintaining fovealization when turning the head or walking, running, etc. requires the interaction between VOR, smooth pursuit and optokinetic system and head-to-trunk vestibulo-vertebral system. Impairment of dynamic cervical stabilization mechanism may lead to impairment of visual field stabilization: the patient may perceive clear oscillopsia when moving or, more frequently, may complain of dizziness. Two tests are easy to perform in a clinical setting:

1. *Head tracking test*. The patient is asked to pursue a target (usually a pen or a finger) moved slowly to and fro by the examiner. She/he has to pursue the target with the eyes (smooth pursuit *eye* tracking), moving only the head trying to maintain eyes as fixed on the target as possible (smooth pursuit *head* tracking). When eye–neck interaction is disturbed, the patient is not able to maintain fixation on the target while moving the head, and corrective saccades are easily observed. The test may be performed in both horizontal and vertical planes. Vertical head tracking is usually more difficult to perform.
2. *Smooth pursuit neck torsion test* [25–27]. The smooth pursuit test is performed with the neck in a neutral position and also with the neck in a torsioned position (45°). The examiner notes if pursuit becomes irregular when performed with the head rotated left- and/or rightward. Head position, and then stretching of neck muscles, is the only variable influencing pursuit performance

3.4.1 Gait

Gait is certainly one of the most complex function to be controlled by the vestibular system that allows a harmonious and coordinate progression of the body into the environment. The prerequisite of gait is human being's capability to shift from bipedal to one-leg stance. Thus the first test to perform is standing on one leg with eyes open (SOLEO) and with eyes closed (SOLEC) [28]. The test consists of measuring the time during which the subject is able to maintain one-leg stance (also called Uemura test). Healthy subjects are able to maintain monopodalic stance for at least 30″ with eyes open and 20″ with eyes closed.

In order to investigate in clinical practice equilibrium control of gait, the patient has to walk quietly in a large room to and fro with eyes open and then with eyes closed. Gait with eyes open provides generic information regarding neurological aspects of gait.

Gait with eyes closed provides specific information regarding human balance control. Not only the direction of body deviation has to be noted but also the qualitative characteristic of gait: the width of the base of support, the position of the arms during gait, the presence of pendular synkinesias and the stability of the head.

A simple way to evaluate equilibrium control, simple but more specific to the balance rehab planning requirements, is the *stepping test*, which is a simplified gait in place [29]. Generally the patient is asked to step for about one minute, which is equal to about 60–80 steps. During this time, with eyes closed, a certain forward progression of the patient is observed. The main characteristics to be noted are:

- Rotation (in degrees), usually due to a vestibular peripheral disturbance
- Translation (in cm), usually due to a leg, hip or pelvis disturbance
- Maintenance of the beginning position or backward displacement, usually due to a low back spine disturbance

The stepping test is also called Unterberg test or Fukuda test. In Fukuda test the patient is asked to extend her/his arms in order to facilitate eventual rotation of the displacement, and the rotation generally correlates the degree of vestibular impairment [30]. In Unterberg test, stepping with arms in natural position, the same characteristic of the gait can be revealed: body sway, coordination of the movement, width of base support, head-to-trunk unsteadiness, etc.

BSR minimal tests to be performed
Romberg test with eyes closed, on a firm surface, on foam, with head backward
Ankle–hip strategies
Standing on one leg with eyes open and closed
Stepping test
Head tracking test

3.5 Cognitive Function

In VDU rehab, three cognitive aspects have to be considered:

1. The perception of the body geometry
2. The capability to navigate into the environment
3. The capability to perform a dual task, that is to say, a cognitive task during a motor task

Perception of the body geometry. The basic tests are the so-called classical cerebellar eprouves: the index-finger-to-nose, the index-finger-to-knee and the heel-to-knee tests. Although they are considered tests for cerebellar function, these simple tests investigate the capability of the subject to recognize the reciprocal position of different body segments; in a certain sense they reflect the inner representation of the body schema.

The internal representation of body geometry may be clinically investigated by means of a *realignment test*: in supine position the patient is correctly aligned along the longitudinal axis, with eyes open; then she/he closes her/his eyes and the examiner moves the head several times placing it in a lateral position, alternating right and left. The patient has to realign the head as correctly as possible, with eyes closed. In this way it is possible to note if the patient presents a correct sense of head–trunk alignment and to note the degrees of dis-alignment.

Other simple evaluation of the subjective vertical and horizontal may be investigated with the patient seated asking to her/him, with eyes closed, to put a pen vertically straight in front of her/his nose (subjective vertical) and horizontally straight in front of her/his eyes (subjective horizontal).

Navigation. Navigation is a function more complex than walking: subjects has to automatically recognize the position of her/his body into a specific environment and to build a reference frame in order to unconsciously calculate distance and position of reference marks, a door, a chair, the walk, etc. On the basis of this framework, the subject may be able to perform a specific movement task into a specific environment and, thanks to working memory, to prepare an automatic map both of the environment and of her/his interaction with the environment itself [31, 32].

The *navigation test* we generally use in rehab is the following:

- The patient is standing with eyes closed (better if he is blindfolded). Then the examiner, without any previous explanation to the patient about the modality and the finality of the test, gives to the patient some simple commands:
  1. One step forward
  2. Another step forward
  3. Turn rightward 90°
  4. Two steps forward
  5. Turns rightward 90°
  6. One step forward
  7. One step forward
  8. Now return to the beginning position

The real orientation test is prompt no. 8: the patient must have in mind the room, the reference marks, her/his path and so on. Thus, the patient might be able to recognize her/his new position and to be able to come back to the beginning position. At the end of the test, the patient has to draw on a sheet her/his path. The patient, on the basis of working memory, has to be also able to draw correctly the path performed.

By means of this simple test, all the processes that lead to navigation in an environment can be evaluated as follows:

- The skill to dynamically recognize the body position in the environment
- The skill to reconstruct and to reproduce a motion experience

In Fig. 3.2 a normal and an abnormal patterns are shown.

Dual-tasking. The "stops walking when talking" (SWWT) has been originally proposed by Lundin-Olsson et al. [33] as a predictor of fall risk. The test is a functional one that investigates a person's ability to execute a secondary task while standing or walking. To perform the test, the examiner starts a routine conversation with the person being tested during a walk of 100 to 200 m and documents whether that person completely stops walking during the conversation. This inability to walk and talk at the same time appeared to be an excellent predictor of falls in cognitively impaired elderly persons.

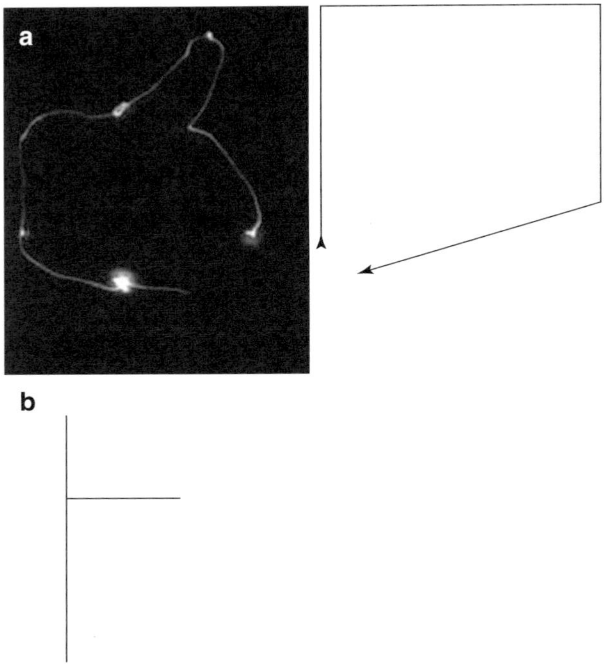

Fig. 3.2 Patient's representation of the path performed during navigation test: (**a**) normal representation; (**b**) pathological representation (Originally published in Cesarani and Alpini [35] published by Springer © 1999)

An abbreviated version of the SWWT test, based on an 8 m walking distance SWWT, has been proposed by de Hoon et al. [34]: the patient is instructed to walk a distance of 8 m twice at her/his own speed with her/his normal walking aid (if needed) without stopping. One examiner walks at the same speed next to the subject. During the first 8 m walk, no question is asked. At 2 m into the second walk, the examiner poses a simple question (what is your age?), which the subject is usually able to answer without stopping. Some patients need to stop before answering, that is to say, their dizziness and/or unsteadiness is connected to the reduced capability to simultaneously manage both movement and attention. We have furthermore simplified SWWT using the stepping test:

The examiner is behind the patient, patient is required to walk in place with eyes open, quietly. The examiner gives the rhythm, one-two, one-two, etc., and after about 30 steps poses the simple question "What is your age?" Some patients need to stop and turn before answering.

Cognitive minimal tests to be performed
Realignment test
Navigation test (even with drawings)
SWWT test

References

1. Brandt T (2003) Vertigo its multisensory syndromes. Springer, London
2. Fife T, Tusa R, Furman J, Zee D, Frohman E, Baloh R et al (2000) Assessment: vestibular testing techniques in adults and children: report of the Therapeutics and Technology Assessment Subcommittee of the American Academy of Neurology. Neurology 55:1431–1441
3. Strupp M, Brandt T (2013) Peripheral vestibular disorders. Curr Opin Neurol 26(1):81–89
4. Smouha E (2013) Inner ear disorders. Neuro Rehabilitation 32(3):455–462
5. Bisdorff A, VonBrevern M, Lempert T, Newman-Toker D (2009) Classification of vestibular symptoms: towards an international classification of vestibular disorders. J Vestib Res 19:1–13
6. Grill E, Bronstein A, Furman J, Zee DS, Müller M (2012) International Classification of Functioning, Disability and Health (ICF) Core Set for patients with vertigo, dizziness and balance disorders. J Vestib Res 22(5–6):261–271
7. Halmagyi GM, Curthoys IS (1988) A clinical sign of canal paresis. Arch Neurol 45:737–739
8. Halmagyi GM (2005) Diagnosis and management of vertigo. Clin Med 5(2):159–165
9. Ulmer E, Chays A, Curthoys IS, Halmagyi GM (2005) Head Impulse test: a analytical device. Ann Otolaryngol Chir Cervicofac 122(2):84–90
10. Halmagyi GM, Weber KP, Aw ST, Todd MJ, Curthoys IS (2008) Impulsive testing of semicircular canal function. Prog Brain Res 171:187–194
11. Ramat S, Zee DS, Minor LB (2001) Translational vestibulo-ocular reflex evoked by a "head heave" stimulus. Ann N Y Acad Sci 942:95–113
12. Syed I, Ahmed W, Selvadurai D (2012) Dix-Hallpike and Epley manoeuvres. Br J Hosp Med (Lond) 73(10):C-149–C-151
13. McClure A (1985) Lateral canal BPV. J Otolaryngol 14:30–35
14. Ulmer E, Chays A, Brémond G (2004) Vibration-induced nystagmus: mechanism and clinical interest. Ann Otolaryngol Chir Cervicofac 121(2):95–103
15. Maigne JY, Maigne R (1991) Trigger point of the posterior iliac crest: painful iliolumbar ligament insertion or cutaneous dorsal ramus pain? An anatomic study. Arch Phys Med Rehabil 72(10):734–737
16. Khasnis A, Gokula R (2003) Romberg's test. J Postgrad Med 49:169–172
17. Lanska D, Goetz C (2000) Romberg's sign: development, adoption, and adaptation in the 19th century. Neurology 55:1201–1206
18. Shumway-Cook A, Horak FB (1986) Assessing the influence of sensory interaction of balance. Suggestion from the field. Phys Ther 66(10):1548–1550
19. Park MK, Kim KM, Jung J, Lee N, Hwang SJ, Chae SW (2013) Evaluation of uncompensated unilateral vestibulopathy using the modified clinical test for sensory interaction and balance. Otol Neurotol 34(2):292–296
20. Fujimoto C, Murofushi T, Chihara Y, Ushio M, Sugasawa K, Yamaguchi T (2009) Assessment of diagnostic accuracy of foam posturography for peripheral vestibular disorders: analysis of parameters related to visual and somatosensory dependence. Clin Neurophysiol 120:1408–1414

21. Black FO, Wall C 3rd, Nashner LM (1983) Effects of visual and support surface orientation references upon postural control in vestibular deficient subjects. Acta Otolaryngol 95(3–4):199–201
22. Nashner LM, Black FO, Wall C 3rd (1982) Adaptation to altered support and visual conditions during stance: patients with vestibular deficits. J Neurosci 2(5):536–544
23. Nashner LM (1983) Analysis of movement control in man using the movable platform. Adv Neurol 39:607–619
24. Magnusson M (1994) Evaluation of brainstem-cerebellar posture control. In: Cesarani A, Alpini D (eds) Equilibrium disorders. Brainstem and cerebellar pathology. Springer, Milan, pp 52–59
25. Tjell C, Rosenhall U (1998) Smooth pursuit neck torsion test: a specific test for cervical dizziness. Am J Otol 19(1):76–81
26. Treleaven J, Gwendolen J, LowChoy N (2005) Smooth pursuit neck torsion test in whiplash-associated disorders: relationship to self-reports of neck pain and disability, dizziness and anxiety. J Rehabil Med 37:219–223
27. Yu LJ, Stokell R, Treleaven J (2011) The effect of neck torsion on postural stability in subjects with persistent whiplash. Man Ther 16(4):339–343
28. Kita I, Sakamoto M, Ryushi T, Aihara Y, Arita H (1998) Dynamics of human cardiorespiratory responses to standing on one leg with eyes closed. Eur J Appl Physiol Occup Physiol 77(1–2):60–65
29. Horak F, Buchanan J, Creath R, Jeka J (2002) Vestibulospinal control of posture. Adv Exp Med Biol 508:139–145
30. Petersen JA, Straumann D, Weber KP (2013) Clinical diagnosis of bilateral vestibular loss: three simple bedside tests. Ther Adv Neurol Disord 6(1):41–45
31. Maguire EA, Burgess N, Donnett JG, Frackowiak RSJ, Frith CD, O'Keefe J (1998) Knowing where, and getting there: a human navigation network. Science 280:921–924
32. Maguire EA, Valentine ER, Wilding JM, Kapur N (2003) Routes to remembering: the brains behind superior memory. Nat Neurosci 6:90–95
33. Lundin-Olsson L, Nyberg L, Gustafson Y (1997) "Stops walking when talking" as a predictor of falls in elderly people [letter]. Lancet 349:617
34. de Hoon EW, Allum JH, Carpenter MG, Salis C, Bloem BR, Conzelmann M, Bischof HA (2003) Quantitative assessment of the stops walking while talking test in the elderly. Arch Phys Med Rehabil 84:838–842
35. Cesarani A, Alpini D (1999) Vertigo and dizziness rehabilitation – the MCS method. Springer, Milan/Heidelberg

Vestibular Rehab: From Cawthorne–Cooksey to Vertigo School

4

4.1 Introduction

The human equilibrium system derives much of its strength and plasticity from the fact that the specific neuronal and growing software is moulded in childhood during the maturation phase, under the influence of permanent information from the world we live in. The software overlying the structural, sensorial and central nervous hardware creates the so-called space concept within the brain. Failures of the sensory inputs as well as of the central balance regulation may lead to various expressions of the illness such as vertigo, nausea and vomiting, blurred vision, nystagmus, head and body instability, changes in cardiac rhythm and metabolic alterations. The system has many inborn possibilities for internal stabilization and compensation; in fact after injuries there are different neurophysiological phenomena involved in the restoration of balance control [1].

The milestones of the early spontaneous static compensation mark the re-establishment of static gaze stability, which provides a common coordinate frame for the brain to interpret residual vestibular information in the context of visual, somatosensory and visceral signals that convey gravitoinertial information. Stabilization of the head orientation and the eye orientation (suppression of spontaneous nystagmus) appears to be necessary [2].

Two modes of neural plasticity occur in the vestibular system following vestibular loss (e.g. due to neuritis): one mode being the limited central compensation for the loss and the second mode being some restoration of peripheral vestibular function [3].

The symptoms of a vestibular lesion, vertigo, dizziness and unsteadiness (VDU), are thought to result from changes in the activity of vestibular sensorimotor reflexes. Since the vestibular nuclei must be intact for recovery to occur, many investigations have focused on studying these neurons after lesions. At present, the neuronal plasticity underlying early recovery from the static symptoms is not fully understood, but rebalancing of excitatory synaptic drive bilaterally is essential for vestibular compensation to proceed [4].

D.C. Alpini et al., *Vertigo Rehabilitation Protocols*,
DOI 10.1007/978-3-319-05482-7_4, © Springer International Publishing Switzerland 2014

4.2 Vestibular Compensation

Vestibular compensation involves multiple, parallel plastic processes at various sites in the brain. Experimental evidence suggests that adaptive changes in the sensitivity of ipsilesional vestibular neurons to the inhibitory neurotransmitters GABA and glycine, changes in the electrophysiological excitability of vestibular neurons, changes in the inhibitory control of the brainstem vestibular networks by the cerebellum, gliosis and neurogenesis in the ipsilesional vestibular nuclei and activity-dependent reorganization of the synaptic connectivity of the vestibular pathways are mechanisms involved in compensation [5].

Rehabilitation specifically acts activating one or more of the neurophysiological phenomena of vestibular compensation. They are as follows [6, 7]:

Restitution can be defined as a complete reparation after a temporarily limited lesion.

Adaptation means that the human equilibrium system can adapt itself to physiologically, as well as pathologically, altered conditions. The central regulatory system can alter the sensitivity of the vestibular, retinal and other receptors used to regulate equilibrium. It comprises all phenomena which ensure that a patient with a persisting peripheral dysfunctional state attains a normal – or near-normal – behaviour in relation to his/her space orientation and balance in rest as well as when executing movements. He/She again maintains his/her erect standing position and has no more "odd" feeling categorized as vertigo or dizziness. Hereto a number of mechanisms contribute, acting at different levels of the central nervous system. The first definition can be applied to adaptation in the strict physiological sense: a change of response during application of a stimulus, as, e.g. a prolonged acceleration which brings about a response decline. Fatigue is characterized by a response decline which develops slowly. It increases with stimulus intensity and progresses indefinitely with time. Such adaptation is characterized by a response decline which develops rapidly at first and thereafter slowly, finally reaching a constant or fully adapted level. Adaptation phenomena in the same time sense are also attributed to a mechanism at the level of the cupola, which is also direction specific. The second definition fits the broader concept of adaptation. The messages sent by the sense organs into the brainstem are more and more suppressed and prevented from reaching the higher centres the longer the steady state in the surrounding world persists. The subject has adapted itself to conditions imposed by the outer world. Yet the slightest change in stimulatory conditions not pertaining to the steady state will alarm.

Habituation is defined by the reduction of the intensity and duration of the subjective vestibular reactions, for example, vertigo and nausea in the case of seasickness. Habituation is a term used in the sense that repeated exposure to a "mismatched" sensory situation (e.g. during caloric testing, postural vertigo, motion sickness conditions) induces such changes in the central processing as to annihilate the undesirable effects and to do so with a prolonged effect. It has been based upon the development of conditioned compensatory reactions to oppose inappropriate responses associated with visuo-vestibular conflicts and exposure to unusual motion environments. The basic characteristics of vestibular habituation, regarding oculomotor aspects, are:

- Acquisition, which is manifested by a progressive decline of VOR response during the period of stimulation.
- Retention, which is manifested by the persistence of modified VOR response after a period of rest. It is cumulative and long persisting.
- Certain specificity for the habituating stimulus transfer, which is manifested by the presence of a modification in responses evoked either by patterns of vestibular stimulation different from those used to provoke habituation or by other sensory stimulation, such as optokinetic stimulation.

Habituation is a specific phenomenon. The possibility of obtaining unilateral habituation by unidirectional vestibular stimulations suggests that habituation is due to selective mechanisms that modify not only the gain but also the dynamic characteristics of the VOR. Unilateral habituation to step stimulation has been shown in the cat. VOR habituation is direction specific. It proves that right and left VOR pathways can be controlled separately in order to obtain a greater system adaptability. Habituation is a central mechanism for which vestibular stimulation is not a necessary condition, since exposure to purely non-vestibular input led to vestibular habituation. The production of nystagmus by the habituating stimulus seems unrelated to the efficacy. The habituating stimulus must produce the same subjective sensation of motion as that produced by true body motion in order to habituate vestibular nystagmus. Habituation represents the simplest type of *negative learning*: stimuli that have lost their significance for the individual are eliminated

Compensation describes another type of central nervous counter-regulation as a result of functional deterioration due to a vestibular or other equilibrium lesion. It utilizes supplementary functions which are added so that an overlay of additionally activated functions covers the underlying equilibrium lesions by means of its neuronal plasticity. However primary lesion continues to exist and can, in the case of a special conflict, manifest itself in the clinical phenomenology. Compensation is a term used in the context of phenomena which are described after unilateral failure of vestibular function. Restricted to the vestibular sphere, it includes those phenomena which cause the imbalance of vestibulo-ocular and vestibulospinal responses seen immediately after an acute unilateral failure of the vestibular system disappear. This compensation at the vestibular level consists in the disappearance of all asymmetries (static and dynamic) in the ocular and vestibulospinal responses. In many cases substitutive interactions by visual and proprioceptive systems are required as well as some more central processes of reorganization of the reflexes in order to reach a sufficient adaptation level. Compensation is a *learning* process. The phenomenon resembles a sensorimotor relearning process implicating the activity of many integrative CNS structures. Active sensorimotor exploration provides the information to detect the errors and to correct them. Repetition of trials promotes the restructure of the motor programmes. Compensation implies reorganization of the remaining structures. Changes induced by the lesion as such would not necessarily lead to functional appropriate adaptation, but rather to randomly formed synapses which may or may not be mismatched to functional needs. This "rewiring" does not result in functionally meaningless outcome, but rather leads to a new and complex circuitry, the activity of which is appropriate for the restoration of normal function. It is a goal-directed process induced by some recognized "error" in the system and directed to its elimination. Thus compensation may be defined as an error-controlled and goal-directed learning process.

These phenomena lead to different levels of recovery. Recovery is essentially due to the integration of different levels of substitution:

- *Sensorial* substitution, in which the movement of the subject is identical to the one before lesion but the subject uses different sets of sensory receptors for triggering and control
- *Functional* substitution, in which the neuronal mechanisms subtending the movement have been changed but still belong to the subsystems normally used by the subject
- *Behavioural* substitution, by which the nervous system calls for new motor behaviours not belonging to its normal repertoire

Knowledge of the recovery phenomena following human balance control disturbance (VDU) is fundamental for planning a correct treatment.

Acute vestibular lesion is a good model to explain the main neurophysiological processes involved in the recovery of equilibrium function. Its evolution has been broadly studied in animals and it can be schematically subdivided into different stages:

- Critical stage: immediately after the lesion, the animal exhibits severe symptoms of imbalance including rapid spontaneous nystagmus, severe head deviation and forced circling and rolling toward the deafferented side.
- Acute stage: it is marked by a rapid partial recovery of asymmetry.
- Compensatory stage: the animal's recovery becomes maximal.

The duration of each period is species dependent as is the level of recovery achieved.

Generally speaking, the evolution of a lesion can be interpreted into three stages of damage:

- The primary damage: the lesion that induces the onset of symptomatology
- The secondary damage: the pathological modification of the compensatory systems
- The tertiary damage: chronicization of pathological adaptive phenomena

Treatment had to be pointed to limit primary damage (usually by means of pharmacotherapy), to reduce secondary damage and to avoid tertiary damage.

According to the *MCS* model, we can simplify the course of the disease hypothesizing that each phenomenon acts separately and consequently from each other.

The first *mechanism* following a vestibular injury is *adaptation*, acting by activation of the internuclear inhibition [8] that is aimed to reduce the activity of the healthy vestibular nuclei. In compensation considered at vestibular level, the commissural fibres play an important role, especially for dynamic compensation. The influence of the remaining labyrinth upon the deafferented nucleus can take place via the commissural fibres, which are the natural means of reciprocal influencing. Another early mechanism is the inhibitory influence of the cerebellum. It has been called the "first line of defence". It is considered a reset to zero as a preliminary requirement to the subsequent recalibration process. This can be considered a *mechanic* phase of compensation. This phase is activated by feedback signals.

Vestibular inhibition is supported by the first compensation phenomenon: sensorial substitution. In particular, vision experience is critical for the acquisition and maintenance of recovery for the abnormally reduced VOR gain created by unilateral vestibular lesion. There has been evidence for the effect of darkness upon the evolution of the lateral head tilt, in the cat, after hemilabyrinthectomy [7, 9]. When put back in the dark at a late postoperative stage, already-compensated animals lose their symmetrical head position. Static visual input is a necessary condition for compensation of both ocular and postural deficits. Vision provides a sensory supply in place of the deficient vestibular supply. This supposes an increased sensitivity of the neurons of the vestibular nuclei for fast changes in the environment. Sensorial substitution is rapidly followed by and it is based on the law of "redundancy." Human balance control is multisensorial based. In this way a vestibular sensorial input deficit may be compensated by reducing inhibition of cervical or other proprioceptive information or increasing visual inputs to the vestibular nuclei. The choice of which sensorial input will substitute the loss input is based on individual preference.

The second phase is recalibration that requires modification of the calibration of the subsystems. It is often accompanied by habituation phenomena. This can be considered the *cybernetic* phase of compensation [10].

The last phase of compensation is radical reorganization of balance control. The law is the equifinality that is behavioural substitution. Sensorial inputs, activity of vestibular nuclei, motor outputs and in general sensorimotor patterns are reorganized to allow the same function: equilibrium. Structural reorganization leads to a total or partial recovery of function and involves plastic structural changes and/or more global functional rearrangements of the neuronal networks, which are generally considered as the main processes underlying behavioural adaptations. This is the *synergetic* phase. This is the ultimate goal of the treatment.

4.3 Vestibular Rehabilitation

Vestibular rehabilitation is a special rehabilitation of motion intolerance and imbalance problems. Vestibular rehabilitation (VR) is an exercise-based treatment programme designed to promote vestibular adaptation and substitution. The goals of VR are (1) to enhance gaze stability, (2) to enhance postural stability, (3) to avoid vertigo and (4) to improve activities of daily living. VR facilitates vestibular recovery mechanisms: vestibular adaptation, substitution by the other eye-movement systems, substitution by vision, somatosensory cues, other postural strategies and

Table 4.1 Cawthorne–Cooksey protocol

In bed or sitting
Eye movements – at first slow, then quick
Up and down
From side to side
Focusing on the finger moving from 3 feet to 1 foot away from face
Head movements – at first slow, then quick, later with eyes closed
Bending forward and backward
Turning from side to side
Sitting
Eye movements and head movements as above
Shoulder shrugging and circling
Bending forward and picking up objects from the ground
Standing
Eye, head and shoulder movements as before
Changing form sitting to standing position with eyes open and then closed
Throwing a small ball from hand to hand (above eye level)
Throwing a ball from hand to hand under knee
Changing from sitting to standing and turning around in between
Moving about (in class)
Circle around centre person who will throw a large ball and to whom it will be returned
Walk across room with eyes open and then closed
Walk up and down the slope with eyes open and then closed
Walk up and down the steps with eyes open and then closed
Any game involving stooping and stretching and aiming such as bowling and basketball

habituation. The key exercises for VR are head–eye movements with various body postures and activities and maintaining balance with a reduced support base with various orientations of the head and trunk while performing various upper-extremity tasks, repeating the movements provoking vertigo and exposing patients gradually to various sensory and motor environments. VR is indicated for any stable but poorly compensated vestibular lesion, regardless of the patient's age, the cause and symptom duration and intensity.

The concept of head, body and coordinated eye exercises as a treatment for vestibular disorders is actually over 70 years. As far back as the mid-1940s, an English otolaryngologist, Sir Terence Cawthorne [11], observed that some patients who experienced dizziness did better or recovered sooner when performing rapid head movements. In cooperation with a physiotherapist, Cooksey [12], they developed a regimen of exercises which, with some modifications, are frequently still used today. The earliest vestibular rehabilitation, thus based on the so-called Cawthorne–Cooksey exercises, was developed to treat patients with labyrinth injury resulting from surgery or head injury. Their value in managing all forms of peripheral vestibular disorders rapidly became apparent, and they now form the mainstay of treatment for this group of patients. Cawthorne–Cooksey [13] protocol is shown in Table 4.1.

4.4 Vertigo School

Generally speaking, the exercises for vestibular rehabilitation can be categorized [14, 15] into two types: (1) physical therapy for vestibular hypofunction and (2) canalith repositioning therapy for benign paroxysmal positional vertigo (BPPV).

This point of view, on one hand, is reductive and, on the other, is wrong.

The eye–head and head–body exercises of Cawthorne–Cooksey protocol, combined with proprioceptive exercises (so-called balance rehabilitation therapy, balance retraining therapy), may be used to improve static and dynamic balance control in the major part of the diseases and disturbances that provoke vertigo, dizziness and/or unsteadiness (VDU).

Furthermore, under the point of view of rehabilitative medicine, physical therapy that promotes functional restoration despite the persistence of the lesion is considered *rehabilitation*, exercises or manoeuvres that solve both the impairment and the "lesion", as in the case of BPPV, in which one has to consider *re-education*. Even if the two terms are used synonymously, they regard two completely different approaches and have completely different goals and outcome expectations. In other words, the aim of *re-education* is *restitutio ad integrum*, while the aim of *rehabilitation* is *restitutio ad functionem*.

Rehabilitation is mainly a *teaching* process that begins in the brainstem and the cerebellum and leads to a radical reorganization of both subcortical and cortical sensorimotor pattern by which the patient *learns* how to manage her/his disease, to cope her/his symptoms, to recover her/his impairment and to avoid disability. Thus, as far as our experience is concerned, the keyword of balance control rehab is *learning*. The other two keywords of rehabilitative medicine, in general, are *efficacy* and *efficiency* Thus, the scope of our approach is to rehab the major part of patients complaining VDU, despite the disease, as effectively and efficiently as possible.

Each pathological condition induces VDU through specific key mechanisms and thus rehab recognizes specific key points for specific treatments. Furthermore, rehab has to be as more customized as possible.

We named our rehab approach Vertigo School because, combining Cawthorne–Cooksey protocol and MCS model, we can prepare disease-specific programmes that can be customized on the basis of the diagnosis of treatment (see Chap. 2). The term *vertigo* is used in this context as generally used by population and thus as generic synonymous of VDU.

Vertigo School approach is inspired by Back School and Neck School principles.

The *Back School* method was developed in 1969 by Mariane Zachrisson Forssell, with the goal of preventing and avoiding recurrent episodes of low back pain. The programme is composed of 4 sessions lasting approximately 45 min, each session being organized by theoretical components, which include anatomy and spinal biomechanics, epidemiology, physiopathology of the most frequent back disorders, posture, ergonomics, common treatment modalities and a practical component (exercises for the maintenance of a "healthy back") [16].

The *Neck School* [17, 18] is based on multimodal treatment emphasizing proprioceptive exercises with both neck lecture and activated home exercise and neck lecture with a recommendation of exercise in patients with chronic nonspecific neck pain.

Our VDU rehab protocols are based on the same *mix of educational and training approach*. Vertigo School is organized into three phases:

1. Counselling
2. Training
3. Home training

4.4.1 Counselling

The role of the doctor in balance control rehab is three folded:

1. To formulate the diagnosis of treatment in order to provide to rehabilitator the main guidelines of treatment of a specific patient
2. To plan the drug treatment of both the symptoms (VDU) and the cause of vestibular disorder that provokes those symptoms in that specific patient
3. To take care of patient in order to correct also lifestyle, if necessary, in order to avoid disability and to stabilize the therapeutic results

When the patient is proposed for a rehabilitation programme, it is necessary to explicate to her/him in the simplest way [19]:

- Which is the role of the vestibular system in the human balance control?
- What is vertigo and dizziness?
- Which are recovery phenomena of a vestibular disorder?
- Which is the natural course of the patient's disturbance (that is to say, the time planning of the disease and its natural recovery)?
- What is vestibular rehab and what is its role in ameliorating both the natural course and the functional recover?
- Which are the patient's general health disturbances that may interfere on both VDU and the recovery?
- Which aspects of her/his lifestyle have to be modified to improve the outcome, to stabilize the results and to avoid relapses?

Regarding lifestyle for each vestibular disturbance, specific indications will be provided into the following dedicated chapter.

Any more, there are some general, but not generic, suggestions that may be provided as in Table 4.2.

4.4.2 Training

Training is generally performed in a gymnasium and rehab may be planned as single patient treatment or as small group (3–4 patients). The diagnosis of treatment leads to single or small-group planning.

Table 4.2 General suggestions to improve global health and thus balance control

Control own Body Mass Index (BMI) BMI is correlated to body fatness and it is calculated as body weight (in kilos) divided by square height (in metres); e.g. a subject weighed 70 k and 1.74 m height has a BMI as follows: 70/(1.74 × 1.74) = 23.1. Normal values are between 18.5 and 24.9 (World Health Organization, WHO)
Perform regular and constant aerobic physical activity: e.g. rapid walking (not running nor jogging) 30′ a day three times/week
Restrict calorie intake (particularly soft drinks)
Restrict red beef meat intake (less than 500 g/week) and to avoid preserved meat
Maintain a diet rich in fruits and vegetables (five servings/day)
Avoid industrial food
Maintain adequate water intake (at least 1.5 l for females and 2 l for males)
Restrict alcohol intake (less than 120 ml for women and 240 ml for men)
Restrict salt intake (less than 5 g/day) in males over 45 years old and females over 50 years (if not a hypotensive subject)
Avoid smoke and, obviously, drug abuse

Although protocols are standardized on the basis of the disorder that provoked VDU in the patient, exercises have to be customized on the basis of diagnosis of treatment that may be reformulated by the therapist as we explained in Chap. 2.

Rehab planning requires two or three sessions a week, 45′ each, for 3 or 4 weeks (10–12 sessions). Exercises progression is organized on the basis of the *MCS* model.

According to the considerations about recovery phenomena, we can state that the therapeutic treatment must be planned according to three different levels:

1. *Mechanic*: enforcement of extensor muscles, mobilization of the main joints like ankle, hip, etc. The patient *acts to* the environment.
2. *Cybernetic*: interaction between ocular and spinal performances. The patient *interacts with* the environment.
3. *Synergetic*: integration of cognitive and movement performances. The patient *learns from* the environment.

The *mechanic phase* (generally three sessions/week) of treatment can be directly resolutive on the primary lesion if it is caused by musculoskeletal impairments, such as in cervical vertigo (see Chap. 9). Due to the hypothesized lithiasic mechanism, also in benign positioning paroxysmal vertigo (see Chap. 8), the combination of *mechanic* treatment like positional manoeuvres and cervico-dorsal treatment may be directly resolutive.

Anyway, musculoskeletal impairments are, more often, secondary to vestibular pathologies, and they result from increased muscle tension, fatigue and pain in the cervical and, sometimes, in the thoraco-lumbar spine. Changes in a patient's internal perception of the vertical can lead to abnormal alignment of body parts with respect to each other and to the base of support. Abnormal alignment may place a patient close to their limits of stability and may alter the movement strategies necessary to move their centre of gravity.

Mechanic exercises are aimed to solve musculoskeletal problems both primary and secondary to prepare patient's muscles, spine and joint for *cybernetic* and *synergetic* exercises.

Exercises performed during this phase will prepare the reorganization of the balance control. Generally speaking, the first step is to prepare the patient to cooperate in a complex programme involving movement, thinking and learning. Musculoskeletal impairments are often provoked or associated with tension and anxiety. Thus, it is very important to begin treatment with simple relaxation exercises. After them, simple exercises pointed to mobilization of the pelvis, of the cervical rachis and the thoraco-lumbar spine have to be planned. In some cases massages can be useful either to relax the patient or to mobilize joints

The *cybernetic phase* (generally three sessions/week) is aimed to correct postural synergies, reorganizing balance control and overcoming functional impairment. Controlling the body's position in space for the purpose of balance requires motor coordination processes that organize muscle throughout the body into coordinated movement strategies. Normal posture control requires the ability to adapt motor strategies to changing task and environmental demands. The inability to adapt movements to changing task demand is a characteristic of many patients. Pathology within the vestibular system can affect the selection of a movement strategy rather than the latency of onset or the temporal and spatial features of the movement synergy itself. Patients with loss of vestibular sensitivity lose the ability to use large hip/trunk movements to control equilibrium, whereas vestibular patients with irritative lesions may use excessive hip/trunk motions for postural sway.

Exercises are provided in three different task conditions: (1) self-initiated postural sway, (2) externally induced postural responses and (3) anticipatory postural adjustments accompanying a potentially destabilizing limb movement.

Reorganization of the balance control is frequently the most important goal to reach in elderly unsteadiness (see Chap. 11) and phobic postural vertigo (see Chap. 13).

The *synergetic phase* (generally three sessions/week) is aimed to reduce incoordination and disorientation and their consciousness, through *learning* new movement strategies and correct orientation. Balance disorders can result from damage within individual sensory systems which provide spatial orientation information and/or from pathologies affecting central sensory structures. In this way, coordination and orientation perception (that is to say, causing vertigo and dizziness) are affected and balance impairment may lead to disability and specific handicap in several ways:

1. A patient's ability to accurately determine the orientation of the body with respect to gravity and the environment may be disturbed.
2. A patient's ability to adapt sensory inputs to changes in task and environmental demand may be impaired.
3. A patient's ability to anticipate instability based on prior experience may be affected.

Generally, the last session of the training period is used to verify the early outcome (see Chap. 15) and to plan home training maintenance (see the following paragraph).

4.4.3 Home Training

Due to the relatively short period of rehab training with the therapist, it is strictly necessary that patient continue exercises at own home just also during training period itself. Exercises are subdivided according to different phases of balance control, from supine to standing to moving, similar to Cawthorne–Cooksey protocol. In each phase, there is a progression from *mechanic* to *synergetic* exercises. Not all exercises have to be performed. Therapist, on the basis of both diagnosis of treatment and patient compliance during training, selects the most suitable exercises. At the end of training period, a shorter protocol aimed to results maintenance will be proposed.

Patient is required to perform exercises twice/day 20–30′ each. Home training cannot ever substitute training performed with the therapist. Table 4.3 shows the overall home training protocol.

Table 4.3 Home training exercise protocol

Supine
Position your right knee against the chest, then extend your leg and position your left knee against the chest. When you position the knee against the chest with the hands, lightly apply traction to the flexed leg
Position your knees to the chest, simultaneously, gently using the hands
Lift your left arm extending over your head and simultaneously position the right flexed leg to the chest, with the aid of your hand. Maintain this position for 10 s and then repeat inverting the arm and leg
Lift your left leg with the extended knee
Lift your right leg with the extended knee
Repeat with the tip of the foot outward
Repeat with the tip of the foot inward
Put a pillow under your leg. Bind a 2 kg weight on your ankle with flexed knee; then extend it alternating the right and left leg
With the flexed legs and the feet on the bed, rotate your pelvis rightward and leftward keeping your knees flexed and your legs united
Lift your pelvis and simultaneously extend your arms over your head. Then position your arms along the body lowering your pelvis
Grasp a stick. Lift your extended arms over your head and then return to primary position
Fixate a target on the ceiling and slowly move your head rightward and leftward
Look for two equidistant targets on the ceiling and then fixate them alternatively first moving only the eyes and then moving only the head. Rotate your head rightward and fixate a target on the lateral wall. Then keep your head straight maintaining the visual fixation. Count until 10 and then rotate your head
Rotate your head leftward and fixate a target on the lateral wall. Then keep your head straight maintaining the visual fixation. Count until 10 and then rotate your head
In quadrupedal position, inspire and arch your back (hyperkyphotic position) positioning your head between your arms. Then expire flexing your head and rotating the pelvis in hyperlordotic position
From supine position move to sitting position fixating a point straight in front of you

(continued)

Table 4.3 (continued)

From supine position move to sitting position fixating a point sited on your right
From supine position move to the sitting position fixating a point sited on your left
In quadrupedal position extend the right arm and the left leg simultaneously. Then repeat with the left arm and the right leg
In prone position lift your left arm and the right leg maintaining your forehead over the bed. Then repeat with the right arm and the left leg
Repeat as above, lifting the head simultaneously
Sitting
Extend your arms and lift your thumbs. Position your arms at about 50 cm, along a horizontal plane, from your eyes, and then fixate alternatively your thumbs. Begin slowly and then increase progressively the velocity of alternating fixation
Extend your arms and lift your thumbs. Position your arms at about 50 cm, along a vertical plane, from your eyes, and then fixate alternatively your thumbs. Begin slowly and then increase progressively the velocity of alternating fixation
Extend your right arm and lift your thumb. Move slowly your arm to and fro, along a horizontal direction and then along a vertical direction. Follow your thumb with eyes only, first slowly and then increasing progressively the velocity of thumb displacement
Repeat as above but simultaneously move the head trying to keep the eyes still
Move your head first slowly and then faster in all directions fixating a target straight in front of you
Look for the three targets sited, in front of you, at your left and at your right, respectively. Fixate the frontal target, then move rapidly your head fixating the right-sited target. Now rotate your head leftward maintaining the fixation of the right-sited target. Fixate the frontal target. Now rapidly move your head leftward and fixate the left-sited target. Then rotate your head rightward maintaining the fixation of the left-sited target
Inhale. Exhaling bend forward positioning your head on the right knee. Wait 10 s. Inhaling return to sitting position. Exhaling bend forward positioning your head on the left knee. Wait 10 s and then inhale and return to sitting position
Inhale. Exhaling bend forward to pick an object on the floor. Inhale and lift it over your head and then fixate it for 10 s. Inhale. Exhaling bend forward and position the object on the floor
Open a book in front of you. Read it moving the book simultaneously to the right and left and then to and fro
Open a book in front of you. Move it away from you extending your arms. Read it. Then bring it near you, slowly, trying to read it. Then move it away. Repeat several times to and fro
Standing
With your hands on a table lift yourself on tiptoes and maintain this position for 30 s
With your hands on a table lift yourself on your heels and maintain this position for 30 s
Fixate yourself in a mirror. Align correctly your position. Maintain equilibrium for 1 min and then close your eyes, visualizing your position in your mind, and remain in that position for at least 1 min
Repeat standing on a soft mattress
Fixate yourself on a mirror. Then oscillate to and fro and to the right and left, around your ankles keeping your pelvis still
Repeat with eyes closed
Repeat standing on a soft mattress
Fixate yourself in a mirror; keeping your feet still, bend your trunk to and fro and to the right and left
Repeat with eyes closed
Repeat standing on a soft mattress

(continued)

Table 4.3 (continued)

Pick a little object and then lift it over your head and fixate it. With your extended arms, move it repeatedly in circles maintaining the fixation of the object		
Repeat with eyes closed		
Repeat standing on a soft mattress		
Pick a little object and lift it over your head. Fixate it. Inhale. Then exhale and bend forward putting the object on the floor. Wait 10 s and then inhaling lift again the object over your head		
Repeat with eyes closed		
Repeat standing on a soft mattress		
Pick a little object and lift it over your head. Fixate it. With your straight arms, move the object repeatedly in circles and, bending your trunk and your knees simultaneously, put it on the floor		
Repeat on a soft mattress		
Open a book in front of you. Read it, moving it simultaneously to and fro and to the right and left		
Repeat on a soft mattress		
Open a book in front of you. Move it away from you extending your arms. Read it. Then bring it near you, slowly, trying to read it. Then, move it away from you extending your arms. Repeat several times to and fro		
Repeat on a soft mattress		
Moving		
Step on the floor with eyes open		
Support yourself on a chair and then step on tiptoes		
Support yourself on a chair and then step on your heels		
Step fixating a target in front of you		
Step with eyes closed		
Step as you move the head to and fro		
Step as you read a book		
Step on a soft mattress		
Go up and down a step, fixating a target according to the following sequences:		
Right foot up	Left foot up	Right foot down
Left foot down	Left foot up	Right foot up
Left foot down	Right foot down	
Repeat with eyes closed		
Go up and down a step, moving your head to and fro, according to the following sequences:		
Right foot up	Left foot up	Right foot down
Left foot down	Left foot up	Right foot up
Left foot down	Foot down	
Repeat with eyes closed		
Along a corridor walk 5 steps forward and backward fixating a target		
Along a corridor walk 5 steps forward and backward staring, without any reference target		
Along a corridor walk 5 steps forward and backward with eyes closed maintaining a 20 cm distance from the wall on the side of your vestibular hypofunction		
Along a corridor walk 5 steps forward and backward moving your head to and fro		
Along a corridor walk 5 steps forward and backward reading a book		

4.5 The Role of Instrumental Rehab

In sudden vestibular loss (see Chap. 5), rehab has mainly aimed to improve sensory substitution. According to the *MCS* model, this aim may be considered as *mechanic*, because rehab is pointed to restore the basic elements (reflexes) of human balance control.

To stimulate sensory substitution, transcutaneous electrical nerve stimulation (TENS) is particularly useful [20]. It is a technique that alters cardiovascular autonomic responses [21], enhances visuospatial abilities [22] and cognitive function [23] and improves vestibulospinal reflexes [24]. *TENS* is a noninvasive technique that provides nerve and/or muscle stimulation by means of surface electrodes. The characteristics, the size and the site of application of the electrodes and the characteristics of the electrical waves play a fundamental role in the neurophysiological effects. TENS means transcutaneous electrical nerve stimulation but this definition can be considered abusive. The excitation of the peripheral motor nerves and the associated muscle activation is caused by the application of an electrical current to the skin, usually in correspondence of the motor points. This kind of stimulation induces depolarization of the motor nerves either in the centrifugal or in the centripetal sense. Furthermore, this kind of stimulation induces an activation of the sensitive nerves of the skin. Thus, it is difficult to divide the motor and the sensitive effects of the TENS. The employed stimulation mode is that used for pain relief. The modulation programme randomly modifies the duration of TENS waves. The mean duration is 100 μs, while the frequency is 80 Hz. Electrodes are small (2 cm^2), placed at the distance of 1 cm from each other. A pair of electrodes stimulates paravertebral muscles at the level of the second cervical vertebra; a pair stimulates the contralateral superior trapezius. The intensity is never able to induce muscle contraction. The frequency used is in the muscle spindles range of vibratory activation (80 Hz). Thus, it is likely that VES activates the same spinal pathways of the cervicospinal reflexes.

During the second (*cybernetic*) phase of training, postural control may be improved by means of visual feedback posturographic-assisted devices.

Haman et al. [25] and Shumway-Cook et al. [26] conducted the first studies that used objective visual feedback (VFB), based on symmetry of postural sway (movement of the COG), for training purposes.

Nowadays, a lot of different posturographic equipment are available and VFB is frequently used to improve postural stability control. VFB provides a ready source of information about postural instability for both the patient and the therapist. The purpose of VFB is to detect and make available to the patient objective information about physiological function or movement that is not ordinarily perceived by the patient. For the therapist the VFB facilitates the design of custom treatments; for the patient it enhances motivation through real-time visual feedback, links perception to movement, internalizes the appropriate alignment or movement pattern, improves volitional control and builds confidence to perform activities of daily living.

The main limitations are as follows:

1. The cost of the equipment
2. The need to perform rehab only as single patient session
3. The incomplete transfer of the acquired skills on the platform into the daily life activities

For the scope of this chapter, despite the various equipment available into the market, we will briefly describe only the Balance Master System (Neurocom, Clackamas, OR, USA, http://resourceonbalance.com), the Tetrax FB system (Tel Aviv, Israel, www.tetraxfb.com) and the Delos System (Turin, Italy, www.delos-international.com).

Balance Master is an equipment that allows, by means of a dual footplate, a visual feedback of COG position, projected on a computer screen facing the patient standing on the platform [27, 28].

Tetrax system is based on the recording of separate CoG of the anterior and posterior part of the 2 ft [29–33].

Delos System is an equipment constituted by an unstable and oscillating platform and an electronic postural proprioceptive station [34] connected to a personal computer with a specific software (DPPS 5.0). The station includes two electronic postural readers (DVC, Delos Vertical Controller), a sensorized bar and a display. The DVCs, applied to the sternum and the head, measure the head and the trunk inclination [35] in the frontal and sagittal plane by means of two-dimensional accelerometer units. VFB is provided by the two accelerometers and the unstable platform. In this way the visual feedback projected on the screen may regard the movements of the table, the trunk or the head or a combination of the three.

4.5.1 Balance Master

When normal subjects maintain a vertically erect position, the CoG is located directly over the area of the base support, slightly above the ankle joints. This position can be maintained without stepping or reaching for support if the sway does not exceed the subject's limits of stability (Fig. 4.1).

Functional stability limits (limits of stability, LoS) have been calculated to be 6.25″ anteriorly and 4.45″ posteriorly for the average adult subject. The angular limits of stability are very nearly the same for all adults regardless of height. The biomechanical properties that determine the LoS are similar for standing in place, walking and sitting without trunk support. For these reasons re-education of the limits of stability in standing in place can be used to rehabilitate the patient to regain normal LoS during walking, too.

Fig. 4.1 Balance Master equipment

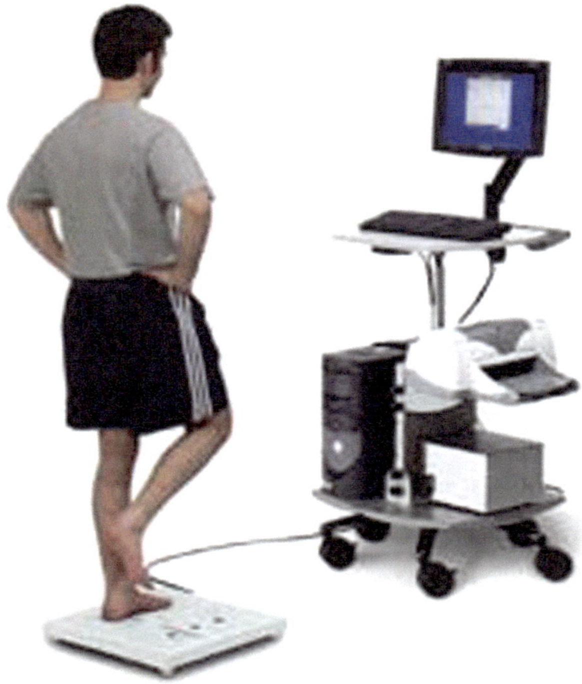

LoS test and exercise require the subject to be able to actively move his/her CoG away from the centre toward a visual target and maintain that position for the required time. The correct execution of the LoS test requires normal combined and integrated ankle–hip strategies (Fig. 4.2).

LoS parameters to be considered are as follows:

Movement time: how many seconds patient takes to reach the desired target (including the reaction time).

Path sway: refers to the percentage of path length.

Target sway: percentage of maximum CoG area maintained on the target.

Patient position: value given in polar coordinates that represents the average position of the COG during the period of target sway assessment. If the target was not reached, the patient position score reflects the point of closest approach to the target.

Distance error: the difference between the patient's average position and the centre of target. This parameter allows one to see how far away from the centre the patient is willing and able to move in a given direction.

LoS misperceptions are common findings in whiplash patients. In these cases training aimed at teaching the appropriate conditions for using ankle movements can have a positive impact. In contrast, weakness of ankle joint muscles, loss of ankle sensation, reduced mobility about the ankles or combinations of these factors prevent the patient from generating effective ankle movements and might be an

PATIENT INFORMATION AND SETTINGS

Patient Name:
Data file
Target/prot. Type: SP06
Therapy Mode: Beep, Feedback
Post-Test Comment:

Age: 30
Ht.: 172 cm
LOS:75%

Test Date. Date 02/16/95
Order #:6
Pacing Speed: 10 sec

Limits of satbility

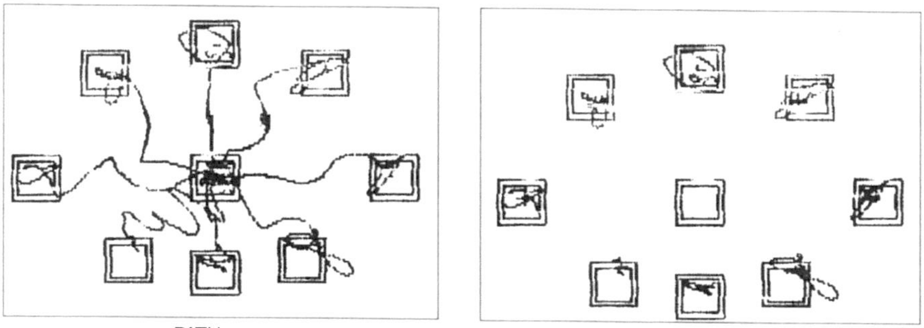

PATH

SWAY AREA

Numeric Summary

Transition		Mvt Time (sec)	Path Sway (% Path Len)	Target Sway (% Max Area)	Patient Position (% LOS)	Patient Position (deg)	Distance Error (% LOS)	Direction Error (deg)
1	(F)	4.28	127.68	N/S	<72.1>	<359.2>	<–2.9>	<–0.8>
2	(RF)	4.00	172.16	0.41	70.8	42.7	–4.2	–2.3
3	(R)	4.04	157.96	N/S	<71.8>	<87.8>	<–3.2>	<–2.2>
4	(RB)	2.94	169.83	0.58	68.6	124.8	–6.4	–10.2
5	(B)	3.74	237.19	0.13	66.8	176.6	–8.2	–3.4
6	(LB)	6.72	347.19	N/S	<60.6>	<230.8>	<–14.4>	<–5.8>
7	(L)	4.50	188.06	N/S	<73.4>	<271.9>	<1.6>	<1.9>
8	(LF)	3.70	158.90	0.20	70.1	314.2	–4.9	–0.8

Fig. 4.2 Example of LoS, a not completely statistical representation (Originally published in Alpini et al. [47] published by Springer © 2014)

abnormal adaptation used by a dizzy patient to minimize head movements and associated stimulation of the neck and vestibular system.

By means of the Balance Master, it is possible to treat patients ranging from 76 to 203 cm in height and from 18 to 138 kg in weight. Each treatment session can be performed according to the LoS, ranging from 25 to 100 % of the predictable LoS, in 5 % increments. The target pacing is 1, 3, 5, 7, 10, 15, 20 s. If trying to promote faster movement, then low pacing settings (1, 2, 5 s) are appropriate. If stability at points in space is desired, then higher pacing settings (10 s or higher) are appropriate so that the patient must "hold" a position (Fig. 4.3).

The duration of each session treatment is 20 min. The frequency generally varies from twice a week to everyday treatment. The frequency of training sessions is dependent on the combination of other rehabilitative treatments such as physical therapy and vestibular electrical stimulation.

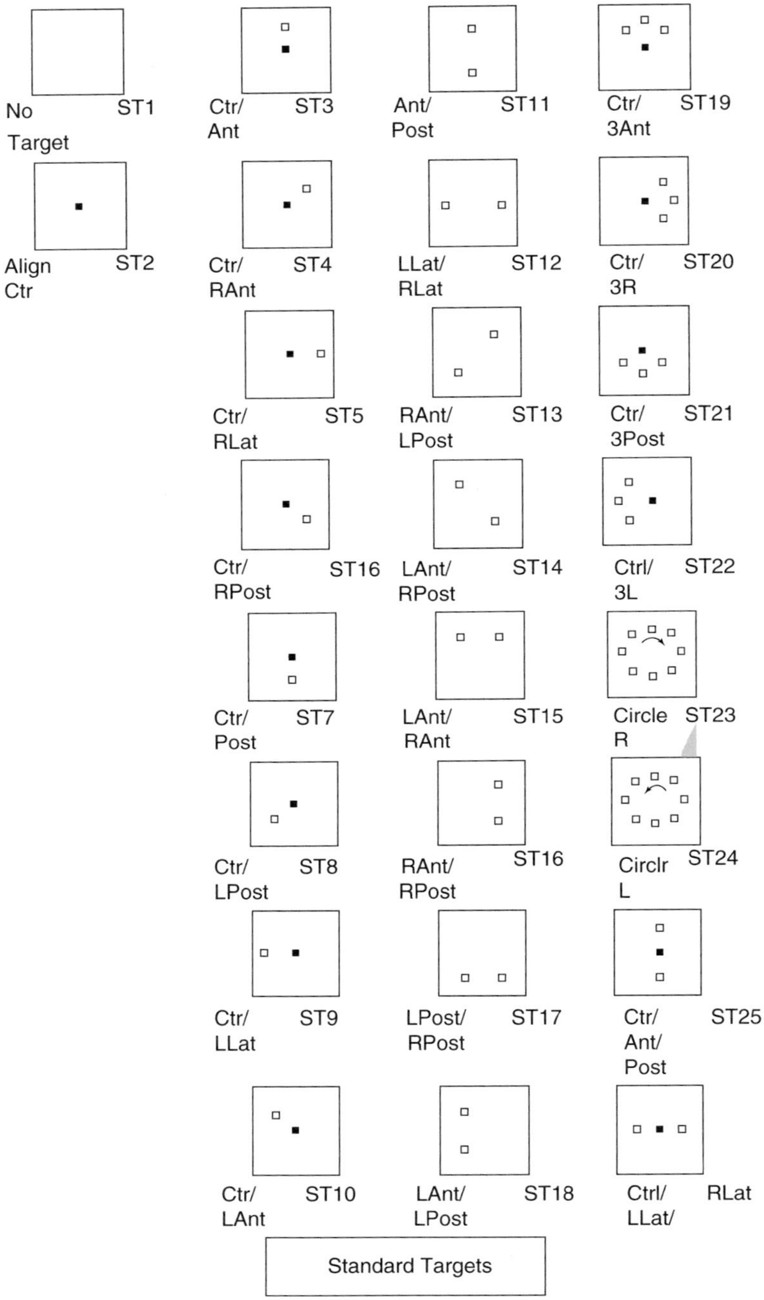

Fig. 4.3 Standard targets available for treatment (Originally published in Alpini et al. [47] published by Springer © 2014)

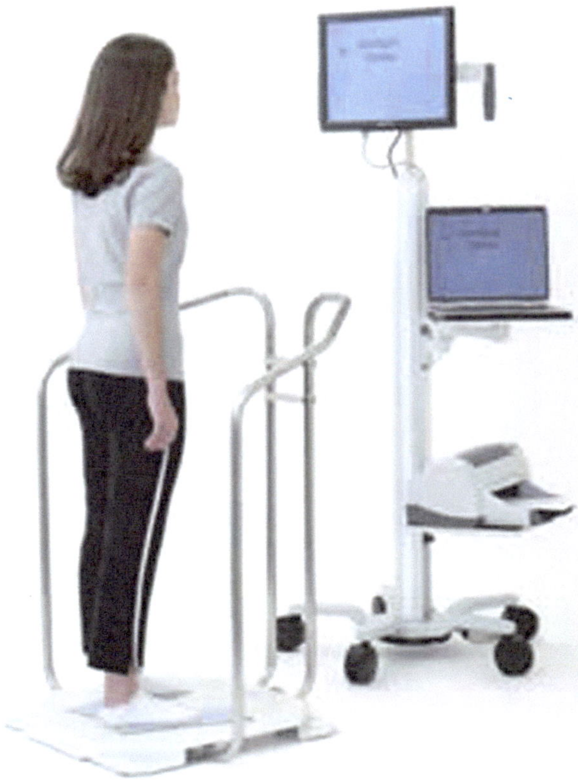

Fig. 4.4 Tetrax FB equipment

4.5.2 Tetrax FB

Tetrax FB works within the principles of simplexity [36], which states that a human body's balance in space is based on the cooperation and interaction of a multiplicity and complexity of many subsystems which are under the control of efficient neurophysiological mechanisms.

It consists of four independent mobile force plates, two for each foot. Each plate contains a strain-gauge force transducer, which is sensitive to vertical force. Tetrax provides independent output from the four balance plates. Subjects are requested to stand quietly on the platforms and control CoG displacements using both feet, toes and heels in a synchronized and coordinated way. "Tetra CoG" has to be moved along visual presented pathways (e.g. a labyrinth; Figs. 4.3 and 4.4) as correctly as possible.

The pressure fluctuations produced by the heels and toes of a subject standing with different positions of the trunk or the head may be visually balanced through the feedback presented on the screen.

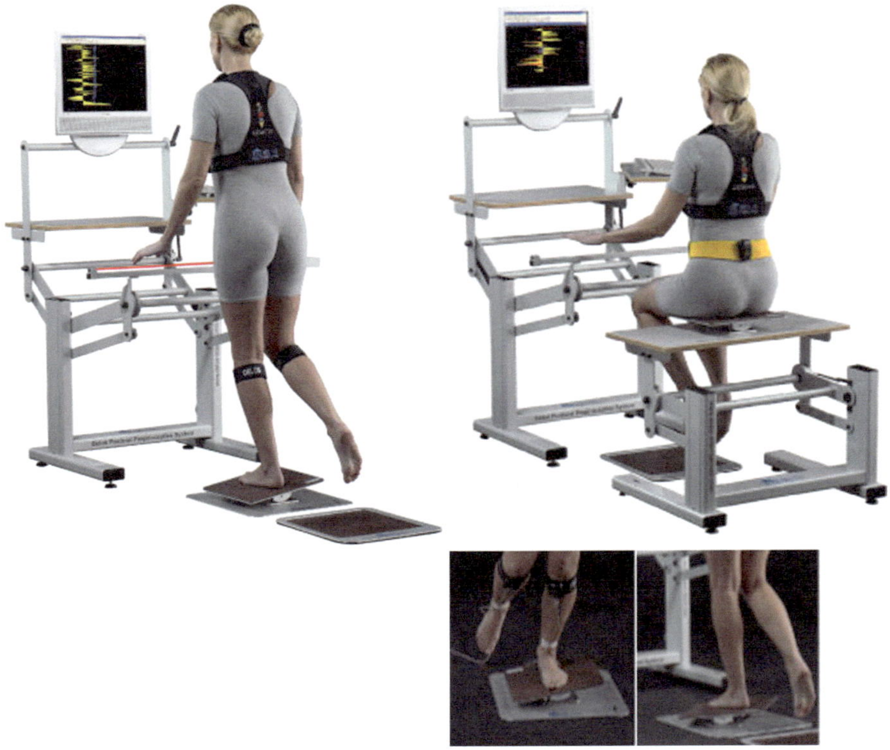

Figs. 4.5 and 4.6 Delos DEB 2 equipment comprising the electronic rocking board and the two accelerometers, on the head and the trunk (Originally published in Alpini et al. [47] published by Springer © 2014)

4.5.3 Delos

It is based on an electronic rocking board, with "a degree of freedom" and visual tracking of the micro-rolling of the point of support. Its exclusive rocking movement, combined with the subcortical visual tracking in real time, creates conditions of instability, capable of activating high-frequency proprioceptive flows both in standing (Fig. 4.5) and sitting position (Fig. 4.6).

The rolling surfaces with variable radii permit the proposal of different levels of instability and the selective activation of the postural strategies. The postural reader measures the subject's levels of stability in static and dynamic monopedalic, bipedalic and seated conditions. It records and visualizes in real time the movements on the frontal and sagittal planes in relation to the vertical axis. The system may use also a wireless electronic rocking board with "3 degrees of freedom" with visualization in real time of the movements on the x, y and z axis, with a 3D view of the trials. It represents the completion of DEB2 proposal, widening the number of biomechanical and postural situations to be managed. The rolling surfaces with variable radii permit the proposal of increasing levels of instability.

Recently the use of Nintendo Wii, a popular video gaming system, has been proposed as both physiotherapist-assisted [37] and home-based [38] exercises. Nintendo Wii balance board is cost-effective and user-friendly [39] and that it has been proposed as an alternative to other popular frequently used systems also in elderly patients [40], but it is limited in its customizability to accommodate different functional levels; thus, in our experience, professional equipment have to be preferred. These kinds of equipment may be useful to improve patient compliance during home training.

In some patients, e.g. vestibular ataxia due to bilateral vestibular loss (see Chap. 7), virtual reality (VR) may be effective [41] to improve behavioural adaptation. VR can be added, at least in some selected patients, during the third phase (*synergetic*) of training.

Virtual reality enables patients to dive into a world of illusion. The perception of the environment is modified by artificial stimuli, generating sensory conflict and altering the gain of the vestibulo-ocular reflex [42]. Repetitive movements of images on the retina produced by virtual reality devices designed to control visual stimuli may induce vestibular response adaptation [43] and adjust the vestibulo-ocular and vestibulospinal reflexes involved in postural control and body balance strategies [44].

Virtual reality technology enables therapists to offer patients a wide range of highly specific stimuli and sensory conflicts of varying degrees of complexity in a safe environment [45, 46].

References

1. Bronstein AM, Brandt T, Woollacott MH (eds) (1996) Clinical disorders of balance, posture and gait. Arnold Ed, London
2. Balaban CD, Hoffer ME, Gottshall KR (2012) Top-down approach to vestibular compensation: translational lessons from vestibular rehabilitation. Brain Res 1482:101–111
3. Allum JH (2012) Recovery of vestibular ocular reflex function and balance control after a unilateral peripheral vestibular deficit. Front Neurol 3:83
4. Peusner KD, Shao M, Reddaway R, Hirsch JC (2012) Basic concepts in understanding recovery of function in vestibular reflex networks during vestibular compensation. Front Neurol 3:17
5. Dutia MB (2010) Mechanisms of vestibular compensation: recent advances. Curr Opin Otolaryngol Head Neck Surg 18(5):420–424
6. Claussen CF (1994) Vestibular compensation. Acta Otolaryngol (Stockh) 513(Suppl):33–36
7. Lacour M, Tighilet B (2010) Plastic events in the vestibular nuclei during vestibular compensation: the brain orchestration of a "deafferentation" code. Restor Neurol Neurosci 28(1):19–35
8. Lewis RF, Nicoucar K, Gong W, Haburcakova C, Merfeld DM (2013) Adaptation of vestibular tone studied with electrical stimulation of semicircular canal afferents. J Assoc Res Otolaryngol 14(3):331–340
9. Zennou-Azogui Y, Borel L, Lacour M, Ez-Zaher L (1993) Recovery of head postural control following unilateral vestibular neurectomy in the cat: neck muscle activity and neuronal correlates in deiters' nuclei. Acta Oto-Laryngol (Stockh) 509(Suppl):19
10. Cousins S, Kaski D, Cutfield N, Seemungal B, Golding JF, Gresty M, Glasauer S, Bronstein AM (2013) Vestibular perception following acute unilateral vestibular lesions. PLoS One 8(5): e61862
11. Cawthorne T (1944) The physiological basis of head exercises. J Chart SocPhysiother 106–107
12. Cooksey FS (1946) Rehabilitation in vestibular injuries. Proc R Soc Med 39:273–278

13. Dix DR (1974) Treatment of vertigo. Physiotherapy 60:380
14. Han BI, Song HS, Kim JS (2011) Vestibular rehabilitation therapy: review of indications, mechanisms, and key exercises. J Clin Neurol 7(4):184–196
15. Herdman SJ (2013) Vestibular rehabilitation. Curr Opin Neurol 26(1):96–101
16. Heymans MW, van Tulder MW, Esmail R, Bombardier C, Koes BW (2011) Back schools for acute and subacute non-specific low-back pain. The Cochrane Collaboration. Wiley, Hoboken, NJ
17. Sweeney T (1992) Neck school: cervicothoracic stabilization training. Occup Med 7(1):43–54
18. Taimela S, Takala EP, Asklöf T, Seppälä K, Parviainen S (2000) Active treatment of chronic neck pain: a prospective randomized intervention. Spine (Phila Pa 1976) 25(8):1021–1027
19. Bronstein AM, Lempert T (2010) Management of the patient with chronic dizziness. Restor Neurol Neurosci 28(1):83–90
20. Cesarani A, Alpini D, Barozzi S (1990) Neck electrical stimulation in the treatment of labyrinth acute vertigo. Riv It Eeg Neurof Cl 13(1):55–61
21. Sanderson JE, Tomlinson B, Lau MS, So KW, Cheung AH, Critchley JA, Woo KS (1995) The effect of transcutaneous electrical nerve stimulation (TENS) on autonomic cardiovascular reflexes. Clin Auton Res 5(2):81–84
22. Vallar G, Rusconi ML, Barozzi S, Bernardini B, Ovadia D, Papagno C, Cesarani A (1995) Improvement of left visuo-spatial hemineglect by left-sided transcutaneous electrical stimulation. Neuropsychologia 33(1):73–82
23. van Dijk KR, Scherder EJ, Scheltens P, Sergeant JA (2002) Effects of transcutaneous electrical nerve stimulation (TENS) on non-pain related cognitive and behavioural functioning. Rev Neurosci 13(3):257–270
24. Osio M, Dezuanni E, Alpini D, Cesarani A, Mangoni A (1995) Low intensity electrical stimulation of neck muscles modifies motor neuron excitability of the Soleus muscles in man. Electroencephalogr Clin Neurophysiol 95(3):P68–P69
25. Hamann KF, Krausen C (1990) Clinical application of posturography. Body tracking and biofeedback training. In: Brandt T, Paulus W, Bles W (eds) Disorders of posture and gait. Thieme, Stuttgart, pp 295–298
26. Shumway-Cook A, McCollum G (1991) Assessment and treatment of balance deficits in the neurologic patients. In: Montgomery P, Connelly B (eds) Motor control. Theoretical framework and practical application, & physical therapy. Chattanooga Corp, Chattanooga, pp 123–138
27. Nashner L (1994) Evaluation of postural stability, movement, and control. In: Hasson SM (ed) Clinical exercise physiology. Mosby, St Louis, p 57
28. Neurocom International Inc (1989) Balance Master operator's manual. Neurocom, Portland
29. Kohen-Raz R, Gentaz R (1993) Posturographic characteristics of patients with lower back pain. Cahiers de Posturologie, Paris
30. Himmelfarb R, Kohen-Raz R, Rapaport J, Bloom A (1992) The application of posturography in the assessment of vertiginous disorders caused by head and neck injuries. In: Proceedings of the international meeting on Whiplash injuries, University of Wales, 1992
31. Kohen-Raz R, Roth V (2000) Posturographic characteristics of whiplash patients. Proceedings of the XII regular meeting of the Barany society. Wurzburg, Germany, 1998. In: Claus CF, Claus-Toni H, Hoffenberth B (eds) Equilibrium research, clinical equilibriometry and modern treatment. Elsevier, Amsterdam
32. Alpini D, Cesarani A, Pugnetti L, Cardini R, Hahn A, Sambataro G (2000) Project to prevent mobility related accidents in elderly and disabled. In: Proceedings of the 3rd international conference on disability, virtual reality and Association technologies, Alghero, pp 249–254
33. Lee KG, Chun MH, Kang SH, Kim BR (2008) The evaluation of effect after biofeedback training using Interactive Balance System in sub-acute stroke patients. Asan Medical Center Korea, XVII. European Stroke Conference, Nice. Poster session: recovery and rehabilitation
34. Delos postural proprioceptive system. 2011. http://www.delosinternational.com/prodotti.asp?sec=scheda&lang=eng

35. Sjostrom H, Allum JH, Carpenter MG, Adkin AL, Honegger F, Ettlin T (2003) Trunk sway measures of postural stability during clinical balance tests in patients with chronic whiplash injury symptoms. Spine 28(15):1725–1734
36. Alain B (2012) Simplexity. Yale University Press, New Haven, USA
37. Levac DE, Miller PA (2013) Integrating virtual reality video games into practice: clinicians' experiences. Physiother Theory Pract 29:504–512
38. Prosperini L, Fortuna D, Giannì C, Leonardi L, Marchetti MR, Pozzilli C (2013) Home-based balance training using the Wii balance board: a randomized, crossover pilot study in multiple sclerosis. Neurorehabil Neural Repair 27(6):516–525
39. Sparrer I, Duong Dinh TA, Ilgner J, Westhofen M (2013) Vestibular rehabilitation using the Nintendo® Wii Balance Board – a user-friendly alternative for central nervous compensation. Acta Otolaryngol 133(3):239–245
40. Taylor MJ, Shawis T, Impson R, Ewins K, McCormick D, Griffin M (2012) Nintendo Wii as a training tool in falls prevention rehabilitation: case studies. J Am Geriatr Soc 60(9):1781–1783
41. Riva G, Rizzo A, Alpini D, Attree EA, Barbieri E, Bertella L, Buckwalter JG, Davies RC, Gamberini L, Johansson G, Katz N, Marchi S, Mendozzi L, Molinari E, Pugnetti L, Rose FD, Weiss PL (1999) Virtual environments in the diagnosis, prevention, and intervention of age-related diseases: a review of VR scenarios proposed in the EC VETERAN project. Cyber Psychol Behav 2(6):577–591
42. Viirre E, Sitarz R (2002) Vestibular rehabilitation using visual displays: preliminary study. Laryngoscope 112(3):500–503
43. Kramer PD, Roberts DC, Shelhamer M, Zee DS (1998) A versatile stereoscopic visual display system for vestibular and oculomotor research. J Vestib Res 8(5):363–379
44. Suarez H, Arocena M, Suarez A, De Artagaveytia TA, Muse P, Gil J (2003) Changes in postural control parameters after vestibular rehabilitation in patients with central vestibular disorders. Acta Otolaryngol 123(2):143–147
45. Akizuki H, Uno A, Arai K, Morioka S, Ohyama S, Nishiike S (2005) Effects of immersion in virtual reality on postural control. Neurosci Lett 379(1):23–26
46. Sparto PJ, Furman JM, Whitney SL, Hodges LF, Redfern MS (2004) Vestibular rehabilitation using a wide field of view virtual environment. Conf Proc IEEE Eng Med Biol Soc 7:4836–4839
47. Alpini DC, Brugnoni G, Cesarani A (2014) Whiplash injuries – diagnosis and treatment, 2nd edn. Springer, Milan, Heidelberg

Part II

Training and Home Training Vestibular Rehab Protocols

5 Sudden Unilateral Vestibular Loss

Unilateral vestibular hypofunction means asymmetrical vestibular functioning, i.e. the sensory input of one side is diminished with respect to that of the other side. A sudden unilateral loss or impairment of vestibular function causes vertigo, dizziness and impaired postural function.

Asymmetrical peripheral functioning can be also detected without the patient complaining of vertigo or instability. Such an asymmetry can be stable, being a sequela of a former lesion. It can be also fluctuant as, e.g. in cases with recurrent attacks of the Ménière's disease. In a more restricted clinical context, unilateral vestibular hypofunction is considered as non-fluctuant unilateral loss, where compensation plays a fundamental role.

The most striking form is the syndrome with sudden loss in which the same signs and symptoms of a post-labyrinthectomy can be observed [1]. The course is characterized by four stages:

1. Stage of irritation: In some cases, the onset of the syndrome may be characterized by a rather vague dizziness. At the moment the spontaneous nystagmus beats toward the affected side, and normal caloric reaction can be observed.
2. Stage of sudden loss of function or paralysis of the system: Typical rotary vertigo is now experienced and spontaneous nystagmus beats toward the normal side. The caloric reaction is absent or reduced at the affected side. Patients are generally visited at the Emergency Room of the hospital during this stage, and hospitalization is common.
3. Stage of central compensation: There is a progressive decrease of vertigo as well as of spontaneous nystagmus [2]. This occurs independently of the persistence of unilateral weakness or areflexia at the affected side which is revealed by caloric stimulations [3, 4]. Provocative manoeuvres (especially head shaking) reveal vertigo and nystagmus.
4. Stage of recovery: When the function of the affected side recuperates, this may lead to a spontaneous nystagmus, reversed in direction, i.e. beating toward the affected side.

D.C. Alpini et al., *Vertigo Rehabilitation Protocols*,
DOI 10.1007/978-3-319-05482-7_5, © Springer International Publishing Switzerland 2014

The most frequent causes of sudden unilateral vestibular loss are:

- Vestibular neuritis o bacterial labyrinthitis (inflammatory lesion) [5]
- Inner ear vascular damage [6]
- Head trauma with consequent concussion of the labyrinth or fracture of temporal bone

After benign paroxysmal positioning vertigo, vestibular neuritis is the second most common cause of peripheral vestibular vertigo. It accounts for 7 % of patients presenting to outpatient clinics that specialize in the treatment of dizziness and has an incidence of 3.5 per 100,000 population [7].

In the cases of vestibular nerve or labyrinth lesion, the *key treatment* is to cure the infection. Evidence suggests that vestibular neuritis is caused by reactivation of a latent Herpes simplex virus type 1 (HSV-1) infection with the vestibular ganglia latently infected with HSV-1 [8–10].

In the case of vascular damage such as in vertebrobasilar insufficiency, the *key treatment* is restoring the arterial blood supply or venous brainstem drainage.

In all the cases, the *key impairment* is acute vertigo in the first days and, immediately after, postural unsteadiness with instability of the visual field, especially when walking, turning or changing position.

The following protocol regards the rehabilitative treatment of patient during the stage of vestibular function sudden loss:

5.1 Hospital Treatment

In the early phase of acute vertigo, symptoms are characterized by nausea and vomiting, rotary vertigo is present in every position of the head and the body with a slight decrease of symptoms lying on the opposite site of the lesion, oscillopsia due to nystagmus, unsteadiness with typically standing and gait deviations toward the affected side. The first mechanism of recovery is internuclear inhibition that can lead to a bilateral reduction of the vestibular responses. Successively, recovery is featured by sensory substitution phenomena.

The *key aims* of rehab are:

1. Reduce antigravitary failure of the affected side
2. Reduce oscillopsia due to nystagmus
3. Activate sensory substitution phenomena
4. Reduce internuclear inhibition
5. Reactivate coordination
6. Reduce spatial disorientation (vertigo)

In the acute phase, drugs are often necessary [11] especially those that reduce neurovegetative symptoms, such as metoclopramide, and those that can potentially activate neurochemical compensation pathways such as benzodiazepine and amantadine [12].

The first step of the rehabilitative treatment of acute vertigo is *TENS* (see Chap. 4 [13–15] (Fig. 5.1).

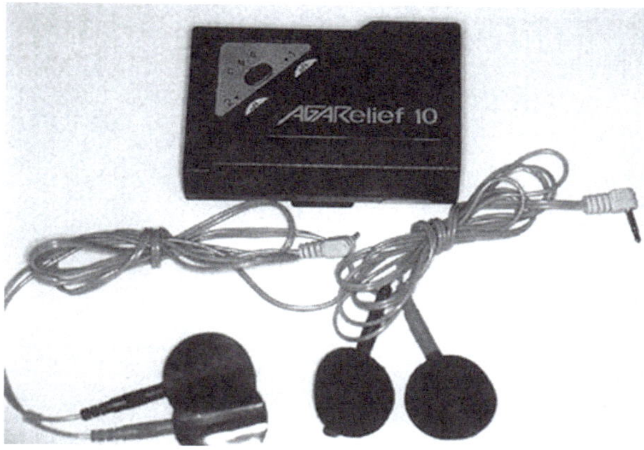

Fig. 5.1 The device used for vestibular electrical stimulation (Originally published in Alpini et al. [20] published by Springer © 1999)

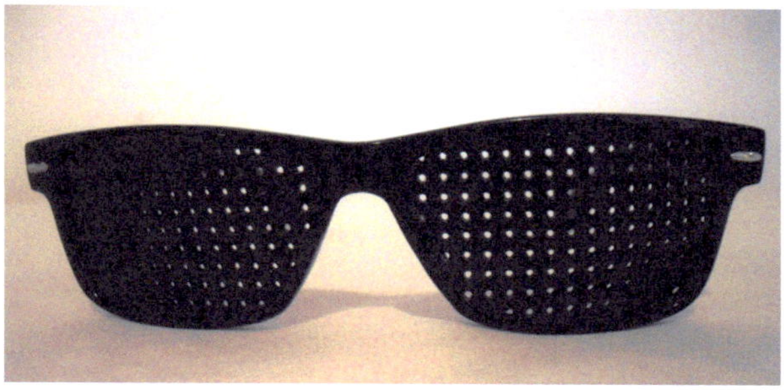

Fig. 5.2 Pinhole glasses, also known as stenopeic glasses: in place of each lens an opaque sheet of plastic with a series of pinhole-sized perforations

One pair of electrodes must be placed on the paravertebral muscles opposite to the affected site (the side of the direction of the spontaneous nystagmus) and one pair in the trapezius muscle of the affected side.

Twice session/day, 45/50′ each have to be performed [16]. During the first 30′ patient remains in bed, possibly in the most comfortable position lying on the healthy side, in the light, trying to keep the eyes open and fixating a target on the opposite position of the visual field (on the side of the affected labyrinth).

Visual field may be stabilized reducing spontaneous nystagmus by means of pinhole glasses [17]. They are also known as stenopeic glasses (Fig 5.2), that is to say, eyeglasses with a series of pinhole-sized perforations filling an opaque sheet of plastic in place of each lens.

Similar to the workings of a pinhole camera, each perforation allows only a very narrow beam of light to enter the eye which reduces the size of the circle of confusion on the retina and increases depth of field. A second effect may appear at the common bridge between each two adjacent holes, whereby two different rays of light coming from the same object (but each passing through a different hole) are diffracted back toward the eye and onto different places on the retina. This leads to an increasing of patient's fixation skill. They are not recommended for people with over 6 diopters of myopia.

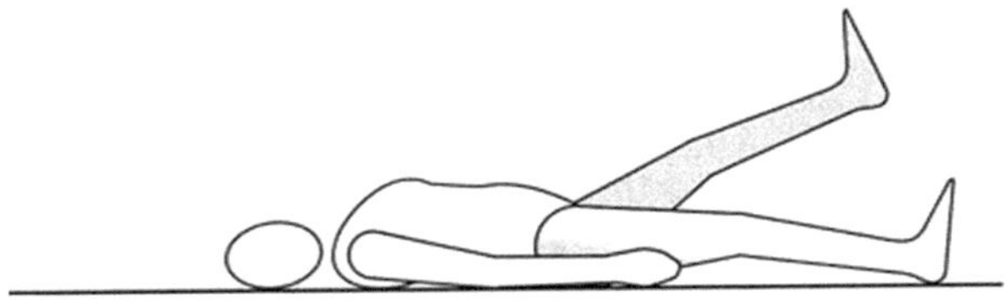

Fig. 5.3 Extension of the left knee in a case of a lesion on the left (Originally published in Alpini et al. [20] published by Springer © 1999)

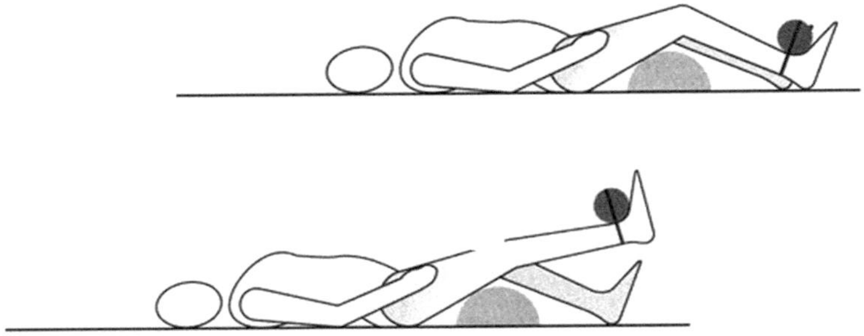

Fig. 5.4 Extension of the right knee, binding a weight to the ankle, in a case of a lesion on the right (Originally published in Alpini et al. [20] published by Springer © 1999)

For about 30′ patient is asked to remain sitting fixating a point through pinhole glasses, maintaining TENS cervical stimulation. Then the patient, under the effect of drugs, must reach the upright position and, accompanied by the therapist, have to begin walking.

Gait has to be performed during TENS, without wearing pinhole glasses, teaching to the patient fixating a target in front of him. After some steps the patient have to return back turning around her-/himself. The sense of rotation must not be casual but it must be in the sense of the health labyrinth. Instructions for re-fixating a target must be furnished.

After the first day of treatment, simple *in-bed exercises* must be performed, twice a day, for at least 20–30 min each session:

1. The patient fixates a target on the ceiling and slowly moves her/his head rightward and leftward.
2. The patient looks for two equidistant targets on the ceiling and then she/he fixates them alternatively first moving only the eyes and then moving only the head.
3. The patient rotates her/his head in the direction of the affected labyrinth and fixates a target on the lateral wall. Then she/he takes her/his head straight maintaining the visual fixation. She/he counts until 10 and then she/he rotates again her/his head.
4. The patient lifts her/his leg of the affected side with the extended knee (Fig. 5.3).
5. She/he repeats with the tip of the foot outward.
6. She/he repeats with the tip of the foot inward.
7. The patient puts a pillow under her/his leg on the affected side, bounding a 2 kg weight on her/his ankle with the flexed knee; then she/he extends it (Fig. 5.4).

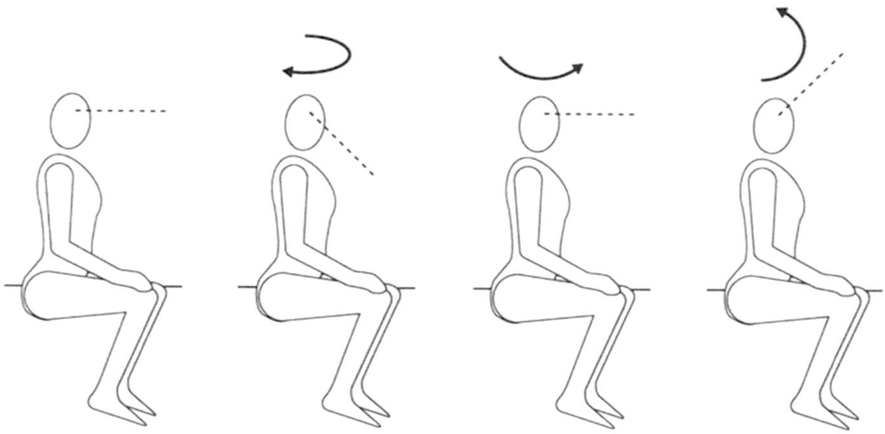

Fig. 5.5 Movements of the head in all directions, fixating a target straight in front of the patient (Originally published in Alpini et al. [20] published by Springer © 1999)

When it is possible to maintain *sitting position,* following exercises (one session a day, about 30′) have to be performed during cervical TENS stimulation:

1. The patient extends her/his arms and lifts her/his thumbs. She/he takes her/his arms at about 50 cm, along a horizontal plane, from her/his eyes and then she/he fixates alternatively her/his thumbs. She/he begins slowly and then increases progressively the velocity of alternating the fixation.
2. The patient extends her/his arms and lifts her/his thumbs. She/he takes her/his arms at about 50 cm, along a vertical plane, from her/his eyes and then she/he fixates alternatively her/his thumbs. She/he begins slowly and then increases progressively the velocity of alternating the fixation.
3. The patient extends her/his right arm and lifts her/his thumb. She/he moves slowly her/his arm to and fro, along a horizontal direction, then along a vertical direction. She/he follows her/his thumb with eyes only, first slowly and then increasing progressively the velocity of thumb displacement.
4. As above, but moving the head simultaneously, trying to maintain the eyes still.
5. The patient moves her/his head first slowly and then faster in all directions fixating a target straight in front of him (Fig. 5.5).
6. The patient looks for three targets placed, respectively, in front of her/him, at her/his left, and at her/his right. She/he fixates the frontal target; then she/he moves rapidly her/his head fixating the right-sited target. Now she/he turns leftward, her/his head maintaining the fixation of the right-sited target. She/he fixates the frontal target. Now rapidly she/he moves her/his head leftward and fixates the left-sited target. Then she/he turns rightward her/his head maintaining the fixation of the left-sited target (Fig. 5.6).
7. The patient is sitting and she/he fixates a target in front of her/him. Then she/he gets down fixating a target on the ceiling. Then she/he gets up, re-fixating the target in front of her/him (Fig. 5.7).

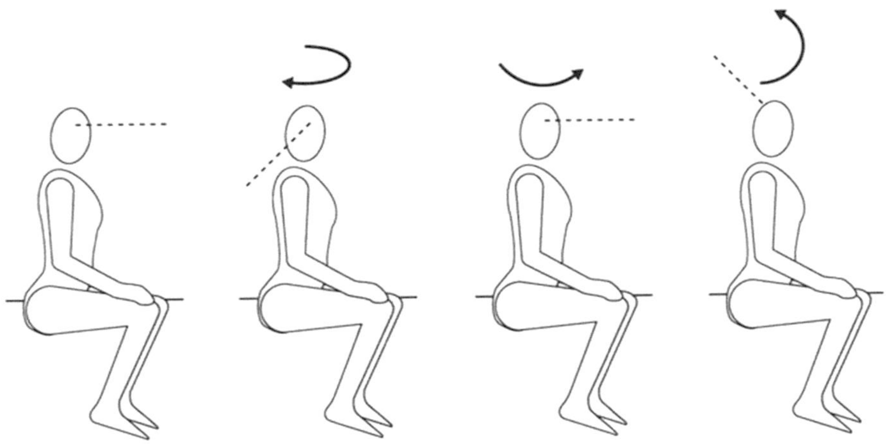

Fig. 5.6 Alternating fixation of three targets (Originally published in Alpini et al. [20] published by Springer © 1999)

8. The patient is sitting on the bed wearing pinhole glasses. The therapist pushes her/him in order to stimulate coordinated equilibrium reactions of the body (Figs. 5.8 and 5.9).
9. The patient is supine on an oscillating plain. The therapist moves the plain to stimulate equilibrium reactions (Fig. 5.10).

When it is possible to maintain *standing position,* following exercises have to be included, always maintaining cervical TENS stimulation in rehab session (once a day, about 45′):

1. The patient is standing and the therapist is at the back. The therapist pulls the patient to stimulate equilibrium reactions (Fig. 5.11).
2. As above, but the therapist is in front of the patient (Fig. 5.12).
3. The patient is on a chair and she/he tries to destabilize her-/himself standing on two legs by the same side of the affected labyrinth, maintaining balance control. Therapist surveys patient's movements in order, preventing falls (Fig. 5.13).

5.2 Home Protocol

When the patient is sufficiently able to walk alone, a home protocol aimed to reach and maintain compensation can be performed. Exercises have been subdivided according to different phases of equilibrium, from supine to standing to moving. In each part, there is a progression from *mechanic* to *synergetic* exercises. The exercises aim to enable the patient to achieve compensation at home as far as possible, reducing the secondary damage and avoiding the tertiary damage. The complete protocol has to be initially performed twice a day for 10 days. After this period the protocol can be reduced to the following exercises, to be performed twice a day for at least 1 month: 8–14, 19–23, 28–32

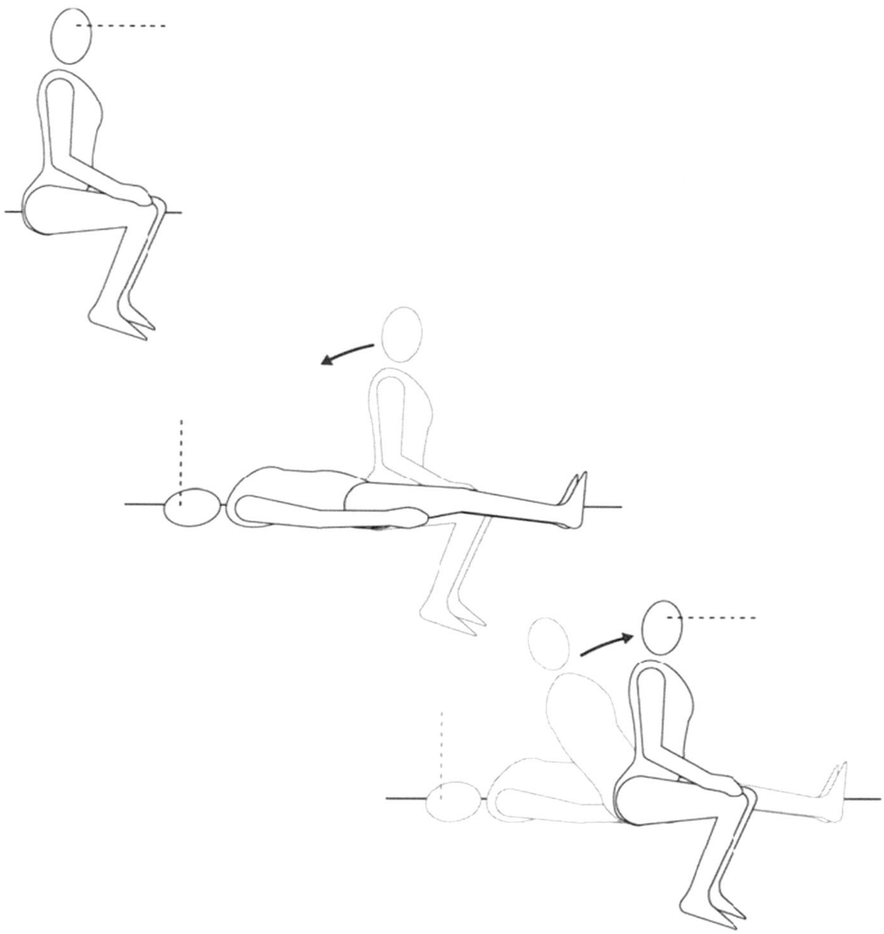

Fig. 5.7 Fixating a target, the patient gets down and gets up (Originally published in Alpini et al. [20] published by Springer © 1999)

Supine

1. Hold your knee, which is the opposite site of the lesion, against the chest; then extend your leg. When you hold your knee against the chest, the hands are gently applying traction to the flexed leg (Fig. 5.14).
2. Take your arm which is the same side as the lesion, extend it over your head and simultaneously hold the controlateral flexed leg to the chest, using your hand for assistance. Maintain this position for 10 s (Fig. 5.15).
3. Lift your leg on the same side as the lesion with the knee extended (Fig. 5.16).
4. Repeat with the tip of the foot outward.
5. Repeat with the tip of the foot inward.

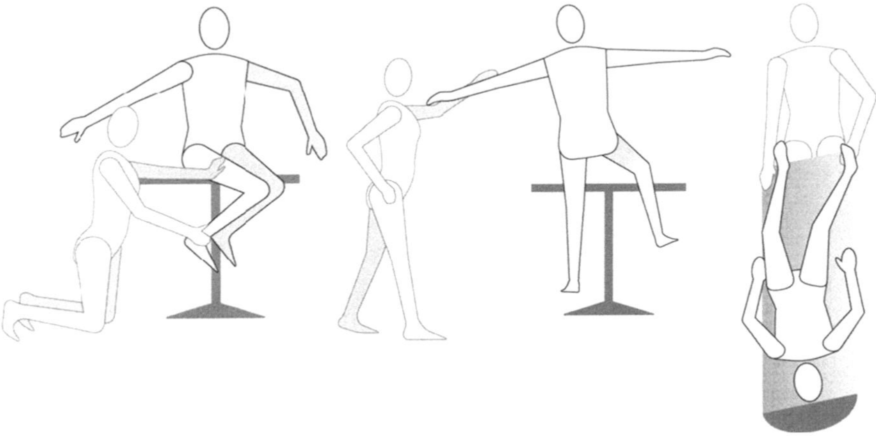

Figs. 5.8, 5.9, and 5.10 Equilibrium reactions to pushing stimulation by the therapist (Originally published in Alpini et al. [20] published by Springer © 1999)

Fig. 5.11 Balance reactions induced by pushing stimulations (Originally published in Alpini et al. [20] published by Springer © 1999)

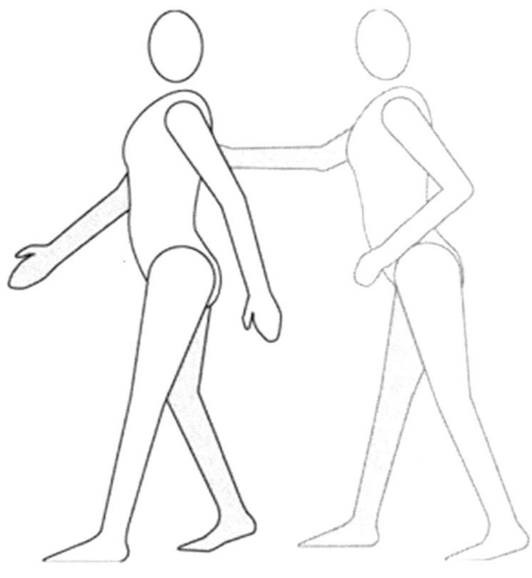

6. Put a pillow under your leg (on the same side of the lesion). Bound a 2 kg weight to your ankle with the knee flexed; then extend it.
7. Lift your pelvis; taking simultaneously, extend your arms over your head. Then drop your arms back along the body and lower your pelvis (Fig. 5.17).
8. Turn your head toward the side of the lesion and fixate a target on the lateral wall. Then straighten your head straight while maintaining the visual fixation. Count 1 up to 10 and then turn your head.

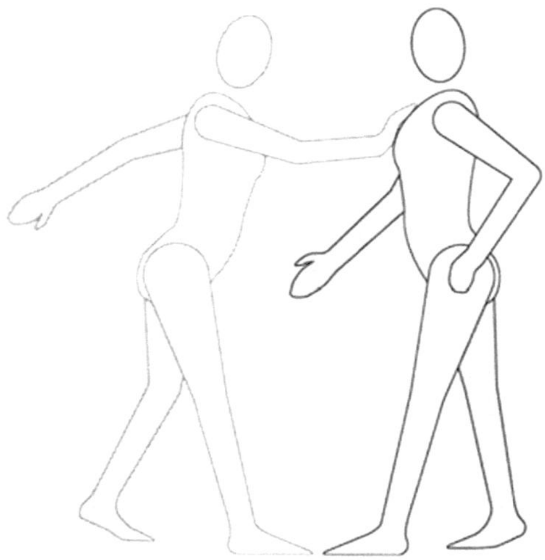

Fig. 5.12 Equilibrium reactions to pushing stimulation by the therapist (Originally published in Alpini et al. [20] published by Springer © 1999)

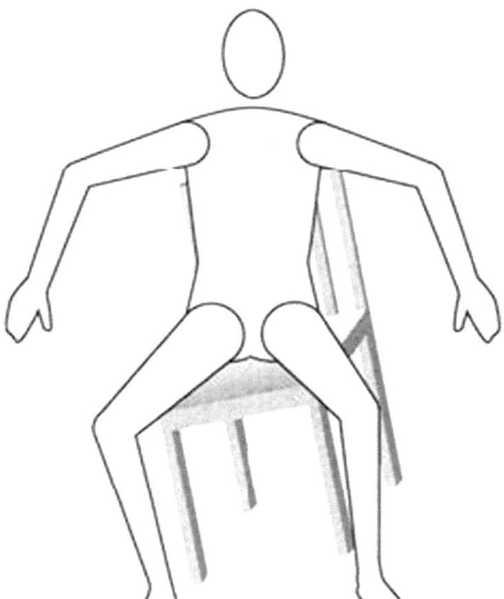

Fig. 5.13 Patient tries to maintain equilibrium in a destabilized position of the chair (Originally published in Alpini et al. [20] published by Springer © 1999)

9. From supine position, move to the sitting position, fixating a point straight in front of you.
10. In prone position, lift your left arm and the right leg, maintaining your forehead over the bed. Then repeat the manoeuvre with the right arm and the left leg (Fig. 5.18).
11. Repeat as above but simultaneously lifting also the head.

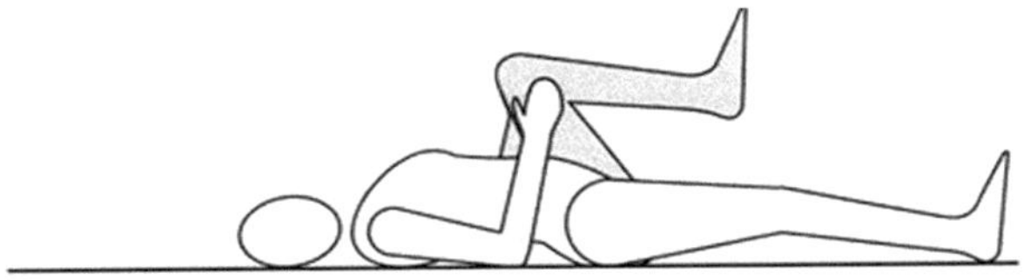

Fig. 5.14 Patient holds the knee against the chest (Originally published in Alpini et al. [20] published by Springer © 1999)

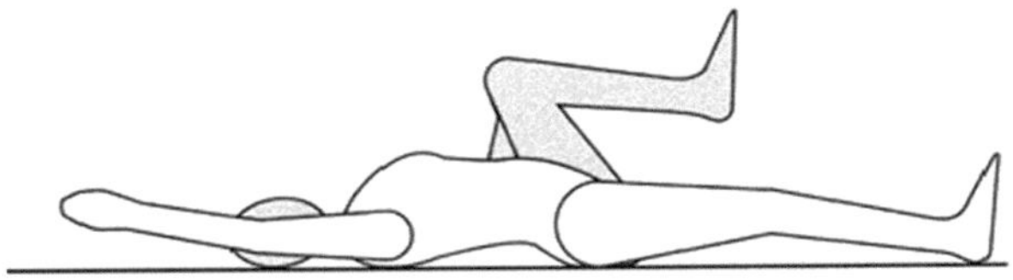

Fig. 5.15 Patient extends the arm on the affected side and at the same time holds the opposite knee against the chest (Originally published in Alpini et al. [20] published by Springer © 1999)

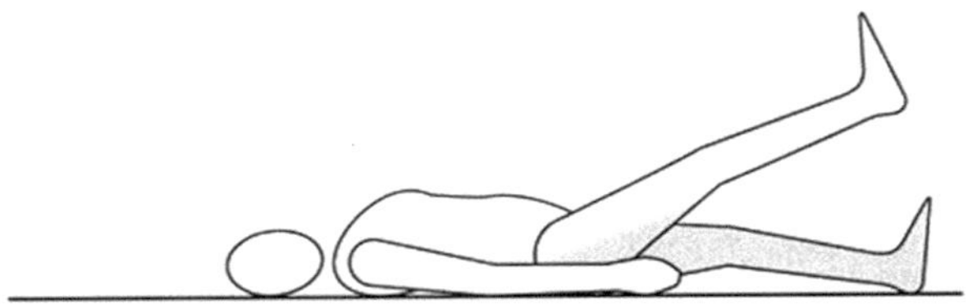

Fig. 5.16 Extension of the leg on the affected side (Originally published in Alpini et al. [20] published by Springer © 1999)

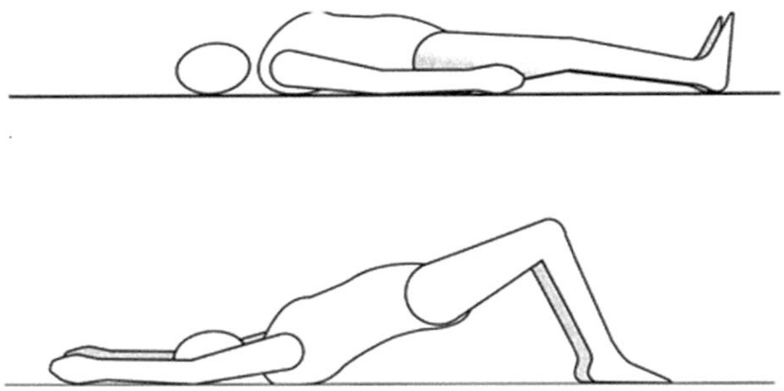

Fig. 5.17 Patient extends the arms, lifting the pelvis (Originally published in Alpini et al. [20] published by Springer © 1999)

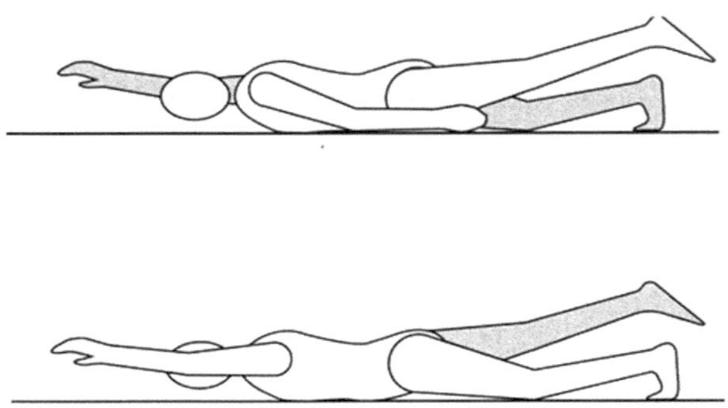

Fig. 5.18 Patient extends the right arm and left leg, in the prone position, and then alternates the arm and leg (Originally published in Alpini et al. [20] published by Springer © 1999)

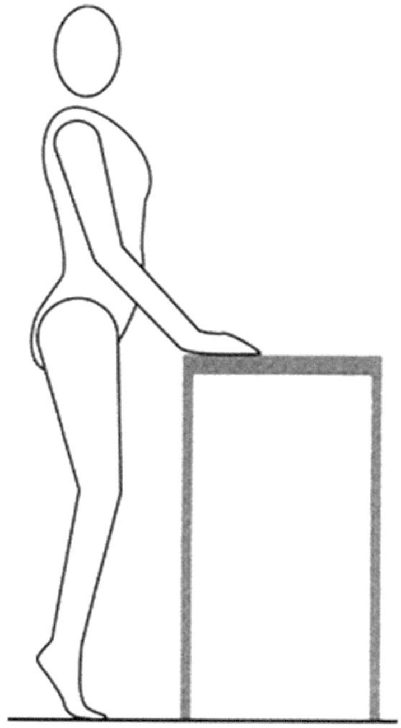

Fig. 5.19 Patient lifts himself standing on tiptoes (Originally published in Alpini et al. [20] published by Springer © 1999)

Sitting

12. Extend your right arm and lift your thumb. Move your arm slowly to and fro, first in a horizontal direction and then in a vertical direction. Follow your thumb with the eyes only, first slowly and then progressively increasing the velocity of thumb displacement.
13. As above, but simultaneously moving also the head while trying to keep the eyes still.
14. Open a book in front of you. Read it moving, simultaneously, the book right and left and then to and fro.

Standing

15. With your hands on a table, lift yourself onto your tiptoes with your weight on the leg on the same side as the lesion; maintain this position for 30 s (Fig. 5.19).
16. With your hands on a table, lift yourself onto your heels, with your weight on the leg on the same side as the lesion; maintain this position for 30 s (Fig. 5.20).
17. Fixate your image in a mirror. Align your position correctly. Maintain equilibrium for 1 min and then close your eyes and continue visualizing your correct position; remain in this position for at least 1 min (Fig. 5.21).
18. Repeat the same exercise standing on a soft mattress.
19. Hold a small object and then lift it over your head and fixate it. With your arms extended, move it in circles of increasing width while maintaining the fixation of the object (Fig. 5.22).
20. Repeat the same with eyes closed.

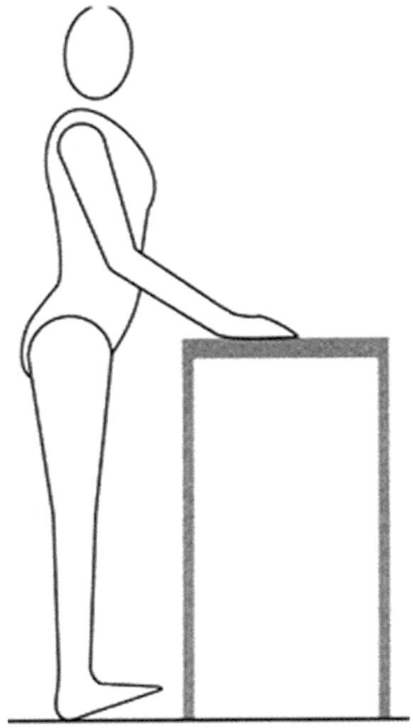

Fig. 5.20 As above, but standing on the heels (Originally published in Alpini et al. [20] published by Springer © 1999)

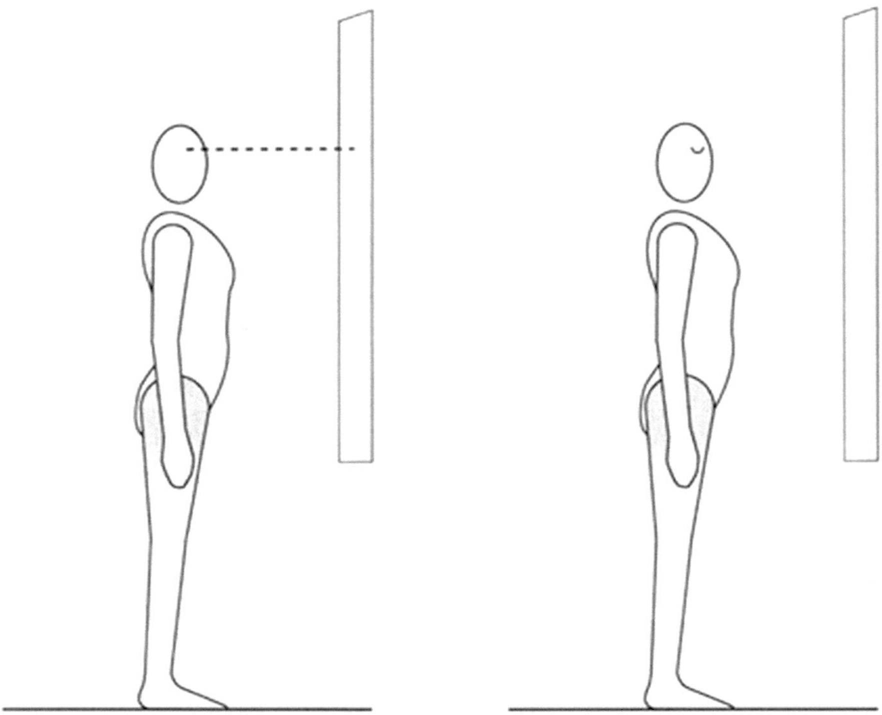

Fig. 5.21 Facing a mirror, the patient aligns himself correctly and then closes her/his eyes, maintaining a correct posture (Originally published in Alpini et al. [20] published by Springer © 1999)

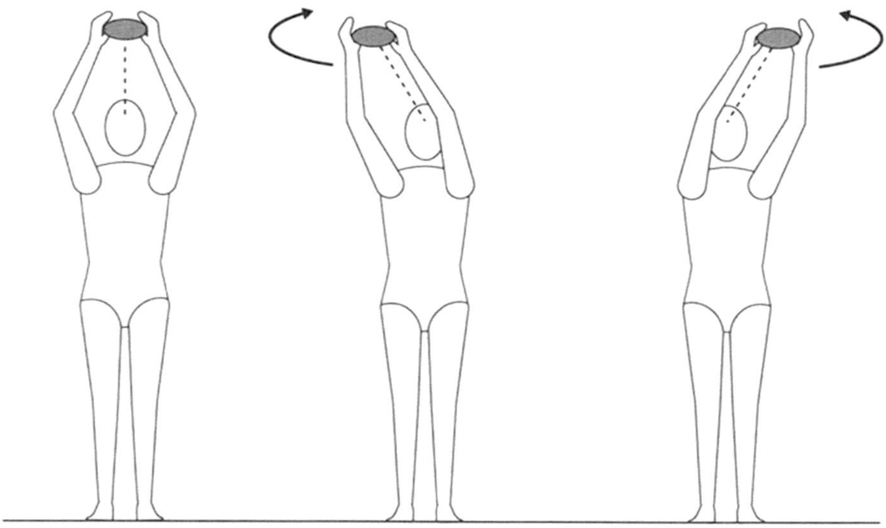

Fig. 5.22 Patient moves an object in circles while fixating it (Originally published in Alpini et al. [20] published by Springer © 1999)

21. Repeat the exercise again standing on a soft mattress.
22. Open a book in front of you. Read it while moving it simultaneously to and fro and from side to side.
23. Repeat the same exercise on a soft mattress.

Moving

24. Stepping on the floor with eyes open.
25. Stepping while fixating a target in front of you (if it is possible wearing pinhole glasses).
26. Stepping with eyes closed.
27. Stepping moving the head to and fro.
28. Stepping reading a book.
29. In a corridor, walk for 5 steps forward and then backward, fixating a target (if it is possible wearing pinhole glasses). Also in a corridor, walk for 5 steps forward and backward staring, without any reference target (without pinhole glasses).
30. In a corridor, walk for 5 steps forward and then backward with eyes closed, remaining a distance of 20 cm. from the wall on the side of your vestibular hypofunction
31. In a corridor, walk for 5 steps forward and then backward while moving your head to and fro.
32. In a corridor, walk for 5 steps forward and then backward reading a book.

5.3 Counselling

As the most frequent cause of sudden vestibular loss is a viral infection, it is important to pay attention to lifestyle, in general, and to stress control, particularly.

The main suggestions are:

- To perform regular and constant aerobic physical activity: e.g. rapid walking (not running neither jogging) 30′/day three times/week
- To maintain a diet rich of fruit and vegetables (five servings/day) especially in autumn and spring
- To avoid industrial food
- To avoid hot chili pepper and, generally, foods containing capsaicin [18]
- To maintain adequate water intake (at least 1.5 l for females and 2 l for males)
- To restrict alcohol intake (less than 120 ml for women and 240 ml for men)
- To avoid smoking and, obviously, drug abuse
- To maintain proper night-and-day rhythm and at least 6–8 h of sleep (melatonin 5 mg at bedtime may be useful)
- To sleep using two pillows in order to maintain the head lifted about 20°

Further, we also suggest prevention of seasonal relapsing by means of vitamins D, C and B (especially B9) and antiherpetic prophylaxis to avoid the possible evolution of viral vestibular neuritis to acoustic neuroma [19].

Note. The contents of this chapter are partially based on: *MCS Protocols* (A. Cesarani, D. Alpini) in: A. Cesarani, D. Alpini (1999) Vertigo and Dizziness Rehabilitation - The MCS Method. Springer, p 128.

References

1. Smouha E (2013) Inner ear disorders. NeuroRehabilitation 32(3):455–462
2. Frenzel H, Tonndorf EE (1957) Nystagmus mobilization with closed eyes and in the darkness and elimination of fixation by spectacles with a lighting device. Pract Otorhinolaryngol (Basel) 19(6):507–517. German
3. Frenzel H (1957) Present stand of vestibular function tests. II. Modern development. Dtsch Med Wochenschr 82(11):372–378. German
4. Frenzel H (1957) Current status of vestibular function tests. Dtsch Med Wochenschr 82(10):337–341; contd. German
5. Brandt T, Dieterich M, Strupp M (2005) Vertigo and dizziness—common complaints. Springer, London
6. Hemenway WG, Lindsay JR (1956) Postural vertigo due to unilateral sudden partial loss of vestibular function. Ann Otol Rhinol Laryngol 65(3):692–706
7. Sekitani T, Imate Y, Noguchi T, Inokuma T (1993) Vestibular neuronitis: epidemiological survey by questionnaire in Japan. Acta Otolaryngol (Stockh) Suppl 503:9–12
8. Arbusow V, Schulz P, Strupp M et al (1999) Distribution of herpes simplex virus type 1 in human geniculate and vestibular ganglia: implications for vestibular neuritis. Ann Neurol 46:416–419
9. Arbusow V, Theil D, Strupp M, Mascolo A, Brandt T (2000) HSV-1 not only in human vestibular ganglia but also in the vestibular labyrinth. Audiol Neurootol 6:259–262
10. Theil D, Derfuss T, Paripovic I et al (2003) Latent herpesvirus infection in human trigeminal ganglia causes chronic immune response. Am J Pathol 163:2179–2184

11. Cesarani A, Alpini D, Monti B, Raponi G (2004) The treatment of acute vertigo. Neurol Sci 25(Suppl 1):S26–S30
12. Ossola B, Schendzielorz N, Chen SH, Bird GS, Tuominen RK, Männistö PT, Hong JS (2011) Amantadine protects dopamine neurons by a dual action: reducing activation of microglia and inducing expression of GNDF in astroglia. Neuropharmacology 61(4):574–582
13. Alpini D, Cesarani A, Barozzi S (1992) Non pharmacological treatment of acute vertigo. In: Claussen CF, Kirtane MV, Schneider D (eds) Diagnostic procedures and imaging techniques used in neurotology. Proceedings of the XVI NES Congress, Dr. Werner Rudat & Co. Nachf. Edition M+P, Hambourg, 1992, pp 337–340
14. Cesarani A, Alpini D, Barozzi S (1990) Electrical stimulation in the treatment of acute vertigo. In: Sacristan T, Alvarez-Vincent JJ, Bartual J, Antoli-Candela F (eds) Otorhinolaryngology, head & neck surgery. Proceedings of the XIV World Congress of Otorhinolaryngology, Madrid, 1989. Kugler & Ghedini Publ., Amsterdam/Berkeley/Milano
15. Cesarani A, Alpini D, Barozzi S (1990) Neck electrical stimulation in the treatment of labyrinth acute vertigo. Riv It Eeg Neurof Cl 13(1):55–61
16. Hu S, Stern RM, Koch KL (1992) Electrical acustimulation relieves vection induced motion sickness. Gastroenterology 102(6):1854–1858
17. Misslisch H, Tweed D, Vilis T (1998) Neural constraints on eye surface, stating that the vectors are confined to a head-fixed motion in human eye-head saccades. J Neurophysiol 79:859–869
18. Vass Z, Dai CF, Steyger PS, Jancsó G, Trune DR, Nuttall AL (2004) Co-localization of the vanilloid capsaicin receptor and substance P in sensory nerve fibers innervating cochlear and vertebro-basilar arteries. Neuroscience 124(4):919–927
19. Burkhart CG (2010) Herpes and acoustic neuromas: is there a cause and effect to observe? Med Hypothes 74:1013–1014
20. Alpini DC, Brugnoni G, Cesarani A (1999) Vertigo and dizziness rehabilitation – the MCS method. Springer, Milan, Heidelberg

6 Uncompensated Unilateral Vestibular Hypofunction

Vestibular unilateral hypofunction is a consequence of the primary damage to the vestibular structures. Incorrect or incomplete compensation can cause secondary and tertiary damages. Natural compensatory phenomena require, without any kind of treatment, a period ranging from 6 to 8 months to reach a good functional recovery. This kind of recovery is not always sufficient to allow performing even everyday life activities in a natural, unconscious and easy manner. Some activities are still difficult such as turning the head rapidly or changing positions of the body, and, frequently, transient vertigo attacks and subcontinuos unsteadiness are observed. Even after some years following an acute episode of vertigo, compensation can turn into transient failure and cause vertigo or dizziness or unsteadiness (VDU).

Incomplete vestibular compensation of any kind of vestibular lesion causes impairment of the most common daily life activities in every patient, but, at least in some subjects, chronic VDU may lead to specific disability and handicap. Disability may be correlated to specific job activities but, more generally, chronic VDU may impact on common life activities through disturbances of the vestibulo-perceptual (VP) system. Cortical vestibular networks presumably mediate perception of whole-body motion. As with all psychophysical systems, decisions ("in which direction am I moving?") are based on the detection of signals (stimuli), such as semicircular canal afferent information, against a background of activity, or noise. As with other psychophysical systems, the VP system has a defined threshold at which a signal becomes recognized relative to the noise level [1, 2]. For the vestibular system, humans possess higher perceptual than VOR thresholds [3]. These higher perceptual thresholds in humans probably reflect the cortical processing of vestibular signals during decision making in direction recognition tasks [4]. Significant cortical changes are observed in patients following acute vestibular lesions [5, 6].

D.C. Alpini et al., *Vertigo Rehabilitation Protocols*,
DOI 10.1007/978-3-319-05482-7_6, © Springer International Publishing Switzerland 2014

The relationship between vestibular function and feelings of unreality was recognized decades ago, when Schilder emphasized its connection with depersonalization [7]. This tendency for abnormal vestibular stimulation to provoke feelings of unreality has also been found in normal healthy subjects undergoing calorics [8, 9]; furthermore, false perceptions of orientation may be a consequence of vestibular disorders [10]. Cousins et al. [11] in fact, provided the functional evidence that higher-order mechanisms, ultimately involving the cerebral cortex, are engaged early in vestibular compensation and vertigo suppression. They showed that vestibulo-perceptual function is significantly affected by vestibular neuritis: VP thresholds are raised and asymmetrical, whereas VP supra-threshold time constants are shortened but symmetrical. In this way, a bilateral suppression of supra-threshold vestibular perception is obtained; this suppression may act as a protective mechanism against vertigo but lead to chronic impairment and disability sometimes with anxiety, panic attack, depersonalization/derealization until phobic postural vertigo (see Chap. 13) [12]. The disorientation due to deficient sensory integration could contribute to derealization that occurs in vestibular patients because their distorted vestibular signals create a misleading frame of spatial reference which mismatches with the other senses, as proposed by [13].

The perceptual dampening is probably the neurophysio-pathological phenomenon that can lead to the transition that a patient with acute vestibular neuritis underwent to phobic postural vertigo within months after disease onset [14].

The following protocol can be adopted also to treat dizziness in Ménière patients (see Chap. 10) during intercritical period. Vertigo attacks cannot be prevented by rehabilitation but often patients complain both sporadic vertigo attacks and continuous unsteadiness. This condition can be treated as a vestibular unilateral hypofunction.

Rehabilitation is the specific treatment of unilateral vestibular hypofunction. In fact, despite the *cause* of hypofunction being known, as after the operation of neurinoma, after an attack of neuronitis, in the postcommotional syndrome, or even when viral or vascular aetiology is confirmed, improvement of the dizziness cannot always be obtained by acting upon these etiologic factors or by administration of some symptomatic drugs. In all these cases with unilateral hypofunction, only the phenomena of the central regulation – the compensation – are able to render these patients free from symptoms and to manage their *impairment,* avoiding *disability*.

Generally speaking, the *key impairment* is due to head dynamic unsteadiness, postural instability and dynamic disequilibrium with fear of new vertigo attacks.

Treatment must be pointed to:

1. Increase extensor tone on the affected side
2. Increase antigravitary paravertebral tone
3. Restore correct ankle–hip strategies dynamic
4. Restore control of head stabilization during movement
5. Restore eye–head coordination
6. Avoid disorientation and transition to phobic postural vertigo (PPV, see Chap. 13)

6.1 Exercises in the Gymnasium

6.1.1 First Week

1. Relaxation exercises such as control of breathing with improving consciousness of abdomen or thoracic breathing. A simple exercise consists in deep inhalation followed, after few seconds, by a forced exhalation pronouncing the word "one". This exercise is repeated 8–10 times.
2. The patient holds her/his right knee against the chest, then she/he extends her/his leg and holds her/his left knee against the chest. When she/he holds the knee against the chest, she/he gently applies traction to the flexed leg with the hands (Fig. 6.1a, b).
3. The patient holds her/his two knees to the chest while simultaneously helping, gently, with the hands (Fig. 6.1c).
4. With the legs flexed and the feet on the bed, the patient rotates her/his pelvis rightward and leftward keeping her/his knees flexed and her/his legs together (Fig. 6.2).
5. The patient lifts her/his pelvis while simultaneously holding her/his arms extended over her/his head. She/he then repositions her/his arms along the body while lowering her/his pelvis (Fig. 6.3).

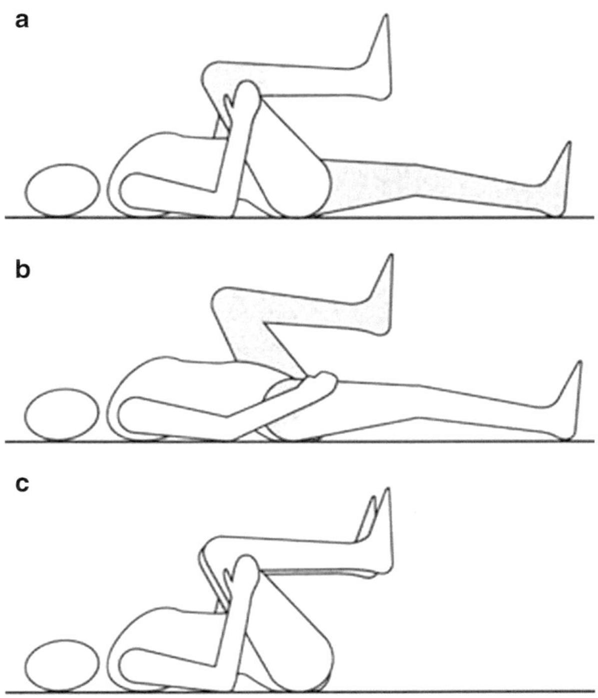

Fig. 6.1 (**a–c**) Exercises holding the knees against the chest (Originally published in Cesarani and Alpini [15] published by Springer © 1999)

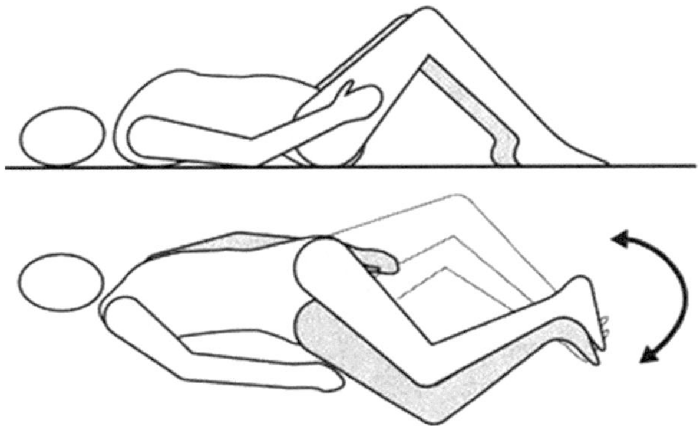

Fig. 6.2 Rotation of the pelvis (Originally published in Cesarani and Alpini [15] published by Springer © 1999)

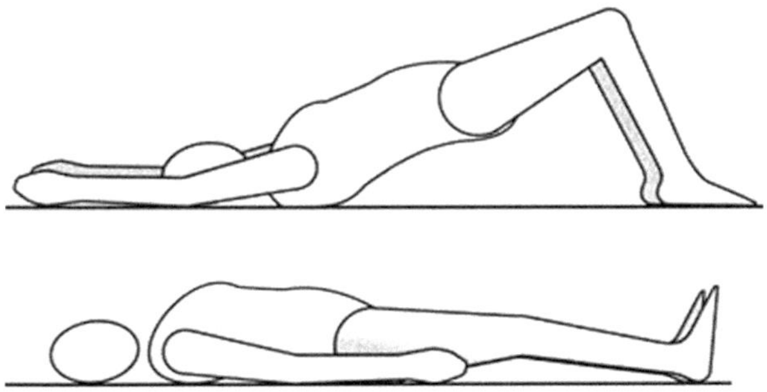

Fig. 6.3 Patient lifts the pelvis and then returns to the supine position (Originally published in Cesarani and Alpini [15] published by Springer © 1999)

6. In the quadrupedal position, the patient inhales and arches her/his back (hyperkyphosis) while holding her/his head between her/his arms. She/he then exhales, flexing the head and rotating the pelvis in hyperlordosis (Fig. 6.4).
7. From supine position, the patient passes to the sitting position, fixating a point straight in front of her/him (Fig. 6.5).
8. The patient, with a pillow under the leg (by the affected side) and with a 2 kg weight bound to the ankle, extends the leg (Fig. 6.6).
9. In the sitting position, the patient grasps a stick with both hands and takes the stick behind her/his shoulder, positioning the stick at the level of cervico-dorsal junction. In this position, she/he pushes the stick against her/his back, exhaling and inhaling rhythmically and slowly. She/he then repeats the exercise, moving the stick forward on the sternum at the level of the sterno-clavear joint. The patient grasps the stick with the hands frontally positioned.

6.1.2 Second Week

The following exercise has to be performed during TENS cervical stimulation, placing electrodes on the trapezius of the affected side and the paravertebral muscles of the opposite side:

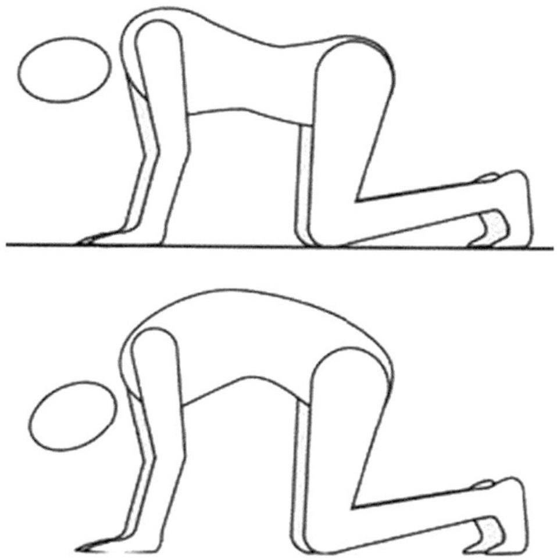

Fig. 6.4 Patient arches the dorsal spine (Originally published in Cesarani and Alpini [15] published by Springer © 1999)

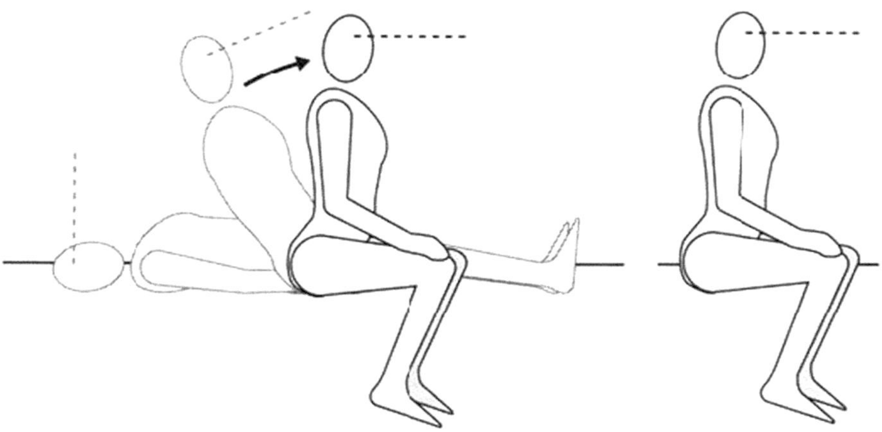

Fig. 6.5 From the supine to the sitting position, fixating a target (Originally published in Cesarani and Alpini [15] published by Springer © 1999)

Standing on a Foam Mattress

1. The patient (if it is possible wearing pinhole glasses) fixates her-/himself in a mirror. Therapist helps her/him to align her/his position correctly. She/he must maintain equilibrium for 1 min with eyes open and then close the eyes and visualize her/his correct position while remaining in this position for at least 1 min.

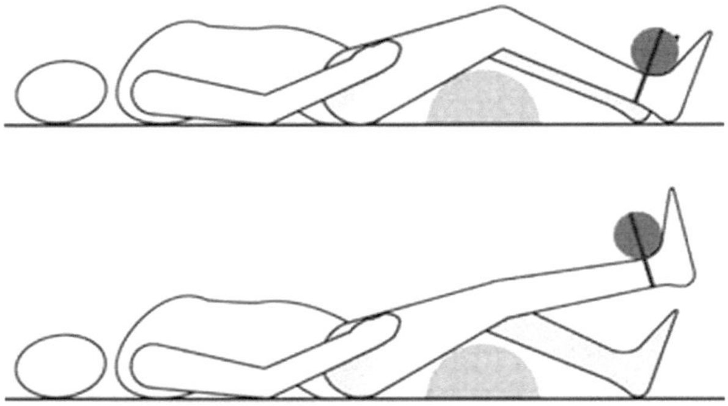

Fig. 6.6 With a weight bound to the ankle, the patient extends the leg on the affected side (Originally published in Cesarani and Alpini [15] published by Springer © 1999)

2. The patient fixates her-/himself in a mirror (Fig. 6.7a). Then she/he oscillates right and left (Fig. 6.7b), around her/his pelvis. She/he then resists the therapist's attempts at destabilizations (Fig. 6.7c) and maintains equilibrium, crossing the legs (Fig. 6.7d).
3. The patient oscillates to and fro around her/his ankles while maintaining fixation in a mirror (Fig. 6.8).
4. The patient holds a small object and then lifts it over the head and fixates it. With her/his extended arms, she/he moves it in circles of increasing width while maintaining the fixation of the object (Fig. 6.9). Standing on an oscillating platform (so-called Balance board) looking a mirror
5. The patient concentrates on a proper posture, using a mirror to see her/his reflection, and thus she/he tries to maintain equilibrium as longer as possible (no more than 1′).
6. The patient transfers her/his weight from one foot to the other with a smooth flowing motion.
7. The patient tries to maintain a proper posture while the therapist destabilizes her/him with gently pushes.

6.1.3 Third Week

The following exercise has to be performed during TENS cervical stimulation placing electrodes on the trapezius of the affected side and the paravertebral muscles of the opposite side:

Standing on a Foam Mattress

1. The patient opens a book in front of her/him and then moves it away from her/him, extending the arms. She/he reads it then moves it closer to her/him, slowly, while trying to read it. Then she/he moves it away.
2. The patient performs steps while fixating a target in front of her/him while wearing pinhole glasses (Fig. 6.10).
3. The patient performs a step while reading a book.

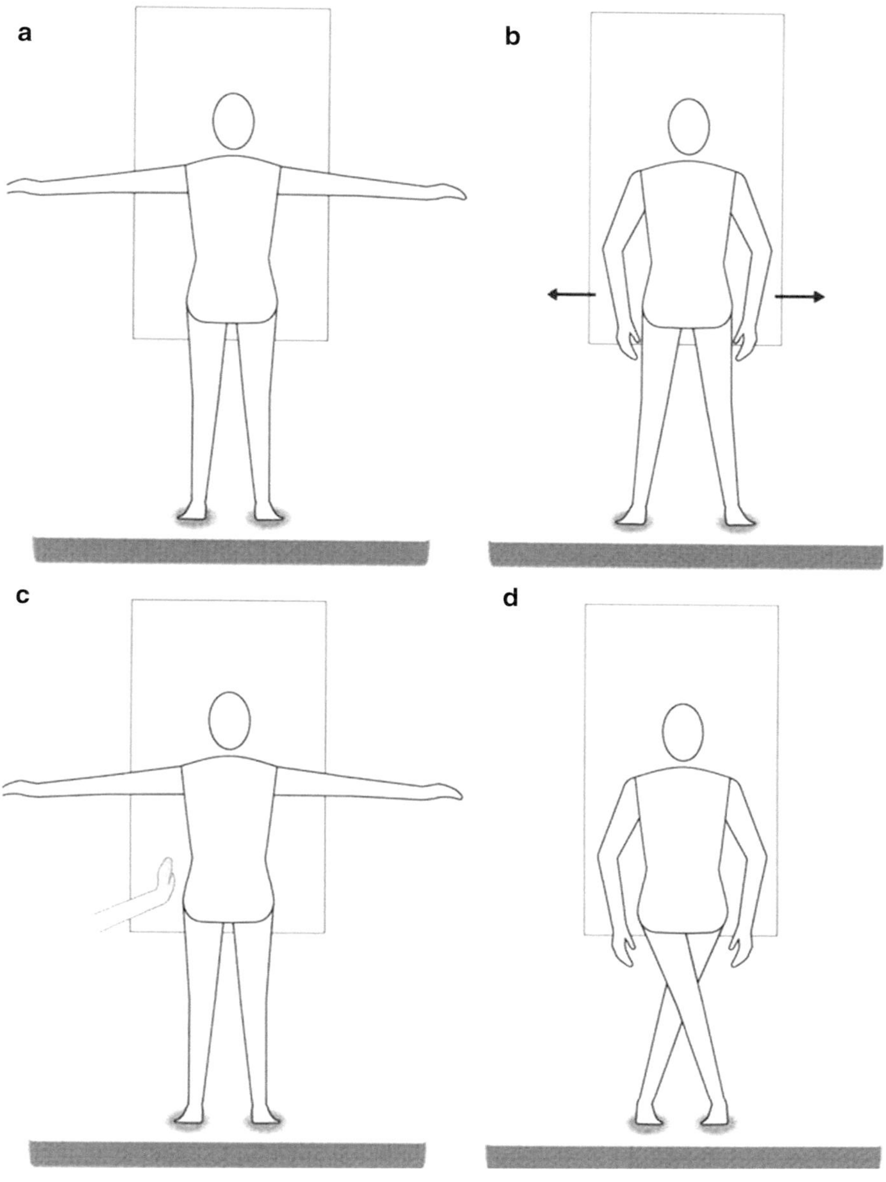

Fig. 6.7 The patient aligns her-/himself looking at a mirror (**a**), then she/he oscillates (**b**), then resists when the therapist destabilizes her/him (**c**) or she/he maintains equilibrium crossing the legs (**d**) (Originally published in Cesarani and Alpini [15] published by Springer © 1999)

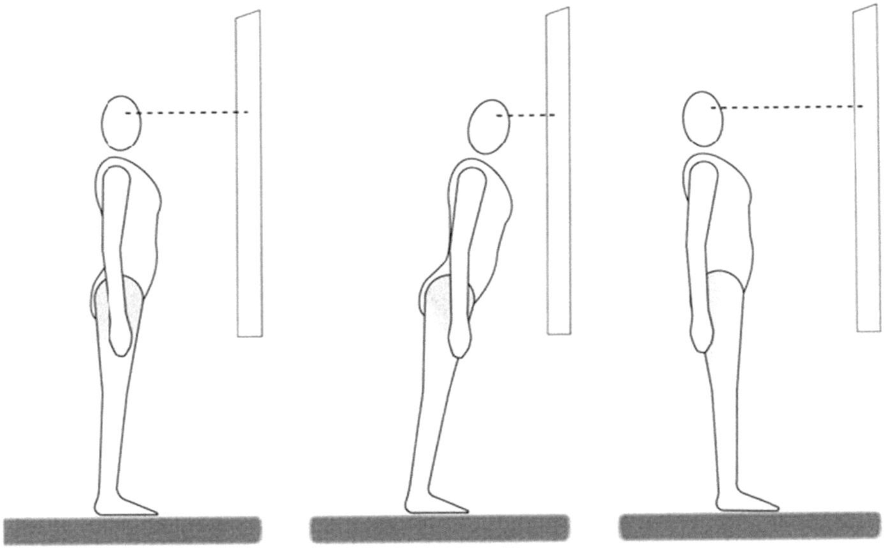

Fig. 6.8 The patient oscillates around her/his ankles, maintaining the pelvis still (Originally published in Cesarani and Alpini [15] published by Springer © 1999)

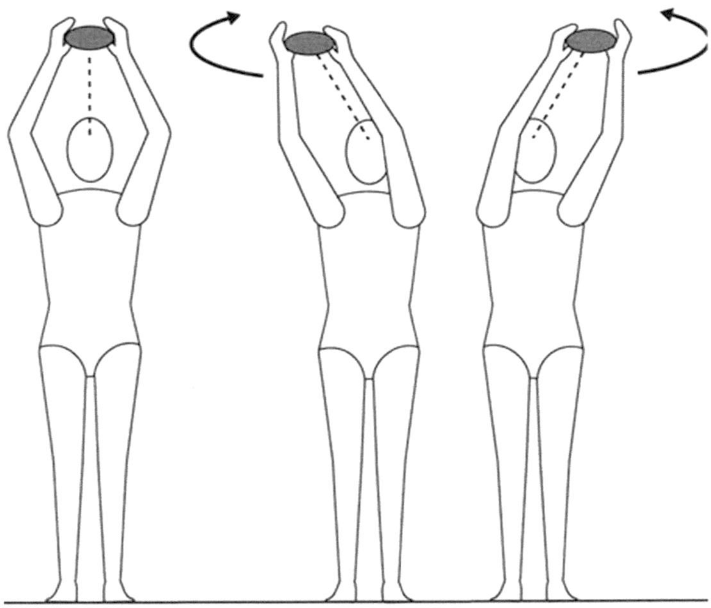

Fig. 6.9 Patient fixates a small object while moving it in circles, standing on a mattress (Originally published in Cesarani and Alpini [15] published by Springer © 1999)

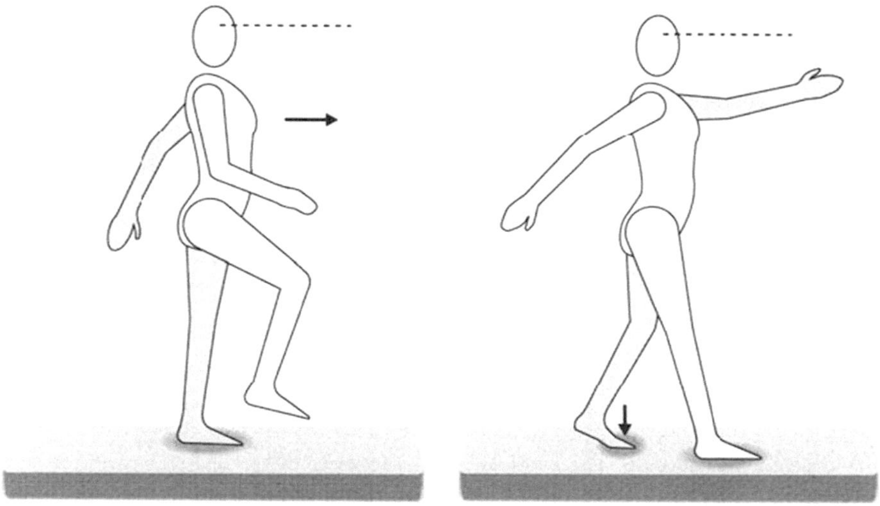

Fig. 6.10 Stepping on a mattress without and with simultaneous oscillations of the arms, fixating a target (Originally published in Cesarani and Alpini [15] published by Springer © 1999)

Standing on an Oscillating Platform (So-Called Balance Board), Looking a Mirror

4. The patient tries to touch some targets (post-its, of different colours) placed in different positions on a facing mirror.
5. The patient maintains equilibrium on one leg, before the leg on the health side and then the leg on the affected side, as longer as possible.

6–7. Exercises 4 and 5 wearing pinhole glasses.

By Visual Feedback Devices

8. The patient is stable on the stabilometric platform, without shoes. The position of the visual targets has to be according to the side of the lesion. In Figs. 6.11 and 6.12, examples of target position for a left vestibular hypofunction are represented.
9. The patient is stable on the platform, with shoes, wearing a lift heel by the same side of lesion. The position of the targets is the same.

Moving

10. The patient walks for 5 steps forward and backward, fixating a target, wearing pinhole glasses.
11. The patient walks for 5 steps forward and backward with eyes closed, remaining a distance of 20 cm. of distance from the wall on the side of the vestibular hypofunction.
12. The patient walks for 5 steps forward and backward, moving her/his head to and fro.
13. The patient walks for 5 steps forward and backward, moving her/his head to and fro, wearing pinhole glasses.

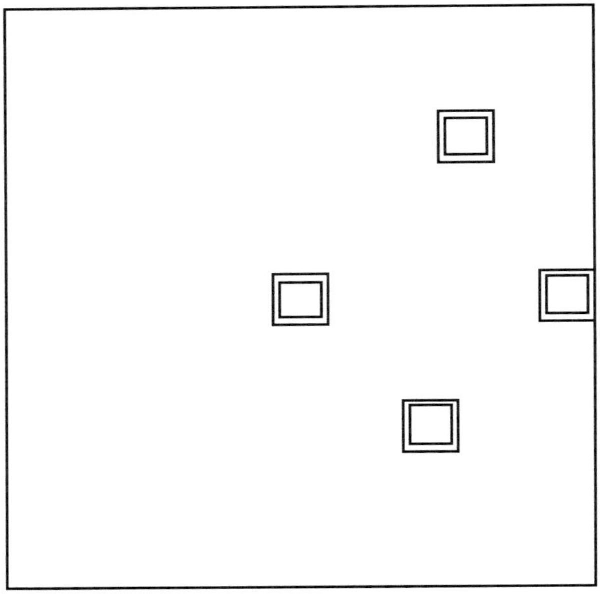

Fig. 6.11 Training for right vestibular hypofunction (Balance Master, reproduced with courtesy of NeuroCom International, Inc, Clackamas, Oregon, USA. Originally published in Cesarani and Alpini [15] published by Springer © 1999)

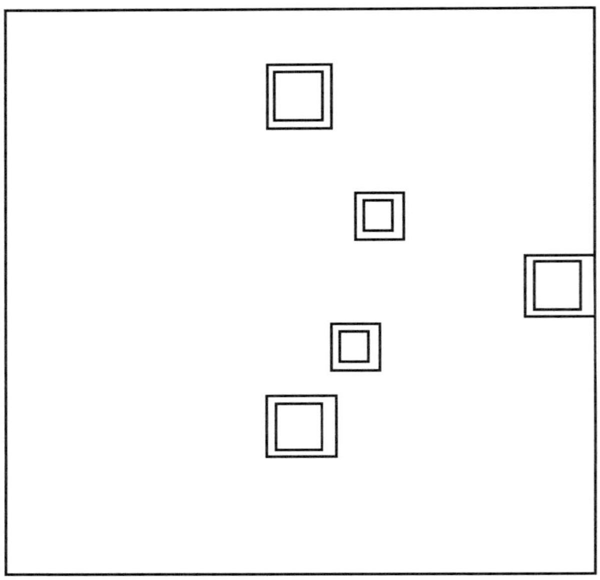

Fig. 6.12 Increasing ankle–hip strategies in right hypofunction (Balance Master, reproduced with courtesy of NeuroCom International, Inc, Clackamas, Oregon, USA. Originally published in Cesarani and Alpini [15] published by Springer © 1999)

Table 6.1 Home protocol

Supine
1. Lift the leg by the same side of lesion with the extended knee.
2. Repeat the exercise with the tip of the foot outward.
3. Repeat the exercise with the tip of the foot inward.
4. Place a pillow under your leg (on the same side as the lesion). Bind a 2 kg weight on your ankle with the flexed knee; then extend it, alternating right and left leg.
5. Lift your pelvis, simultaneously extending your arms over your head. Then reposition your arms along the body, lowering your pelvis.
6. From supine position, shift to sitting position, fixating a point straight ahead.
Sitting
7. Extend your right arm and lift your thumb. Move your arm slowly to and fro in a horizontal direction and then in a vertical direction. Follow your thumb with eyes only, first slowly and then increasing progressively the velocity of thumb displacement.
8. As above, but simultaneously moving the head trying to keep the eyes still.
9. Look for three targets sited, respectively, in front of you, at your left and at your right. Fixate the frontal target; then move your head, rapidly fixating the right-hand target. Now turn your head leftward while maintaining the fixation of the right-hand target. Fixate the frontal target. Now rapidly move your head leftward and fixate the left-hand target. Then turn your head rightward while maintaining the fixation of the left-hand target.
10. Extend your right arm and lift your thumb. Move your arm slowly to and fro, first in a horizontal direction and then in a vertical direction. Follow your thumb with eyes only, first slowly and then increasing progressively the velocity of thumb displacement.
11. As above, but also moving the head simultaneously while trying to keep the eyes still.
Standing
12. Standing on a soft mattress, fixate yourself in a mirror. Align your position correctly. Maintain equilibrium for 1 min and then close your eyes and visualize your correct position; remain in this position for at least 1 min.
13. Hold a small object and then lift it over your head and fixate it. With your arms extended, move it in circles of increasing width while maintaining the fixation of the object. Then close your eyes and continue making the circles.
14. Standing on a soft mattress, open a book in front of you. Read it while simultaneously moving it to and fro and from side to side.
Moving
15. Stepping with eyes closed.
16. Stepping, moving the head to and fro.
17. In a corridor, walk for 5 steps forward and backward with eyes closed, remaining a distance of 20 cm from the wall on the side of your vestibular hypofunction.

6.2 Home Protocol

The aim of home protocol is to maintain the results obtained with the therapist. Exercises have been subdivided according the sequence of equilibrium (Table 6.1). Only the most effective exercises have been comprehended into this protocol because the patient has to repeat them twice or three times a day.

6.3 Counselling

It is important to pay attention to lifestyle, in general, and to stress control, particularly.

The main suggestions are:

- To control own Body Mass Index (BMI).
- BMI is correlated to body fatness and it is calculated as body weight (in Kilos) divided by square height (in metres); e.g. a subject weighed 70 kg and 1.74 m height has a BMI as follows: 70/(1.74 × 1.74) = 23.1. Normal values are between 18.5 and 24.9 (World Health Organization, WHO).
- To perform regular and constant aerobic physical activity: e.g. rapid walking (not running neither jogging) 30′/day three times/week.
- To maintain a diet rich of fruit and vegetables (five servings/day) especially in autumn and spring.
- To avoid industrial food.
- To avoid chili foods (see also Chap. 5).
- To maintain adequate water intake (at least 1.5 l for females and 2 l for males).
- To restrict alcohol intake (less than 120 ml for women and 240 ml for men).
- To avoid smoking and, obviously, drug abuse.
- To sleep using two pillows in order to maintain the head lifted about 20°.

Note The contents of this chapter are partially based on: *Uncompensated Unilateral Vestibular Hypofunction* (A. Cesarani, D. Alpini) in: A. Cesarani, D. Alpini (1999) Vertigo and Dizziness Rehabilitation – The MCS Method. Springer, p 141.

References

1. Green DM, Swets JA (1966) Signal detection theory and psychophysics. Wiley, New York
2. Merfeld D (2011) Signal detection theory and vestibular thresholds: I. Basic theory and practical considerations. Exp Brain Res 210:389–405
3. Seemungal BM, Gunaratne IA, Fleming IO, Gresty MA, Bronstein AM (2004) Perceptual and nystagmic thresholds of vestibular function in yaw. J Vestib Res 14:461–466
4. Haburcakova C, Lewis R, Merfeld D (2012) Frequency dependence of vestibulo-ocular reflex thresholds. J Neurophysiol 107(3):973–983
5. Helmchen C, Klinkenstein J, Machner B, Rambold H, Mohr C et al (2009) Structural changes in the human brain following vestibular neuritis indicate central vestibular compensation. Ann N Y Acad Sci 1164:104–115
6. Dieterich M, Brandt T (2008) Functional brain imaging of peripheral and central vestibular disorders. Brain 131:2538–2552
7. Schilder P (1964) The image and appearance of the human body. Studies in the constructive energies of the psyche. Wiley, New York
8. Cappon D, Banks R (1961) Orientational perception. A review and preliminary study of distortion in orientational perception. Arch Gen Psychiatry 5:380–392
9. Cappon D, Banks R (1965) Orientational perception. II. Body perception in depersonalization. Arch Gen Psychiatry 13:375–379
10. Cappon D (1969) Orientational perception: 3. Orientational percept distortions in depersonalization. Am J Psychiatry 125:1048–1056

11. Cousins S, Kaski D, Cutfield N, Seemungal B, Golding JF et al (2013) Vestibular perception following acute unilateral vestibular lesions. PLoS ONE 8(5):e61862. doi:10.1371/journal.pone.0061862
12. Brandt T (1996) Phobic postural vertigo. Neurology 46:1515–1519
13. Yen Pik Sang F, Jauregui-Renaud K, Green DA, Bronstein A, Gresty AM (2006) Depersonalisation/derealisation symptoms in vestibular disease. J Neurol Neurosurg Psychiatry 77:760–766
14. Brandt T, Strupp M, Novozhilov S, Krafczyk S (2012) Artificial neural network posturography detects the transition of vestibular neuritis to phobic postural vertigo. J Neurol 259:182–184
15. Cesarani A, Alpini D (1999) Vertigo and dizziness rehabilitation – the MCS method. Springer, Milan, Heidelberg

7 Vestibular Ataxia (Bilateral Vestibular Hypofunctionpathy)

Bilateral loss of vestibular inputs affects far fewer patients than unilateral inner ear damage [1]. Bilateral vestibular hypofunction (BVH) produces a variety of clinical problems, including impaired balance control, inability to maintain stable blood pressure during postural changes, difficulty in visual targeting of images and disturbances in spatial memory and navigational performance. The cardinal symptoms are motion-dependent postural vertigo with unsteady gait and stance, particularly in darkness and on uneven ground (vestibulospinal functional impairment), together with oscillopsia and blurred vision when walking or moving the head (impairment of the vestibulo-ocular reflex). Patients with BVH are typically symptom-free when sitting or lying.

BVH involves circumscribed atrophy of the hippocampus with impairments of spatial memory and navigation and is the most frequent cause of motion-dependent postural vertigo in older patients.

There are many possible causes of BVP; the three most frequently identified are:

- Ototoxic aminoglycosides
- Bilateral Menière's disease [2]
- Meningitis

Antibiotic treatment with aminoglycosides is the most frequently determined cause of bilateral vestibulopathy. This class of drugs should therefore be used very sparingly, particularly since their ototoxic effect has a latency of several days.

One connection between BVH and degenerative cerebellar diseases has now been clearly established as cerebellar ataxia, neuropathy and vestibular areflexia syndrome (CANVAS) [3].

CANVAS comprising BVH in combination with sensory axonal polyneuropathy, cerebellar ataxia and oculomotor disturbances is responsible for around 30 % of the cases previously classified as idiopathic [4].

Despite a multitude of visits to the doctor, BVH is usually diagnosed too late, which amplifies the patient's symptoms.

The key impairments are head dynamic instability with oscillopsia, postural instability with unsteadiness and cognitive (navigation) problems.

D.C. Alpini et al., *Vertigo Rehabilitation Protocols*,
DOI 10.1007/978-3-319-05482-7_7, © Springer International Publishing Switzerland 2014

Recovery is strictly dependent on compensation and thus rehab plays the major role in the therapeutic planning. Experiments in animals have shown that non-labyrinthine inputs to the vestibular nuclei are rapidly amplified following the onset of BVH, which may explain the recovery of postural stability and orthostatic tolerance that occurs within 10 days. However, the loss of the vestibulo-ocular reflex and degraded spatial cognition appear to be permanent in animals with BVH. Current concepts of the compensatory mechanisms in humans with BVH are largely inferential. Translation of animal studies of compensation for BVH into therapeutic strategies and subsequent application in the clinic is the most likely route to improve treatment [5].

In addition to physical therapy, prosthetic devices have been proposed to treat individuals with bilateral loss of vestibular inputs. The relative efficacy of this treatment paradigm, and whether it can be combined to facilitate recovery, is yet to be ascertained [6].

Rehab with gait and balance training helps the patient adapt to the functional deficit by maximizing the potential for visual and sensorimotor compensation. Treatment must be pointed to:

1. Increase dynamic head stabilization
2. Increase antigravitary paravertebral tone
3. Restore correct ankle–hip strategies dynamic
4. Restore eye–head coordination
5. Decrease oscillopsia
6. Avoid disorientation

7.1 Exercises in the Gymnasium

7.1.1 First Week

1. Relaxation exercises such as control of breathing with improving consciousness of abdominal or thoracic breathing. A simple exercise consists of deep inhalation followed, after few seconds, by a forced exhalation pronouncing the word "one". This exercise is repeated 8–10 times.
2. In the quadrupedal position, the patient inhales and arches her/his back (hyperkyphosis). She/he then exhales and rotates her/his pelvis in hyperlordosis. A small laser pointer (Fig. 7.1) is fixated on the patient's head; during both phases, the head is maintained straight in order to point the laser spot on a target placed on the wall.
3. A small laser pointer is fixated on the patient's head. From supine position, the patient shifts to sitting position, pointing the laser spot on a target straight in front of her/him (Fig. 7.2).
4. In the sitting position, the patient grasps a stick with both hands and takes the stick behind her/his shoulder, positioning the stick at the level of the cervico-dorsal junction. In this position she/he pushes the stick against her/his back, exhaling and inhaling rhythmically and slowly. She/he then repeats the exercise, moving the stick forward on the sternum at the level of the sterno-clavear joint.

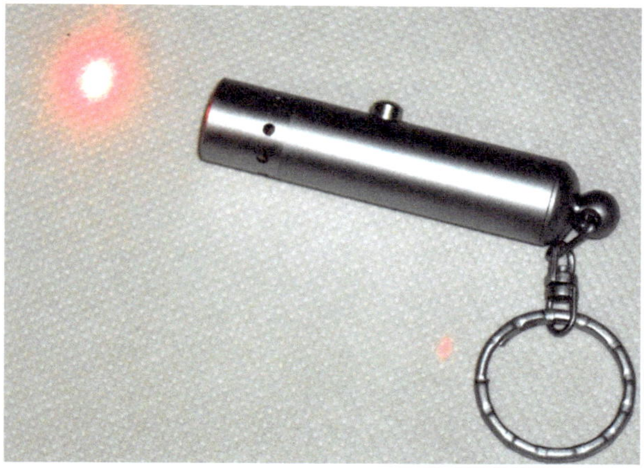

Fig. 7.1 A low-cost laser pointer easy to fixate on the patient's head through a Velcro band

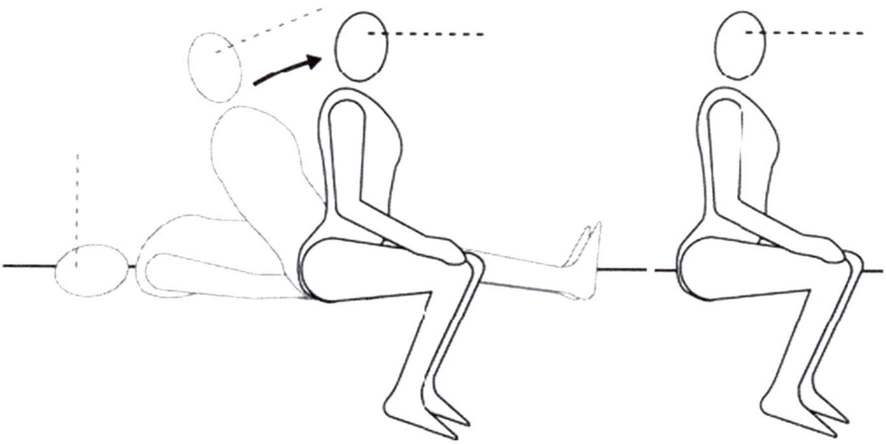

Fig. 7.2 From the supine to sitting position fixating a target (Originally published in Cesarani and Alpini [15] published by Springer © 1999)

The patient grasps the stick with the hands frontally positioned. The patient maintains the fixation of a target placed on the wall, wearing pinhole glasses.

5. The patient is standing on both legs and wearing pinhole glasses. The patient fixates her-/himself in a mirror. The therapist helps the patient to align her/his position correctly. She/he must maintain equilibrium for 1 min with eyes open and then close her/his eyes, visualizing her/his correct position while remaining in this position for at least 1 min.
6. The patient is standing on one leg, wearing pinhole glasses. The patient fixates her-/himself in a mirror. The therapist helps her/him to align her/his position correctly. She/he must maintain equilibrium for session of at least 10 s each. After 5–7 repetitions on one leg, the same exercise is performed with the patient standing on the other leg.

7.1.2 Second Week

The following exercises have to be performed during TENS cervical stimulation, placing the electrodes on the paravertebral muscles of both sides and magnifying lenses (Fig. 7.3) to obtain visual image magnification [6].

1. The patient is standing on a soft mattress and fixates her-/himself in a mirror. The therapist helps her/him to align her/his position correctly. She/he must maintain equilibrium for 1 min with eyes open and then close her/his eyes, visualizing her/his correct position while remaining in this position for at least 1 min.
2. The patient fixates her-/himself in a mirror (Fig. 7.4a). Then she/he oscillates right and left (Fig. 7.4b), around her/his pelvis. She/he then resists the therapist's attempts at destabilizations (Fig. 7.4c) and maintains equilibrium by crossing the legs (Fig. 7.4d).
3. The patient oscillates to and fro around her/his ankles while maintaining fixation in a mirror (Fig. 7.5).
4. The patient repeats exercises 2 and 3, standing on a soft mattress.
5. The patient holds a small object and then lifts it over her/his head and fixates it. With his arms extended, she/he moves it in circles of increasing width while maintaining the fixation of the object (Fig. 7.6).

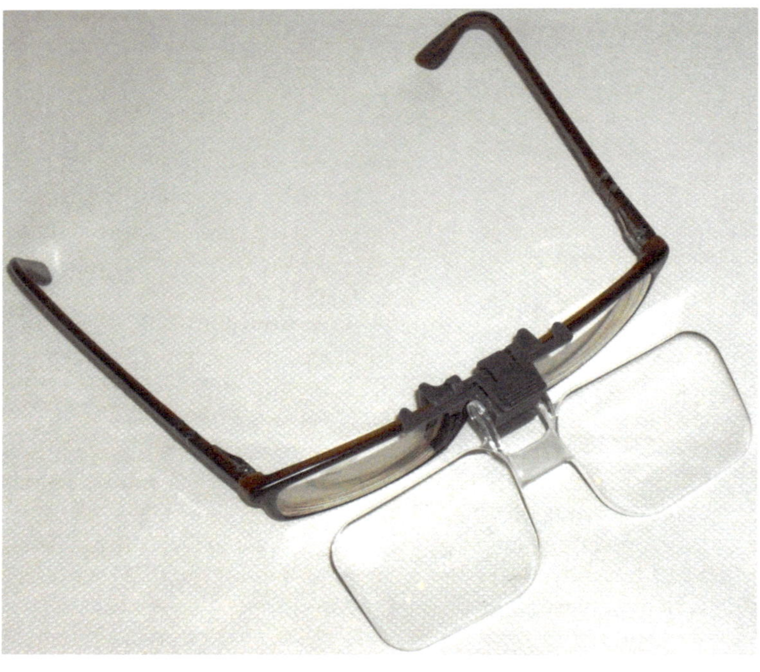

Fig. 7.3 Magnifying lenses to be applied to the patient's glasses or to a neutral lens glasses

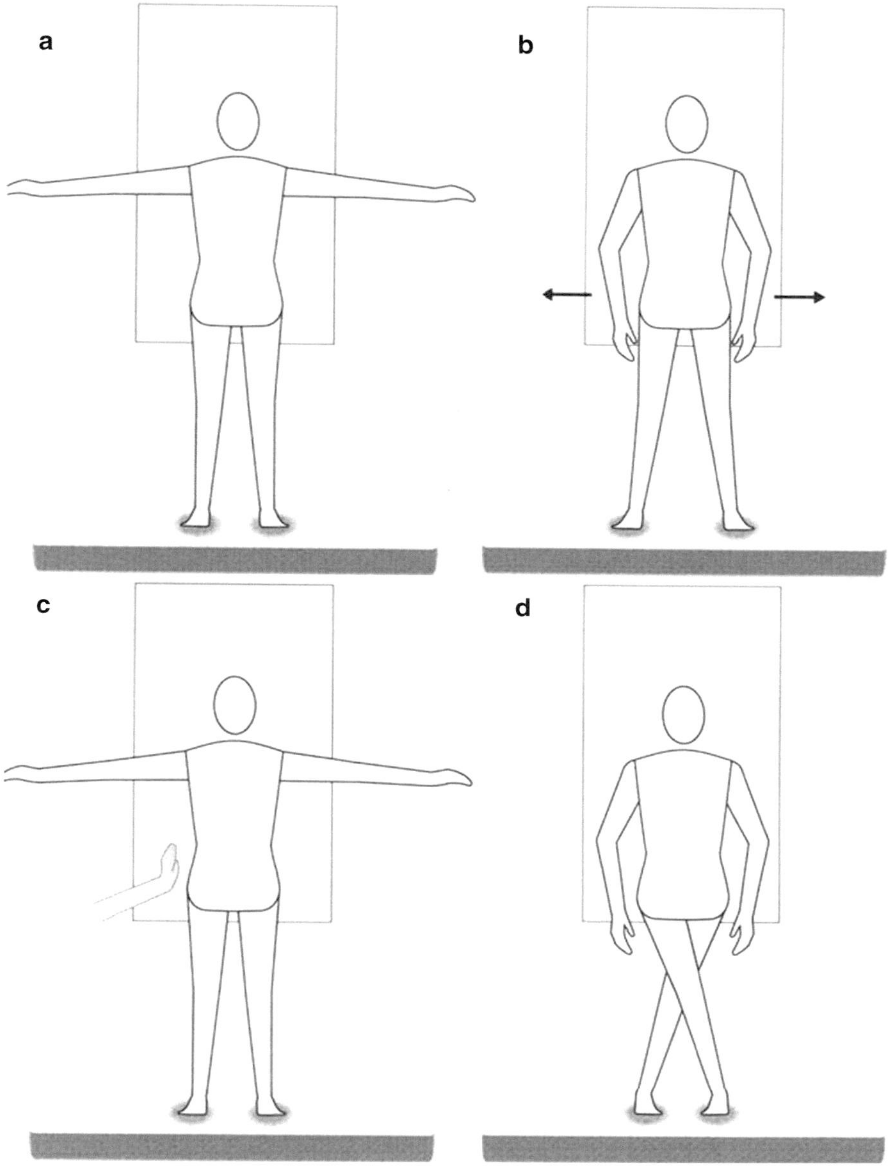

Fig. 7.4 The patient aligns himself looking at a mirror (**a**), then he oscillates (**b**), then resists when the therapist destabilizes him (**c**) or he maintains equilibrium by crossing the legs (**d**) (Originally published in Cesarani and Alpini [15] published by Springer © 1999)

6. The patient is standing on a soft mattress looking in the mirror. The patient concentrates on a proper posture using a mirror to see her/his reflection, and thus, she/he transfers her/his weight from one foot to the other with a smooth flowing motion of the pelvis trying to maintain her/his head as stable as possible.

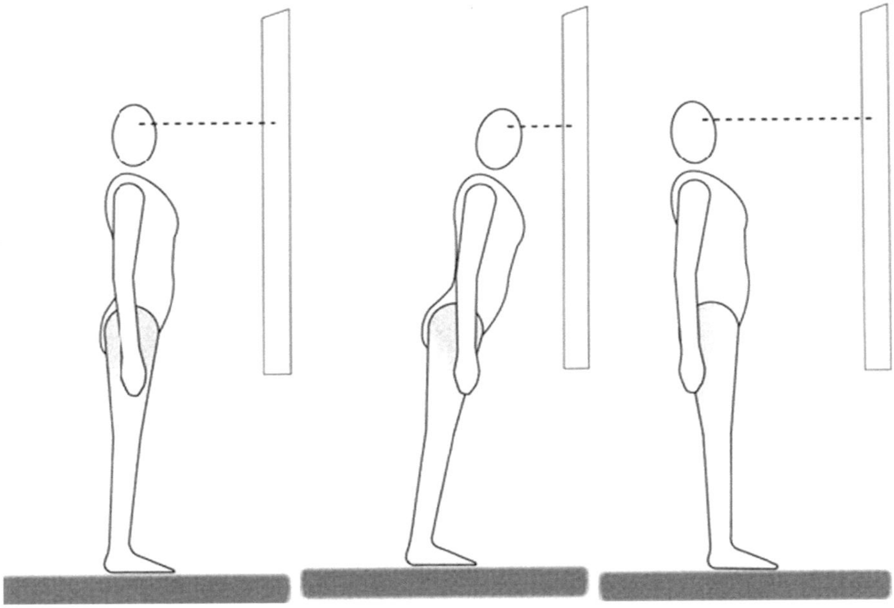

Fig. 7.5 The patient oscillates around his ankles, maintaining the pelvis still (Originally published in Cesarani and Alpini [15] published by Springer © 1999)

7. The patient tries to maintain proper posture while the therapist destabilizes her/him with gentle pushes.
8. The patient is standing on a soft mattress; she/he opens a book in front of her/him and then moves it away from her/him by extending the arms. She/he reads it then moves it closer to her/him, slowly, while trying to read it. Then she/he moves it away.
9. The patient walks while fixating a target on the wall in front of her/him (Fig. 7.7).
10. The patient walks while reading a book.

7.1.3 Third Week

Standing on an oscillating platform (so-called balance board) during TENS bilateral cervical stimulation, the patient concentrates on head stabilization using as feedback a laser spot pointed on a target placed on the wall.

1. The patient tries to maintain equilibrium as longer as possible (no more than 1′)
2. The patient transfers her/his weight from one foot to the other with a smooth flowing motion.
3. The patient tries to maintain proper posture while the therapist destabilizes her/him with gentle pushes

In this phase, exercises performed using an electronic rocking board with visual feedback like the Delos equipment (see Chap. 4) is particularly useful. Also in this case bilateral cervical TENS stimulation is provided.

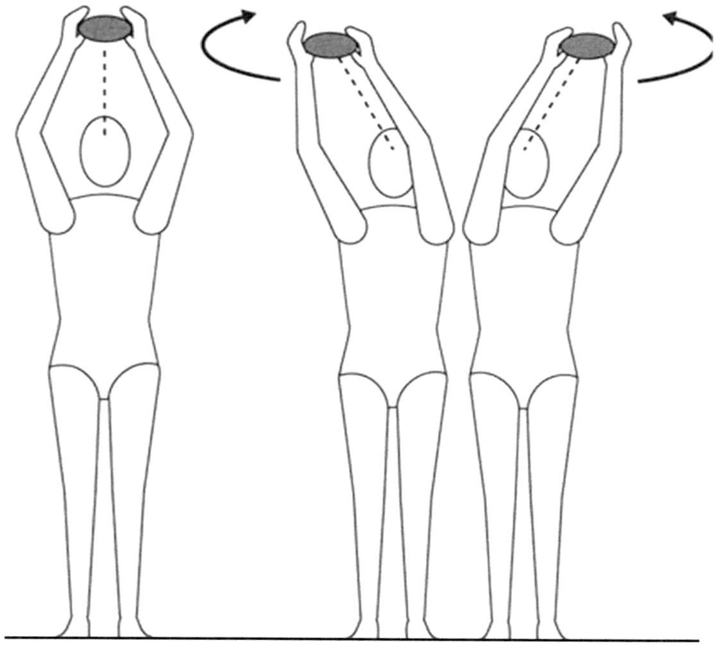

Fig. 7.6 The patient fixates a small object while moving it in circles, standing on a mattress (Originally published in Cesarani and Alpini [15] published by Springer © 1999)

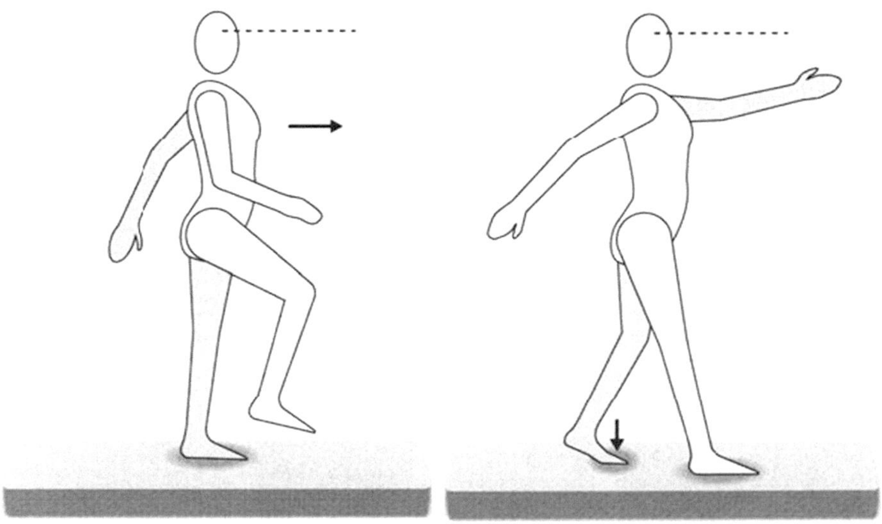

Fig. 7.7 Stepping on a mattress without and with simultaneous oscillations of the arms, fixating a target (Originally published in Cesarani and Alpini [15] published by Springer © 1999)

7.2 Virtual Reality

It is well known [7] that repeated visual stimulations, through activation of the optokinetic circuits, may improve vestibular compensation. Virtual reality (VR) and augmented reality (AR) appear as a technologically advanced optokinetic vestibular stimulation [8, 9].

The recent advances in virtual reality (VR) technology make it available for use in the clinical field. This creates appropriate surroundings to facilitate achievement of important goals which are impossible to achieve in a regular treatment set. This new technology (VR) can be used to train realistic everyday tasks in the clinic and to combine complex abilities to fulfil complicated tasks. Without the dangers of the real world, VR exercises might be used to motivate patients to act and to comply in more demanding situations in an interactive immersive environment. For this purpose, commercial low-cost video game equipment has been proposed [10, 11].

Immersion and a high sense of presence are necessary to obtain enduring results [12, 13]. Commercial video games are user friendly but with a low grade of immersion and presence. For this reason, we adopt the Self-Experienced Virtual Reality [14] as in ice skaters' training.

BVH patient's training requires maintaining static and dynamic balance during observation of a video reproducing visual and auditory stimuli recorded during simple motion activities.

Both "objective" and "subjective" views are recorded while the patient is moving. The "objective" view is provided by the therapist that films the patient by means of a digital camera while the "subjective" view is recorded by means of an outdoor sport action camera fixed on the patient's head (Fig. 7.8).

Alternatively, a digital photocamera fixed on the head of the patient trough Velcro bands may be used [8].

Videos are collected when the patient:

(a) Walks for 5 waks forward and backward with eyes open
(b) Walks for 5 waks forward and backward with eyes closed
(c) Walks forward for 5 waks and then turns leftward walking back for another 5 waks and turns rightward walking forward for another 5 waks
(d) Walks in circle before clockwise and then counterclockwise
(e) Walks along an 8-shaped pathway

Video stimulation will be then provided using a notebook or a TV screen (at least a 15″ screen is necessary). The screen is heighted at the level of the subject's eyes' horizontal line. The room is darkened to increase immersion. Videos improve both static and dynamic balance. Alternating objective and subjective views of each video are projected.

7.2.1 Static Balance

The patient stands on the floor in front of the screen and a laser pointer is mounted on her/his head. The patient is required to point the laser spot on a target placed on the upper edge of the screen.

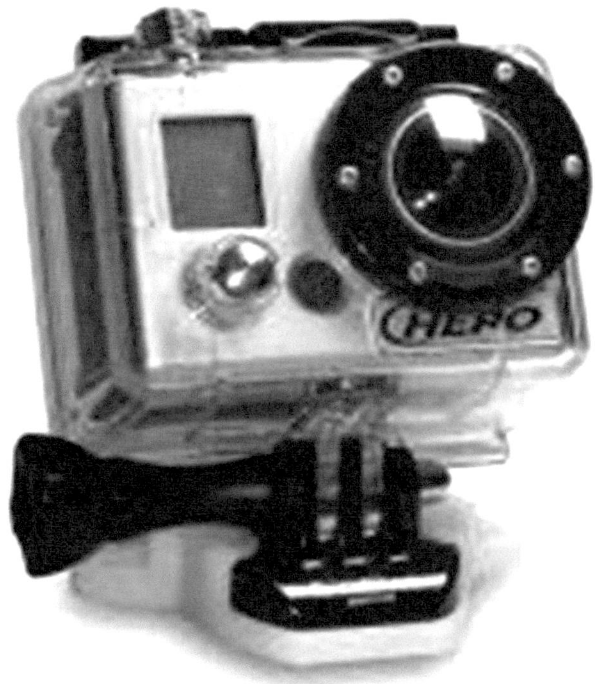

Fig. 7.8 An outdoor sport action camera, usually fixed directly on the head of the patient

1. The patient has to maintain steady the laser spot while standing on both legs for at least 30 s.
2. The patient is required to repeat the exercise standing on one leg. She/he has to try to stand on one leg at least 10″. Then she/he repeats the exercise standing on the other leg.
3. The same exercises are performed while standing on a soft mattress.

7.2.2 Dynamic Balance

The patient stands upright on a balance board in front of the screen.

1. The patient is required to maintain balance. The therapist helps the patient to avoid falls.
2. When the patient is able to maintain balance for at least 30 s during video projection, a laser pointer will be mounted on the patient's head, and stabilization of the laser spot on a target placed on the upper edge of the screen will be required.

7.3 Home Protocol

The aim of the home protocol is to maintain the results obtained with the therapist. The patient has to repeat the exercises at least twice a day. A small laser pointer, magnifying lenses and a DVD reader are necessary.

1. The laser pointer is fixated on your head. In the quadrupedal position, inhale and arch your back (hyperkyphosis). Then exhale and rotate the pelvis in hyperlordosis. During both phases, the head is maintained straight in order to point the laser spot on a target placed on the wall.
2. The laser pointer is fixated on your head. From the supine position, shift to sitting position, pointing the laser spot on a target straight in front of you.

Sitting Wearing Magnifying Lenses

3. Extend your right arm and lift your thumb. Move your arm slowly to and fro in a horizontal direction and then in a vertical direction. Follow your thumb with your eyes only, first slowly and then increasing progressively the velocity of thumb displacement.
4. Repeat as above but simultaneously moving also the head trying to keep the eyes still.
5. Look for three targets sited, respectively, in front of you, at your left and at your right. Fixate the frontal target, then move your head rapidly, fixating the right-hand target. Now turn your head leftward while maintaining the fixation of the right-hand target. Fixate the frontal target. Now rapidly move your head leftward and fixate the left-hand target. Then turn your head rightward while maintaining the fixation of the left-hand target.
6. Extend your right arm and lift your thumb. Move your arm slowly to and fro first in a horizontal direction and then in a vertical direction. Follow your thumb with your eyes only, first slowly and then increasing progressively the velocity of thumb displacement.
7. Repeat as above but moving simultaneously also the head while trying to keep the eyes still.

Standing and Wearing Magnifying Lenses

8. Standing on a soft mattress, fixate yourself in a mirror. Align your position correctly. Maintain equilibrium for 1 min and then close your eyes and visualize your correct position; remain in this position for at least 1 min.
9. Hold a small object and then lift it over your head and fixate it. With your arms extended, move it in circles of increasing width while maintaining fixation of the object. Then close your eyes and continue making the circles.
10. Standing on a soft mattress, open a book in front of you. Read it while simultaneously slowly moving it to and fro and from side to side.
11. Walk moving the head to and fro.
12. In a corridor, walk for 5 waks forward and backward your eyes open.

During Video "Objective" Projection

13. Maintain equilibrium in front of the screen while standing on the floor and then standing on a soft mattress.
14. Maintain equilibrium while stepping on the floor and then standing on a soft mattress.

7.4 Counselling

It is important to pay attention to lifestyle. The main suggestions are:

- To control own body mass index (BMI)
  BMI is correlated to body fat and it is calculated as body weight (in kilos) divided by the square of the height (in metres); e.g. a subject weighing 70 kg and 1.74 m in height has a BMI as follows: 70/ $(1.74 \times 1.74) = 23.1$. Normal values are between 18.5 and 24.9 (World Health Organization, WHO)
- To perform regular and constant aerobic physical activity: e.g. rapid walking (not running neither jogging) 30′/day three times/week
- To maintain a diet rich of fruit and vegetables (five servings/day) especially in autumn and spring
- To avoid industrial food
- To avoid chilli foods, generally, and capsaicin intake (see also Chap. 5)
- To maintain adequate water intake (at least 1.5 l for females and 2 l for males)
- To restrict alcohol intake (less than 120 ml for women and 240 ml for men)
- To avoid smoking and, obviously, drug abuse

References

1. Strupp M, Brandt T (2013) Peripheral vestibular disorders. Curr Opin Neurol 26(1):81–89
2. Requena T, Espinosa-Sanchez JM, Lopez-Escamez JA (2014) Genetics of dizziness: cerebellar and vestibular disorders. Curr Opin Neurol 27:98–104
3. Petersen JA, Wichmann WW, Weber KP (2013) The pivotal sign of CANVAS. Neurology 81(18):1642–1643
4. Benítez Del Rosario JJ, Santandreu Jiménez ME, Lousa Gayoso M. Cerebellar ataxia with neuropathy and bilateral vestibular areflexia syndrome (CANVAS) in an imbalance patient. Acta Otorrinolaringol Esp. 2013 Apr 12. pii: S0001-6519(13)00024-1. doi: 10.1016/j.otorri.2013.01.002.
5. McCall AA, Yates BJ (2011) Compensation following bilateral vestibular damage. Front Neurol 2:88
6. Cushman JD, Aharoni DB, Willers B, Ravassard P, Kees A, Vuong C, Popeney B, Arisaka K, Mehta MR (2013) Multisensory control of multimodal behavior: do the legs know what the tongue is doing? PLoS One 8(11):e80465
7. Viirre E, Draper M, Gailey C, Miller D, Furness T (1998) Adaptation of the VOR in patients with low VOR gains. Vestib Res 8(4):331–334
8. Vitte E, Sémont A, Berthoz A (1994) Repeated optokinetic stimulation in conditions of active standing facilitates recovery from vestibular deficits. Exp Brain Res 102:141–148
9. Gottshall KR, Sessoms PH, Bartlett JL (2012) Vestibular physical therapy intervention: utilizing a computer assisted rehabilitation environment in lieu of traditional physical therapy. Conf Proc IEEE Eng Med Biol Soc 2012:6141–6144
10. Meldrum D, Glennon A, Herdman S, Murray D, McConn-Walsh R (2012) Virtual reality rehabilitation of balance: assessment of the usability of the Nintendo Wii(®) Fit Plus. Disabil Rehabil Assist Technol 7(3):205–210
11. Sparrer I, Duong Dinh TA, Ilgner J, Westhofen M (2013) Vestibular rehabilitation using the Nintendo® Wii Balance Board – a user-friendly alternative for central nervous compensation. Acta Otolaryngol 133(3):239–245
12. Riva G, Rizzo A, Alpini D, Attree EA, Barbieri E, Bertella L, Buckwalter JG, Davies RC, Gamberini L, Johansson G, Katz N, Marchi S, Mendozzi L, Molinari E, Pugnetti L, Rose FD, Weiss PL (1999) Virtual environments in the diagnosis, prevention, and intervention of

age-related diseases: a review of VR scenarios proposed in the EC VETERAN Project. Cyberpsychol Behav 2(6):577–591
13. Akizuki H, Uno A, Arai K, Morioka S, Ohyama S, Nishiike S (2005) Effects of immersion in virtual reality on postural control. Neurosci Lett 379(1):23–26
14. Tornese D, Botta M, Mattei V, Alpini DC (2011) Self-experienced virtual reality to improve vestibulo-oculomotor performances in ice dancers. A pilot study. Sport Sci Health 6:45–50
15. Cesarani A, Alpini D (1999) Vertigo and dizziness rehabilitation – the MCS method. Springer, Milan, Heidelberg

Benign Paroxysmal Positional Vertigo

8

Benign paroxysmal positional vertigo (BPPV) is the most common cause of vertigo [1]. The lifetime prevalence of BPPV is 2.4 %, and the 1-year incidence is 0.6 % [2]. In the majority of cases, the aetiology of idiopathic BPPV is still nowadays unclear. Secondary BPPV is less common and may result from several pathological conditions such as head trauma, surgery, infection, vertebrobasilar insufficiency or inner ear diseases [3, 4].

BPPV is recognized to be a pure inner ear problem that results in short-lasting, but severe, room-spinning vertigo generally provoked by movement of the head or changing position in bed. It was described in Barany's (1907) works [cited in 5], but it gained its definite clinical through the report of Dix and Hallpike [6].

The principal complaint is the occurrence of sudden attacks of vertigo precipitated by certain head positions. The attacks can be induced by rolling over bed, to one side and to both sides; by sudden movement of the head; by extending the neck; by looking upward, as reaching for an object from the top shelf in the kitchen; by bending the head backward for hair washing; by lying down beneath a car; or by throwing the head backward to paint a ceiling. The patient sometimes recognizes that the onset of the vertigo is associated with this critical position and will say he or she does his or her best to avoid it.

The initial occurrence is usually experienced on awakening in the morning, which is considered characteristic, or during the night. Many patients are frightened by the intense vertigo and try to shut out the sensation by closing their eyes. Nausea, often accompanied by anxiety, even vomiting, may follow the attack in few cases. In rare cases, the nausea persists for hours. Vertigo is of short duration (<1 min), but because of the intensity of the vertiginous sensation, a longer duration can be assigned to the attack.

Generally speaking, two main kinds of BPPV can be recognized:

1. Vertigo elicited by the so-called Dix–Hallpike manoeuvre [6] accompanied by a typical horizontal-rotary geotropic nystagmus while the patient is supine during simultaneous rotation and hyperextension of the head. Nystagmus appears immediately or few seconds after the execution of the manoeuvre (*latency*); it increases *paroxysmally* for few seconds and *exhausts* in less than 1′, and it is

D.C. Alpini et al., *Vertigo Rehabilitation Protocols*,
DOI 10.1007/978-3-319-05482-7_8, © Springer International Publishing Switzerland 2014

decreased by the following repetition of the same manoeuvre (*fatigability* due to habituation phenomena). In some cases, no nystagmus is observed, but the patient complains of vertigo with the same characteristic of latency, paroxysm, exhaustion and fatigability.

2. Vertigo and pure horizontal nystagmus provoked by rolling the head from side to side while the patient is recumbent. In this case (so-called Pagnini–McClure manoeuvre [7, 8]), two kinds of nystagmus can be observed, geotropic or ageotropic nystagmus. Generally, this kind of BPPV is long-lasting and may appear without latency.

The characteristic presentation of this disorder involves repeated episodes of transient illusion of spinning, triggered by head motion in the plane of the involved semicircular canal (SCC). Cupulolithiasis and canalolithiasis [9] have both been proposed as pathophysiologic biomechanical models underlying BPPV.

According to the *cupulolithiasis* model, originally described by Schucknecht [10], substances having a specific gravity greater than the endolymph, and thus subject to movement with changes in the direction of gravitational forces, come into contact with the cupula of the posterior semicircular canal (in the case of vertigo induced by Dix–Hallpike manoeuvre) or of the lateral semicircular canal (in the case of vertigo elicited by Pagnini–McClure manoeuvre). The change of position of the labyrinth during movement of the head provokes the displacement of the cupula by direct influence of these heavy substances on it. According to the *canalithiasis* model, during head movements, free-floating particles move within the affected SCC stimulating the cupula in a pathological way.

Signs (nystagmus) and symptoms (nausea, vertigo, etc.), manifest during provocative tests for the disorder, fall into two main categories: tonic and phasic. Tonic responses include maintained ocular nystagmus that is initiated immediately upon reorientation of the head relative to gravity. This condition, typically associated with the pathological presence of a heavy particulate mass adhered to a cupula, is correlated to cupulolithiasis model [9]. In contrast, phasic symptoms occur with a delayed onset and subside over time. These responses are typically attributed to the canalithiasis model [9].

On the basis of these models, manoeuvres aimed to the "liberation" of the cupula or the canal from heavy particles (generally residual of otoconia metabolism) have been proposed, and most cases of BPPV can be treated using physical therapy, Semont's [11] liberatory manoeuvre in the case of cupulolithiasis, Epley's [12] canalith-repositioning procedure (CRP) and Lempert's "barbecue manoeuvre" [13] in the case of canalolithiasis.

In these years various modifications of these three "basic" manoeuvres have been proposed, but for the scope of this book, we prefer to present only them and our personal treatment of BPPV.

8.1 Semont's Manoeuvre

The patient lies on the affected side for at least 3 min (in Fig. 8.1a, a left PPV is represented). Then the head is rotated upward about 105° in order (according to the cupolithiasis model) to allow the displacement of the heavy particles at the basis of

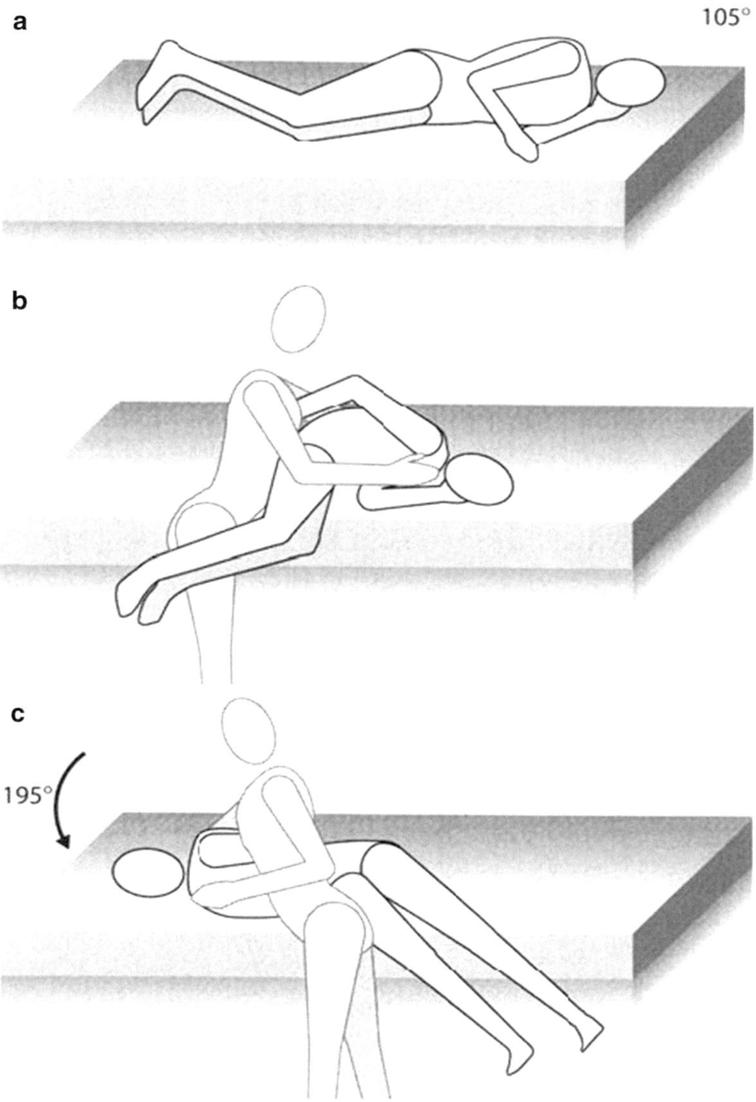

Fig. 8.1 (**a–c**) Semont's manoeuvre (Originally published in Cesarani and Alpini [36] published by Springer © 1999)

the posterior semicircular canal with downward deflexion of the cupula. Then the therapist takes firmly the head of the patient (Fig. 8.1b), and decisively he or she brings the patient on the opposite side with a contemporary rotation of the head downward about 195° (Fig. 8.1c). Usually, in this position, after few seconds, a "liberatory" nystagmus toward the affected side appears. When nystagmus and vertigo disappear, the patient returns slowly in sitting position

8.2 Epley's Manoeuvre

According to the original description of the technique, the patient is premedicated with transdermal scopolamine the night before or diazepam 5 mg. Nowadays, premedication is usually not necessary; even in very anxious patients, administration of diazepam 5 mg per os 2–3 h before treatment may be useful.

The patient is seated on an examining table (Fig. 8.2a) so that when the patient is brought to the supine position, the head extends beyond the bed. The operator is located directly behind the patient and an assistant at the patient's side.

According to the original description of the technique, throughout the positioning manoeuvres, oscillations of the skull are optionally induced. The handheld oscillator with a frequency of approximately 80 Hz does not actually touch the head but acts through the operator's hand applied to the ipsilateral mastoid process.

The patient lies downward with a slight hyperextension of the head and a contemporary 105° rotation toward the affected side (in the case of the figures, the left, Fig. 8.2b). In this position, nystagmus and vertigo appear. The patient remains in each position 6–13 s but may extend to more than 30 s. Then the head is rotated on the opposite side toward the healthy labyrinth for 90° (Fig. 8.2c). Simultaneous to head rotation, also the trunk and the legs rotate toward the healthy side (Fig. 8.2d). In this position, usually, a "liberatory" nystagmus is observed. Then the patient completes the rotation of the legs and returns in sitting position keeping the head turned toward the opposite side with respect to the affected labyrinth (Fig. 8.2e).

8.3 Lempert's Manoeuvre

This manoeuvre represents an adaptation of Epley's posterior canal repositioning procedure, and it aims to shift heavy particles (according to the canalolithiasis model) ampullofugally toward and beyond the horizontal canal opening into the utricle. The manoeuvre consists of 270° head rotation around the supine patient's longitudinal axis; the rotation is performed in rapid steps of 90°. The patient is in recumbent position. Then the head is rotated toward the affected side (Pagnini–McClure position). In this position, nystagmus is elicited. When vertigo and nystagmus disappeared, the therapist performs a complete rotation of the head and the body of the patient in step of 90° until a complete 270° rotation. Head positions are maintained for between 30 and 60 s until all nystagmus has subsided.

In the case of geotropic nystagmus, the first rotation of the head is toward the opposite side, while in the case of ageotropic nystagmus, the first rotation of the head is in the direction of the affected ear.

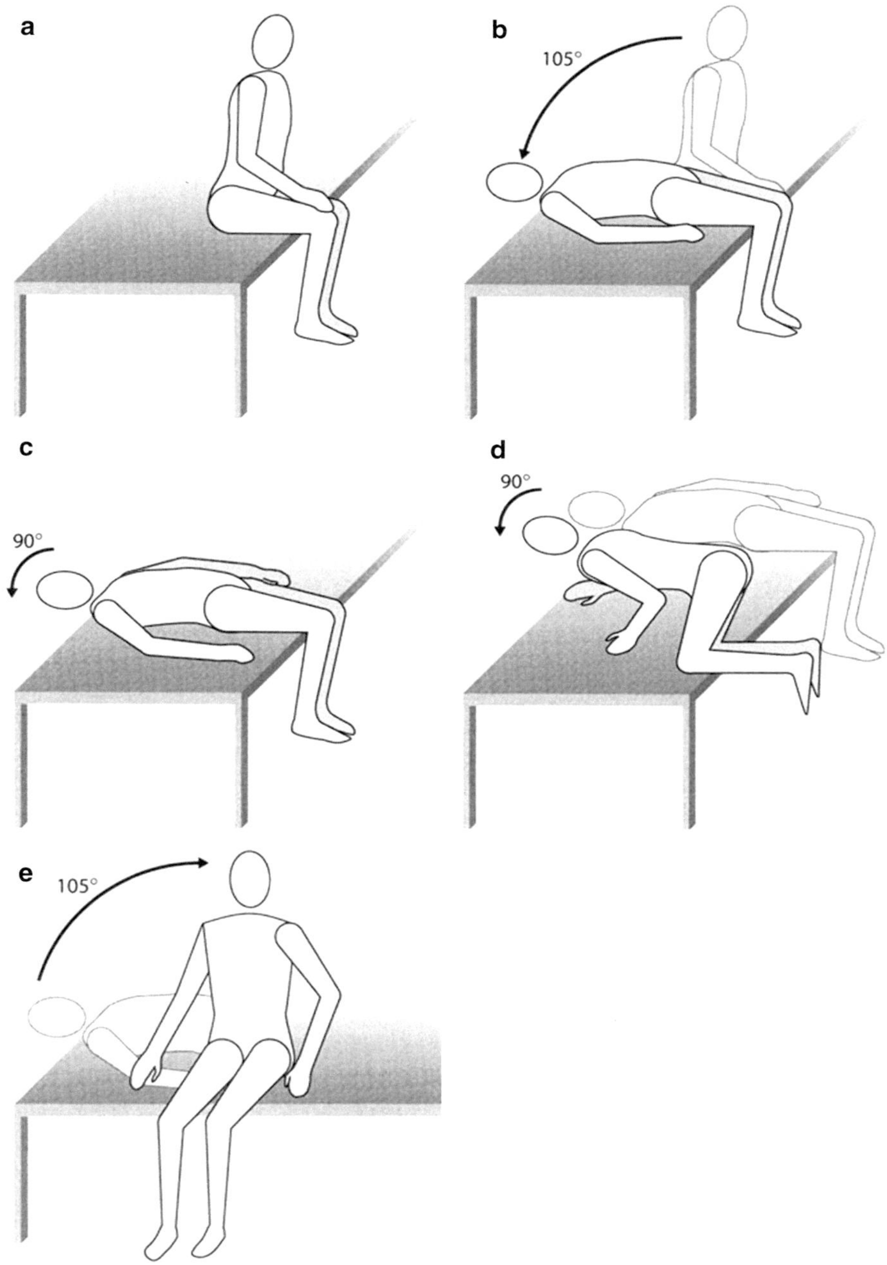

Fig. 8.2 (**a**–**e**) Epley's manoeuvre (Originally published in Cesarani and Alpini [36] published by Springer © 1999)

8.4 BPPV Treatment in Elderly and/or Difficult Patients

Although the described manoeuvres have been shown to have therapeutic benefits, they require sequential procedures involving moving the patient's head and body into unnatural positions, making them sometimes unsuitable for patients with cervical or back disorders, especially for older patients.

In this kind of patients, it is thus better to use more conservative procedures like the supine to prolonged lateral position (SPLP) [14] or the rolling over manoeuvre (ROM) [15].

SPLP contained two steps. First, the patient was instructed to start in an upright sitting position and then lie down supinely on the bed and maintain this position for 3 min. During this step, it was proposed that the trapped otolithic particles would move away from the ampulla (ampullofugal), drift toward the common crus by crossing the horizontal SCC plane and stay in the superior arm of the posterior SCC. In the second step, the patient was asked to sleep on their healthy side by turning their head and body from the previous supine position toward the healthy side laterally. This process allowed the particles to slip through the common crus into the utricle. To facilitate their movement back into the utricle and to prevent any floating particles in the utricle from being trapped in the posterior SCC again, a prolonged side lateral position (minimum duration 30 min) was suggested at bedtime, with or without a pillow support.

ROM involves moving the patient from supine to nose-up position to a right ear-down position and maintaining this position for 10 s, before subsequently returning the head to a nose-up position, which is maintained for further 10 s. The patient is then moved to the left ear-down head position which is maintained for 10 s. The patient repeats these manoeuvres 10 times in a set and 2 sets in a day, before getting up in the morning and before sleeping in the night.

ROM can be performed either by neck rotation or by whole-body movements without any cervical torsion. This is very suitable for whiplash patients, especially in the early phases of trauma.

8.5 Personal Approach to BPPV

The heavy particles attached to the cupula or free-floating into the canals may be derived by residual of otoconia metabolism, otoconia fragments displaced by a head or a whiplash trauma, inflammatory material or any other pathological particles produced during the course of a systemic (i.e. autoimmune thyroiditis, diabetes, hyperuricaemia, etc.) or an inner ear disorder (i.e. vestibular neuronitis, Ménière's disease, etc.). In all the cases, through the natural course of endolymph renewal or by means of liberatory manoeuvres, these particles are expelled to the inner ear venous system and thus to the cervical venous system. The cervical venous drainage is composed of the internal jugular veins anteriorly and the vertebral venous system posteriorly. The latter is composed of the external and internal vertebral venous plexuses, which are anastomosed by way of the intervertebral and basivertebral veins [16]. The venous vertebral system is composed of plexuses along all the spine from the skull until the lumbar region, and thus, in our experience, combining "liberatory" manoeuvres with manual techniques and some suggestions (see Sect. 8.5.3) aimed to facilitate the drainage of the inner ear improve the efficiency of BPPV treatment.

8.5.1 Physical Therapy

The first step is to restore the spinal biomechanics through the manual medicine techniques that act mainly as high-level reflex therapy [17]. Manipulation of the rachis may improve vascular reflexes of the neck and visceral reflexes of the stomach with consequent reduction of the neurovegetative symptoms. All the manual treatments are performed with the patient sitting on the examination bed.

Then the proper liberatory manoeuvre is performed. Thus, the physical therapy of BPPV comprehends the following steps:

1. High-velocity low-range epigastric supported manipulation of the middle thoracic joint (Th7–8 segment) (Fig. 8.3) in extension

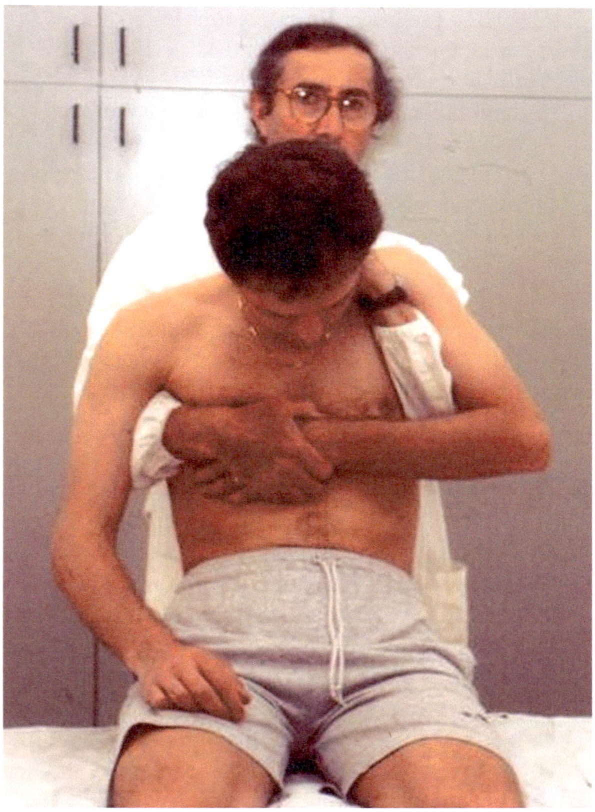

Fig. 8.3 High-velocity low-range manipulation of the middle thoracic joint (Th7–8 segment)

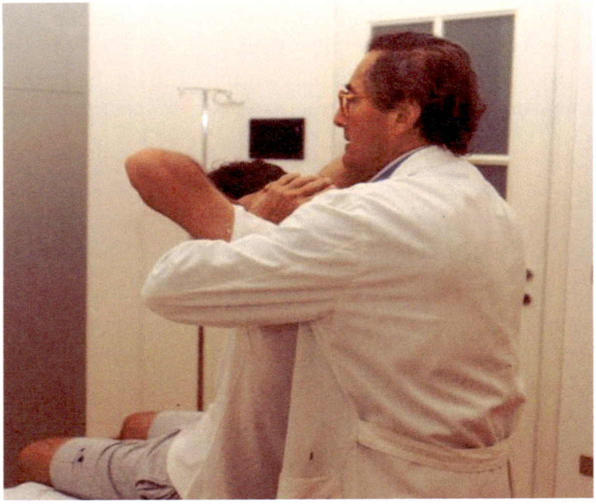

Fig. 8.4 High-velocity low-range manipulation of the cervicothoracic (C7–Th1–2 segment)

2. High-velocity low-range sternum supported manipulation of the cervicothoracic (C7–Th1–2 segment) in extension (Fig. 8.4)
3. Treatment of the cervical soft tissues (Fig. 8.5)
4. Proper liberatory manoeuvre:
   - Semont's manoeuvre in the case of a tonic response during Dix–Hallpike provocative test
   - Epley's manoeuvre in the case of a phasic response during Dix–Hallpike provocative test
   - Lempert's manoeuvre in the case of response to Pagnini–McClure provocative test

When it is not possible to perform a liberatory manoeuvre, we suggest to the patient the supine to prolonged lateral position (SPLP) in the case of Dix–Hallpike elicited BPPV or the rolling over manoeuvre (ROM) in the case of Pagnini–McClure elicited BPPV.

8.5.2 Home Protocol

After 48 h from liberatory manoeuvre, we propose to the patient to perform at bedtime for about 10 days some exercises that are the combination of the supine to prolonged lateral position (SPLP) and the rolling over manoeuvre (ROM):

1. Start in an upright sitting position and then lie down supinely on the bed and maintain this position for 30″ after the end of symptoms.
2. Rotate, slowly and with eyes open, the head from supine nose-up position to a right ear-down position and maintain this position for 10 s.
3. Then move, slowly and with the eyes open, the head to the left ear-down head position and maintain this position for 10 s.

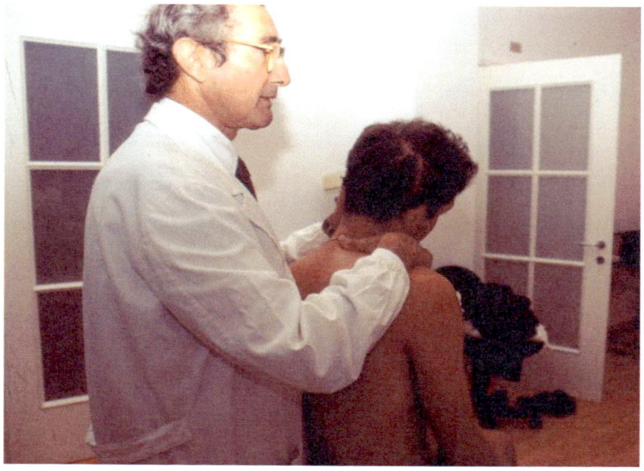

Fig. 8.5 Treatment of the cervical soft tissues

4. Repeat these manoeuvres 10 times.
5. Lie on your symptomatic side and maintain this position for 30″ after the end of symptoms.
6. Turn the head and body laterally from the previous position toward the healthy side maintaining a prolonged side lateral position (minimum duration of 30 min) with a pillow support.

8.5.3 Counselling

The *key lesion* of BBPV is endolymph alteration or otolithic membrane damage, and thus, even the treatment of choice is physical as described above, some attention has to be paid in relapsing BBPV or in some particular patients. In fact, BPPV presents usually as a single episode during the course of the life, even if the attacks may last several days or weeks when the patient is not adequately treated, but sometimes BPPV episodes relapse in the same patient after several years, and sometimes BBPV assumes the characteristics of a relapsing, even if remitting, disease.

In this case, the *possibility that BPPV is secondary* to a previous (even years) disease of the inner ear has to be taken in account. BPPV may be secondary to head trauma, vascular lesion of the labyrinth [18], viral vestibular neuritis [19], Ménière's disease [20] and otosclerosis [21].

Despite the general agreement about the biomechanical model of labyrinth lithiasis, the pathogenesis of idiopathic BPPV is not yet completely understood. In 2008, Mariani et al. [22] performed a 5-year retrospective statistical analysis of 575 patients showing a significant correlation between frequency of BPPV attacks and air pollution (PPM10 and NO2) peaks. They found an inverted correlation between BPPV and temperature and sun irradiation, while they didn't find correlation with

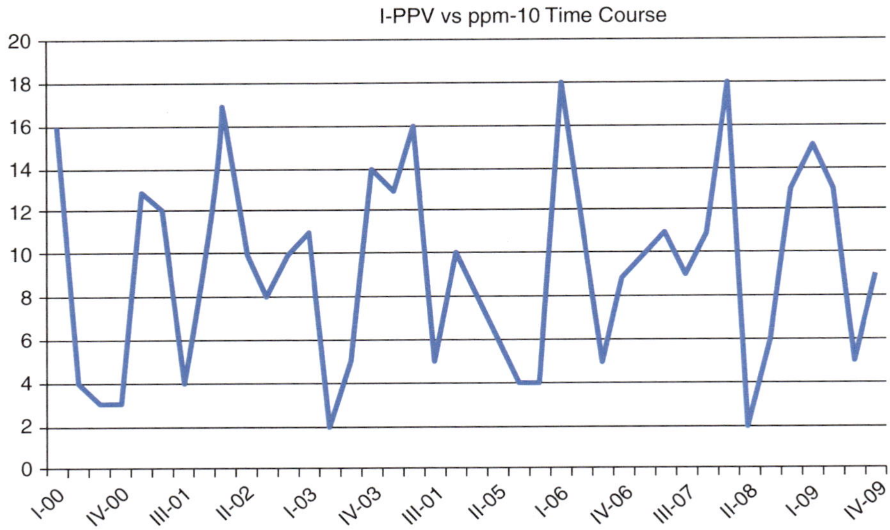

Fig. 8.6 BPPV events observed in the period 2000–2009. Events are distributed according to the season with winter having increased attacks (I trimester of each year, I-00, I-01, etc.) and progressive decrease in spring and summer (III trimester of each year, III-00, III-01, etc.) all along the 10-year period of observation

air pressure. The authors adopted a descriptive statistics to show the trend of the two more correlated variables (temperature and PPM10 particles): When particles increased, there was a major incidence of patients suffering from BPPV, and when temperature decreased, particles increased and, thus, when the temperature decreased, events increased.

Analysis showed that BPPV is a cyclic phenomenon and that it could be correlated to pollution. As far as the author's knowledge is concerned, no other papers have been yet published regarding correlation between PPV and environmental phenomena, but in 2011 Alpini et al. [23] confirmed these observations along a 10-year course regarding NO2 and ultrafine particles (ppm10).

Figures 8.6, 8.7 and 8.8 show the distribution along 10 years of idiopathic cases of BPPV observed in a single otoneurological laboratory regarding patients from a homogenous geographic area (so-called Great Milan, Italy) and the correlation with NO2 and PPM10.

Increasing water intake is fundamental to facilitate clearance of both absorbed pollution particles and, in general, lithiasic endolymph particles.

It is well known that idiopathic BBPV is more frequent in females and that it affects prevalently the right side [24, 25].

Female prevalence has been correlated by Vibert et al. [26] to osteopenia and osteoporosis. The diagnosis of osteopenia or osteoporosis was confirmed by a bone mineral density measurement made with dual x-ray absorptiometry of the spine and hip (T-score). Results showed osteopenia or osteoporosis 75 % of considered cases.

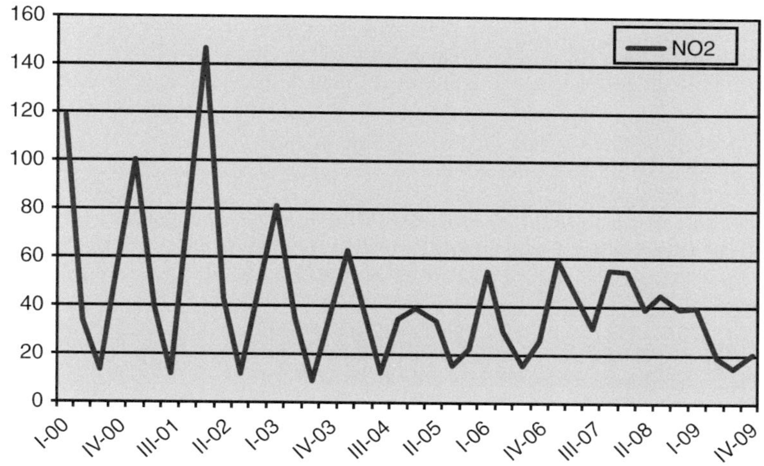

Fig. 8.7 Trimester trend of events from 2000 to 2009 correlated to nitric monoxide (NO2) in Greater Milan area. Trends of two curves are very similar

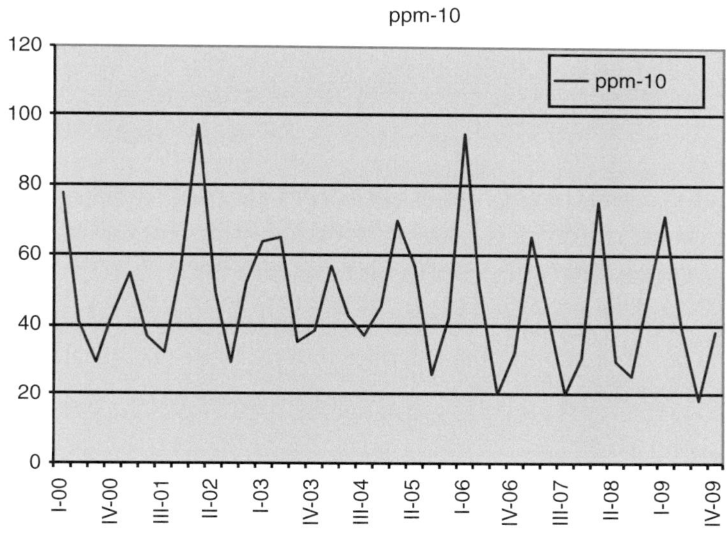

Fig. 8.8 Trimester trend of events from 2000 to 2009 correlated to ultrafine particle pollution (ppm10) in Greater Milan area. Trends of two curves are very similar

The T-scores were compared to those of 83 healthy women. The patients with BPPV had a significantly lower ($p < 0.026$) T-score. The authors hypothesized an influence of calcium metabolism dysregulation on otolith metabolism with increased trend to otoconia debris formation.

Thus, we suggest for a female around the menopausal age to have a *dual x-ray absorptiometry* of the hip and to *take serum vitamin D* because it takes part in the

Table 8.1 BPPV counselling

To increase water intake (at least 2 l for females and 2.5 l for males)
To elevate the head during bed rest (two pillows or lifting the bed), the so-called inclined bed therapy
To restrict alcohol intake (less than 120 ml for women and 240 ml for men)
To avoid smoke and, obviously, drug abuse
To restrict red beef meat intake (less than 500 g/week)
To take into account the possibility of secondary BPPV in case of recurrent cases
To investigate for a subclinical autoimmune thyroiditis especially in case of young females
To investigate bone metabolism and dose serum vitamin D in case of females around or after menopause
To regulate carbohydrate and calorie intake in the case of positive personal or family history of diabetes or glucose intolerance (particularly soft drinks)

regulation of calcium and phosphorus found in the body and plays an important role in maintaining proper bone metabolism [27, 28].

Right-side prevalence was discussed by Cakir et al. [29]. They found that the ear affected by BPPV was to be consistent with the right head-lying side during bed rest in 86 %. Thus, they concluded that habitual lateral head positioning during bed rest could be a major factor leading to the development of BPPV in the ipsilateral ear.

Thus, we suggest to our patient to maintain during bed rest an elevated head position (so-called inclined bed therapy), at least for 5–7 days after physical treatment.

Furthermore, all BBPV patients have to reduce *alcohol* intake, avoid *smoking* [30] and reduce *red meat* consumption [31].

Another metabolic disorder correlated to BPPV that may be corrected by means of diet is diabetes [32]. Thus, in patients affected with diabetes or with a family history of glucose intolerance and/or diabetes, a modification of *carbohydrate consumption* is suggested.

Finally, in all recurrent BPPV patients, a subclinical autoimmune thyroiditis [33, 34] has to be taken into account and properly investigated and treated even if in euthyroid phase [35] (Table 8.1).

References

1. Prokopakis EP, Chimona T, Tsagournisakis M, Christodoulou P, Hirsch BE, Lachanas VA, Helidonis ES, Plaitakis A, Velegrakis GA (2005) Benign paroxysmal positional vertigo: 10-year experience in treating 592 patients with canalith repositioning procedure. Laryngoscope 115:1667–1671
2. von Brevern M, Radtke A, Lezius F, Feldmann M, Ziese T, Lempert T, Neuhauser H (2007) Epidemiology of benign paroxysmal positional vertigo: a population based study. J Neurol Neurosurg Psychiatry 78:710–715
3. Korres SG, Balatsouras DG, Papouliakos S, Ferekidis E (2007) Benign paroxysmal positional vertigo and its management. Med Sci Monit 13:CR275–CR282
4. Levrat E, van Melle G, Monnier P, Maire R (2003) Efficacy of the Semont maneuver in benign paroxysmal positional vertigo. Arch Otolaryngol Head Neck Surg 129:629–633
5. Frenzel H (1961) Pathologico-anatomical and pathologico-physiological basis of positional nystagmus. Acta Otolaryngol Suppl 159:73–77. German

6. Dix MR, Hallpike CS (1952) The pathology, symptomatology and diagnosis of certain common disorders of the vestibular system. Ann Otol 61:987–1016
7. Pagnini P, Nuti D, Vannucchi P (1989) Benign paroxysmal vertigo of the horizontal canal. ORL J Otorhinolaryngol Relat Spec 51:161–170
8. Parnes LS, McClure JA (1992) Free-floating endolymph particles: a new operative finding during posterior semicircular canal occlusion. Laryngoscope 102:988–992
9. Rajguru SM, Ifediba MA, Rabbitt RD (2004) Three-dimensional biomechanical model of benign paroxysmal positional vertigo. Ann Biomed Eng 32:831–846
10. Schuknecht HF (1969) Cupulolithiasis. Arch Otolaryngol 90:765–778
11. Semont A, Sterkers JM (1980) Reeducation vestibulaires. Les Cahiers D' Orl 15:305
12. Epley J (1992) The canalith reposition procedure: for the treatment of benign paroxysmal vertigo. Otolaryngol Head Neck Surg 107:399–404
13. Lempert T (1994) Horizontal benign positional vertigo. Neurology 44:2213–2214
14. Shih CP, Wang CH (2013) Supine to prolonged lateral position: a novel therapeutic maneuver for posterior canal benign paroxysmal positional vertigo. J Neurol 260(5):1375–1381
15. Sugita-Kitajima A, Sato S, Mikami K, Mukaide M, Koizuka I (2010) Does vertigo disappear only by rolling over? Rehabilitation for benign paroxysmal positional vertigo. Acta Otolaryngol 130(1):84–88
16. Schaller B (2004) Physiology of cerebral venous blood flow: from experimental data in animals to normal function in humans. Brain Res Rev 46:243–260
17. Maigne R., Nieves WL (2005) Diagnosis and treatment of pain of vertebral origin, 2nd edn. Pain management. Informa Healthcare, 568 p
18. Lindsay JR, Hemenway WG (1956) Postural vertigo due to unilateral sudden partial loss of vestibular function. Ann Otol Rhinol Laryngol 65:692–708
19. Gacek RR (2013) A perspective on recurrent vertigo. ORL J Otorhinolaryngol Relat Spec 75(2):91–107
20. Balatsouras DG, Ganelis P, Aspris A, Economou NC, Moukos A, Koukoutsis G (2012) Benign paroxysmal positional vertigo associated with Meniere's disease: epidemiological, pathophysiologic, clinical, and therapeutic aspects. Ann Otol Rhinol Laryngol 121(10):682–688
21. Crossland G, De R, Axon P (2004) Far advanced otosclerosis and intractable benign paroxysmal positional vertigo treated with combined cochlear implantation and posterior semicircular canal occlusion. J Laryngol Otol 118(4):302–304
22. Mariani P, Pelagatti M, Hahn A, Alpini D (2008) Epidemiology of paroxysmal positioning vertigo: correlation with seasons, climate, and pollution. Int Tinnitus J 14(2):168–174
23. Alpini DC Mariani P Mattei V (2011) Paroxysmal positioning vertigo (Ppv) and pollution: a ten years correlation. Archives of sensology and neurootology in science and practice-ASN, vol 6. http://neurootology.org. ISSN 1612 – 3352
24. Caruso G, Nuti D (2005) Epidemiological data from 2270 PPV patients. Audiological Med 3(1):7–11
25. Neuhauser HK, von Brevern M, Radtke A, Lezius F, Feldmann M, Ziese T, Lempert T (2006) Epidemiology of vestibular vertigo: a neurotologic survey of the general population. Neurology 67(8):1528
26. Vibert D, Kompis M, Hausler R (2003) Benign paroxysmal positional vertigo in older females may be related to osteoporosis and osteopenia. Ann Otol Rhinol Laryngol 112:885–889
27. Jeong SH, Kim JS, Shin JW, Kim S, Lee H, Lee AY, Kim JM, Jo H, Song J, Ghim Y (2013) Decreased serum vitamin D in idiopathic benign paroxysmal positional vertigo. J Neurol 260:832–838
28. Büki B, Ecker M, Jünger H, Lundberg YW (2013) Vitamin D deficiency and benign paroxysmal positioning vertigo. Med Hypotheses 80(2):201–204
29. Cakir BO, Ercan I, Cakir ZA, Civelek S, Turgut S (2006) Relationship between the affected ear in benign paroxysmal positional vertigo and habitual head-lying side during bedrest. J Laryngol Otol 120(7):534–536
30. Sunami K, Tochino R, Tokuhara Y, Yamamoto H, Tomita S, Koshimo N, Yamane H (2006) Effects of cigarettes and alcohol consumption in benign paroxysmal positioning vertigo. Acta Otolaryngol 126(8):834–838

31. Lin YT, Lin HW, Huang YC, Ho WT, Li YC, Chen TJ (2013) Association between gout and vertigo in a Taiwanese population. J Clin Neurosci 20:857–861, pii: S0967-5868 (12)00464-X
32. Yoda S, Cureoglu S, Yildirim-Baylan M, Morita N, Fukushima H, Harada T, Paparella MM (2011) Association between type 1 diabetes mellitus and deposits in the semicircular canals. Otolaryngol Head Neck Surg 145(3):458–462
33. Modugno GC, Pirodda A, Ferri GG, Montana T, Rasciti L, Ceroni AR (2000) A relationship between autoimmune thyroiditis and benign paroxysmal positional vertigo? Med Hypotheses 54:614–615
34. Papi G, Corsello SM, Milite MT, Zanni M, Ciardullo AV, Di Donato C, Pontecorvi A (2009) Association between benign paroxysmal positional vertigo and autoimmune chronic thyroiditis. Clin Endocrinol (Oxf) 70:169–170
35. Padberg S, Heller K, Usadel KH, Schumm-Draeger PM (2001) One-year prophylactic treatment of euthyroid Hashimoto's thyroiditis patients with levothyroxine: is there a benefit? Thyroid 11(3):249–255
36. Cesarani A, Alpini D (1999) Vertigo and dizziness rehabilitation – the MCS method. Springer, Milan, Heidelberg

9 Cervicogenic Vertigo and Dizziness

Cervicogenic balance disorders (CBD) were first described as "cervical vertigo" by Ryan and Cope in 1955 [1]. Other terms used for the same disorder are proprioceptive vertigo, cervicogenic vertigo and cervical dizziness [2, 3].

Although the diagnosis has remained controversial since its introduction, several observations have led to the proposal of a plausible pathophysiologic mechanism:

- The deep intervertebral muscles in the cervical spine possess a high density of muscle spindles and are assumed to play an important role in postural control [4–6].
- Cervical afferents are known to be involved in the cervico-collic reflex, the cervico-ocular reflex and the tonic neck reflex, which work in conjunction with other reflexes influenced by the visual and vestibular systems to stabilize the head, the eyes and posture.
- Vestibular and proprioceptive inputs are linearly combined for computing egocentric, body-centred coordinates [7–11].
- Anaesthetic injections to the upper cervical dorsal nerve roots can produce dizziness and nystagmus [12, 13].
- Electrical [14] or vibratory [15] stimulation to the cervical muscles has also been shown to induce a sensation of tilting or falling.

Brandt and Bronstein [3] proposed a mechanism where changed firing characteristics of cervical somatosensory receptors due to neck pain lead to a sensory mismatch between vestibular and cervical input, resulting in cervical vertigo. This mechanism seems to agree with the most recent findings about vestibular–somatosensory convergence in head movement control [16–18].

Cervicogenic balance disorders may be caused by a specific lesion mechanism like whiplash injury. More frequently, no apparent cause is revealed. Spontaneous neck pain may present or not. A case history of cervicoartrosis or neck dysfunction, in general, may be present or not.

In the case of a CBD due to whiplash, the patient has to be treated as explained in Chap. 12.

D.C. Alpini et al., *Vertigo Rehabilitation Protocols*,
DOI 10.1007/978-3-319-05482-7_9, © Springer International Publishing Switzerland 2014

Generally, vertigo or dizziness due to a cervicogenic mechanism appears suddenly, after a more or less brisk movement of the head or of the body, usually in the sitting position, frequently after some time spent watching television or working at a PC. After the onset, symptoms may be caused by any kind of movement of the head/body, and even if cervical vertigo may be confused with benign paroxysmal positioning vertigo, the specific tests explained in the Chap. 8 lead to the correct diagnosis.

The *key impairment* of CBD is head and neck motion intolerance not provoked by a whiplash mechanism nor a labyrinth lithiasis. The *key lesion* is the oversensitivity of spinal proprioceptors and a mismatch with vestibular cues [19].

Accurate case history and proper clinical examination are usually the *diagnostic key*, but sometimes instrumental diagnosis is necessary to confirm and to help adequate therapeutic planning.

Instrumental diagnosis is aimed to evaluate cervical role on static postural control (static posturography), dynamic head-to-trunk stabilization (cranio-corpo-graphy) and cervico-oculomotor interaction (smooth pursuit neck torsion test, SPNTT) (see also Chap. 3). Cervical x-rays and neuroimaging (CT, MRI) are useless for this kind of diagnosis.

9.1 Static Posturography

The upright position is controlled by three distinct sensorial cues: visual, somatosensorial (from spine proprioceptors and pressure sensors in the feet) and vestibular (mainly from otolithic maculae). Posture is more stable when all the sensory systems operate and the head is aligned with the trunk. Routinely, posturography (PG) recording is performed under two basic conditions, patient standing on the platform with eyes open (EO) and with eyes closed (EC). Besides these basic tests to verify the presence of a latent postural disorder, cervical destabilizing tests are usually employed to identify a cervical origin of the dizzy symptoms. Through tests performed with rotation ("cervical dynamic activation" [20, 21], "head turned" [22] and retroflexion of the head [23]), it is possible to obtain some information about cervical destabilizing inputs. However, positive results obtained with the abovementioned tests must be evaluated within the entire clinical context, because they cannot be considered as pathognomonic.

9.2 Cranio-corpo-graphy

Head destabilization seems to be the specific target to investigate equilibrium disturbances in whiplash patients and thus in CBD. Since 1968, cranio-corpo-graphy (CCG) has been used as a simple procedure to evaluate head-to-trunk stabilization in vestibular disorders [24] (Fig. 9.1).

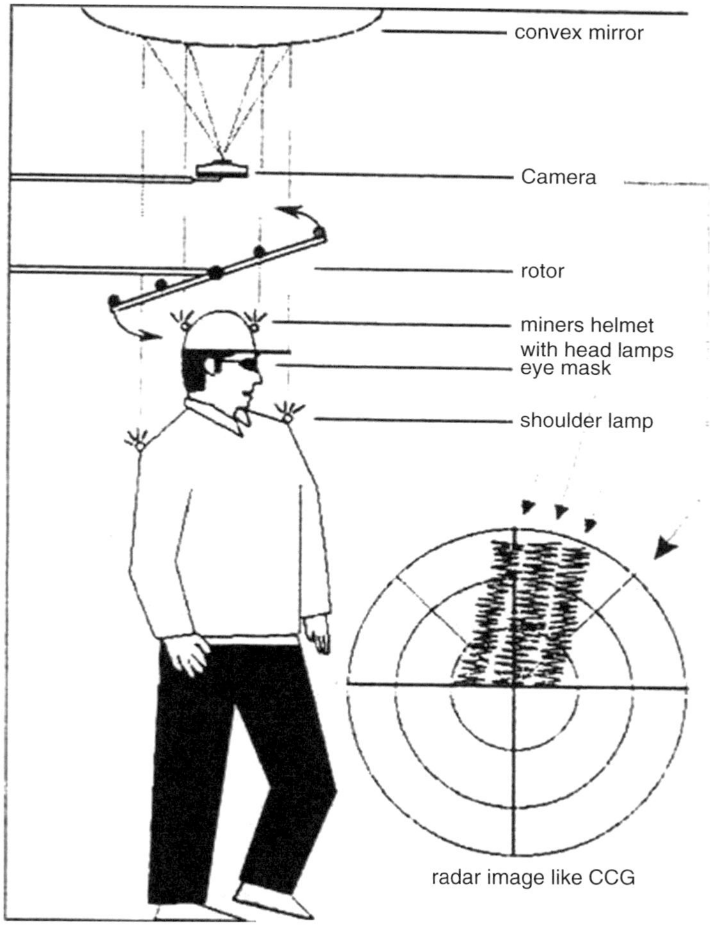

Fig. 9.1 A schematic representation of cranio-corpo-graphy. Subjects walk in place in a dark room, and movements of the light bulbs placed on the head (helmet) and shoulder impress the film in an instant Polaroid camera in order to obtain four light traces on a black imagine

It has proved to be one of the most efficient, quick, objective and quantitative tests for screening equilibrium function for nearly 20 years, and the West German Labour Security Surveillance Board introduced it for occupational medical ability testing in 1983. Cranio-corpo-graphy (CCG) has been successively digitalized (dCCG) on the basis of the optoelectronic technology [25]. Digital cranio-corpo-graphy (dCCG) was a non-invasive assessment based on a 50 Hz CCD camera for acquiring the position of four markers placed on the subject who walks in place (Fukuda stepping test) (Fig. 9.2).

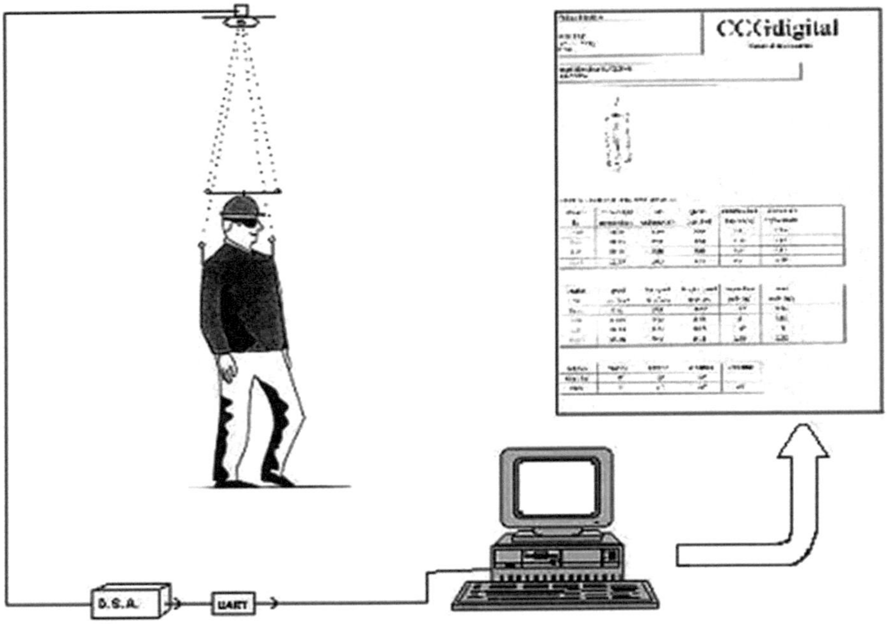

Fig. 9.2 Two passive reflective markers (*front* and *rear*) are set at the extremities of a stick attached to a worker's hardhat, while two markers (*left* and *right*) are attached on rigid shoulder supports

Investigations performed with dCCG suggested that the most specific parameter able to discriminate between normal and pathological cervico-cephalic control is the ratio between head and trunk displacements. It is also possible to detect directly head and trunk sagittal (Y) and lateral (X) movements using a commercial equipment that uses two accelerometers that are 2D-sensitive (e.g. Delos, Turin, Italy) [26], respectively, fixed to the occiput and to the sternum in order to record sagittal and lateral displacements of the two body segments (Fig. 9.3).

The equipment records 20″ body segment movements each test. Head-to-trunk stabilization (ratio between X and Y head and trunk displacements) during walking-in-place is thus calculated: a ratio <1 indicates stabilization of the head with respect to the trunk. Normal values range from 0.6 to 0.8. Values around 1 are considered borderline, while ratios >1 are pathological (Fig. 9.4).

9.3 Smooth Pursuit Neck Torsion Test (SPNT)

In 1998 Tjell and Rosenhall [27] firstly described a specific oculomotor test, named *smooth pursuit neck torsion test* (SPNTT), successively improved by Treleaven et al. [28].

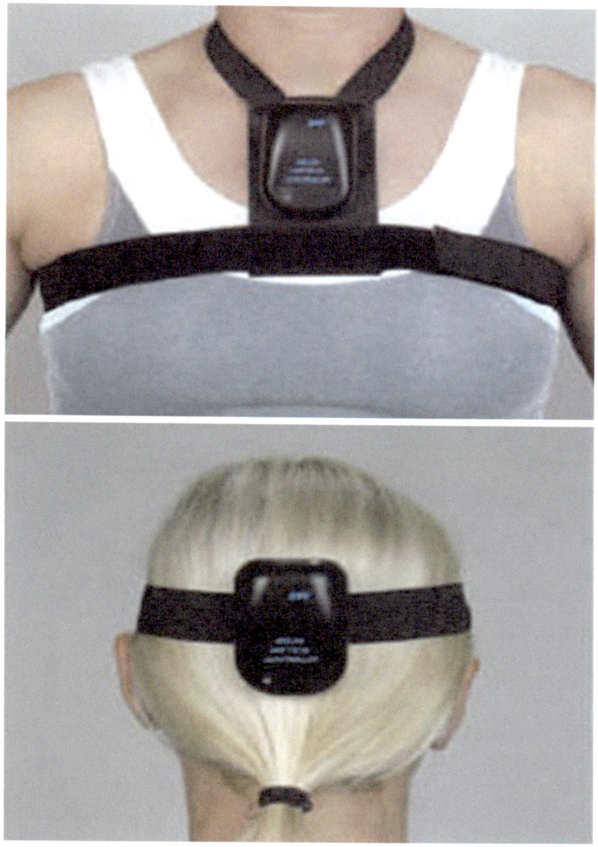

Fig. 9.3 An accelerometer is fixed on the head and the other on the trunk in order to record sagittal and lateral displacements of the two body segments. Software calculates mean displacement velocities of the segments (°/s) and the ratio between head and trunk displacements

The test is performed with the patient sitting on a chair free to rotate. SPNTT compares the gain of eye movements following a target (smooth pursuit) with the head in neutral position and with the body turned 45° right- and leftward (neck torsion). In this way the head counteracts the body rotation, but the eyes remain and labyrinths are not stimulated. To avoid "cervical bias," it is necessary to slowly rotate the chair and to use a headrest to avoid neck fatigue and head sway. Any modification of smooth pursuit performance may only be due to cervical inputs, both proprioceptive and nociceptive.

Generally the test is performed using electrooculography (EOG) that measures and records eye movement while following a moving target. The target consists of a light spot projected into a TV screen through a visual angle of 30°. The smooth pursuit (SP) gain is calculated with the neck in a neutral position and also with the neck in a torsioned position. The difference between the gain in neutral and the average values in torsion equalled the smooth pursuit neck torsion difference ((*SPNT-diff*): gain[neutral] – (gain[left] + gain [right])/2).

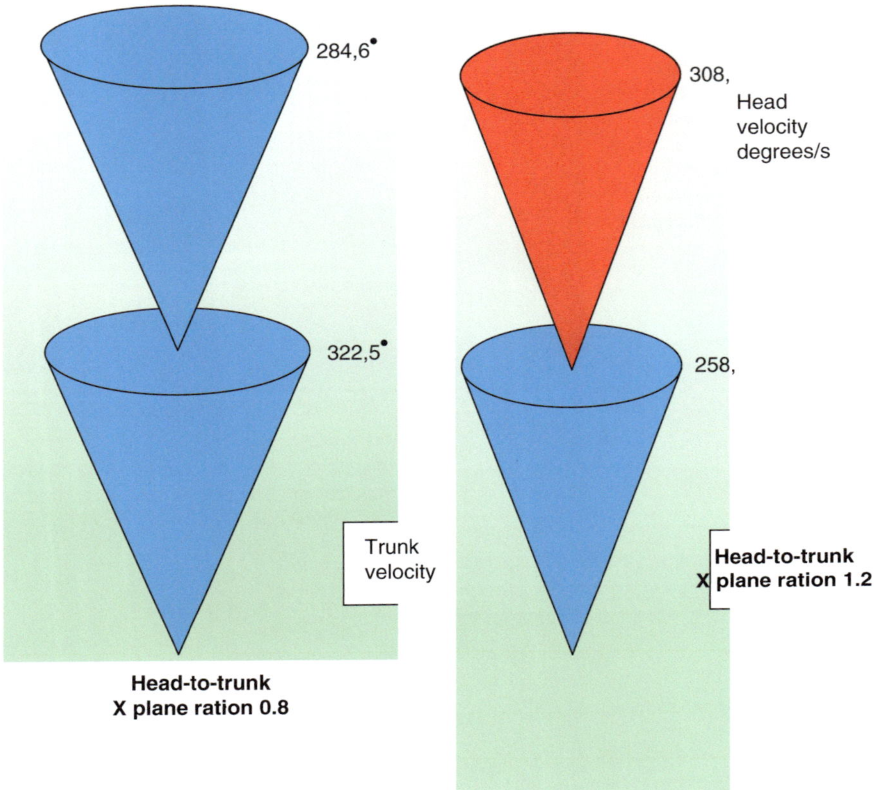

Fig. 9.4 Head and trunk sway are represented as superimposed cones. In normal, (*left*) cervico-cephalic control the head cone is smaller than the trunk cone, and head-to-trunk ratio is less than 1, while in a patient with pathological cervico-cephalic control (*right*), the pattern is reversed

The *SPNT-diff* thus equals 0 if the smooth pursuit eye movement performance did not differ between the neutral and the rotated positions.

Electrooculography may be used also to perform the *Head Tracking Test* (*HTT*) explained in Chap. 3. In this case the more efficient the cervico-ocular interaction, the lesser the movements of the eyes, that is to say, the lower the gain of smooth pursuit.

9.4 Treatment

The specific treatment is based on manual therapy interventions just like cervical pain and cervicogenic headache [29–31]. Physiotherapy and counselling consolidate the therapeutic result.

The treatment is a four-step programme as follows:

1. Removing cervico-cephalic sensorimotor disturbances by means of manual medicine techniques [32, 33] including also vertebral manipulations performed by the physician
2. Amelioration of lifestyle through adequate counselling based on case history, accurate examination of the neck and the spine [34] and, eventually, some specific cervical function questionnaires like the Core Outcome Measurement Index for neck pain (COMI-neck), a short, multidimensional outcome instrument [35]
3. Leading the patient to an awareness of her/his own body and learning breath and neck tension control through physical exercises performed with a physiotherapist
4. Maintaining the results through home exercises

9.4.1 Manual Medicine

Manual medicine (MM) is a medical discipline based on the use of palpation and operator-directed techniques to aid in the diagnosis and treatment of musculoskeletal disorder. Manual medicine treatment includes the use of but is not limited to thrust/impulse (also the so-called high-velocity low-amplitude, HVLA) spinal manipulation, soft tissue mobilization (also the so-called low-velocity high-amplitude, LVHA), myofascial release and functional release. Manual medicine identifies a specific manipulable lesion, which is treated with an appropriate manipulative technique to resolve the condition [32]. The goal of manipulation is to restore maximal pain-free movement of the musculoskeletal system in postural balance.

Manual medicine is as old as medicine itself. It was practiced in Thailand 4,000 years ago and used in ancient Egypt. Hippocrates, the founder of modern medicine, used traction and leverage techniques to treat spinal disorders. In the nineteenth century "bone setters" were popular in Europe and the United States. Dr. Edward Harrison, in 1784; Andrew Taylor Still, in 1874; and D.D. Palmer, in1896, began what is known today as manual medicine, osteopathy and chiropractic, respectively. In the twentieth century James Mennell and Edgar Cyriax began the modern use of manual medicine in Europe. Manual medicine has found application in orthopaedic, neurologic, rheumatologic, physical medicine and rehabilitation.

Standardization of the appropriate diagnostic course to identify specific manipulable lesion is mainly due to Robert Meigne's researches [33]. This author defined the so-called painful minor intervertebral dysfunction (PMID) as the basis of the treatment diagnosis of a spinal musculoskeletal disorder [34].

The identification of PMIDs at different spine levels allows a specific conservative and manual treatment of the biomechanic dysfunctions that lead to cervicogenic balance disorders (CBD).

On the basis of clinical and instrumental evaluation of the patient affected with CBD, appropriate combination of different manual techniques may be planned.

Generally speaking, a proper treatment may be stepped as follows:

1. *Soft tissue* treatment, that is to say, delicate massage of superficial and deeper layers of the muscle and connective tissue of the shoulders and the neck in order

to enhance function, decrease muscle reflex activity and inhibit motor-neuron excitability.

It includes manoeuvres directed toward the muscles and fascia throughout the body. It involves a doctor or therapist using his/her hands to stretch or relax dysfunctional soft tissue structures. While these techniques can be applied almost anywhere, they are especially useful for the paraspinal musculature that surrounds each vertebra of the spine [36].

2. *Spinal mobilization* (*LHVA*), a type of passive movement of a spinal segment or region.
   Spinal mobilization has been described as a gentle, often oscillatory, passive movement applied to a spinal region or segment to gently increase the passive range of motion of that segment or region [37].
3. *Muscle energy technique* [38], a direct and active technique; meaning it engages a restrictive barrier and requires the patient's participation for maximal effect.
   As the patient performs an isometric contraction, Golgi tendon organ activation results in direct inhibition of the agonist muscles, a reflexive reciprocal inhibition occurs at the antagonistic muscles, and, as the patient relaxes, the agonist and antagonist muscles remain inhibited allowing the joint to be moved further into the restricted range of motion.
4. *Spinal manipulations* (*HVLA*), a therapeutic intervention performed on spinal articulations [39]. Due to the intrinsic risk of these manoeuvres, this kind of intervention has to be performed only by well-trained doctors and never by physiotherapists.

Generally speaking, spinal manipulation consists of forced passive mobilization which stretches the joint elements beyond their physiological or pathological barrier up to the limit of their passive movement [38]. It is called "high speed" or "with impulse". This kind of controlled brisk movement causes a sort of proprioceptive shock at the medulla centres. This discharge is therefore able to reset neuromuscular and vegetative control at the level of the treated segment. Even if therapeutic spinal manipulations, always performed only by a trained medical doctor, are based on the golden Meigne rule of "no pain and reverse movement", a certain degree of complications is always possible especially with regard to cervical manipulations. Serious complications after manipulation of the cervical spine are estimated to be 0.25–2 in a million manipulations. Neck manipulation is believed to account for 6–9 % of cervical artery dissections. Vascular accidents are responsible for the major criticism of spinal manipulative therapy. However, this procedure, in experienced hands, gives beneficial results with few adverse side effects [40]. Manipulation techniques should be used to resolve PMID treating the active (spontaneously painful) and the inactive ones (non-spontaneously painful) when localized in specific zones: the most significant inactive PMID.

Due to biomechanics of the postural control, it is therefore advisable to begin treatment searching for the PMID, even the inactive ones, at the lumbosacral and mid-lumbar passage, at L3–L4, thus proceeding with their treatment (Fig. 9.5).

The next step is the treatment of the thoracolumbar segment (Fig. 9.6) and the mid-thoracic (T7–8, Fig. 9.7) region.

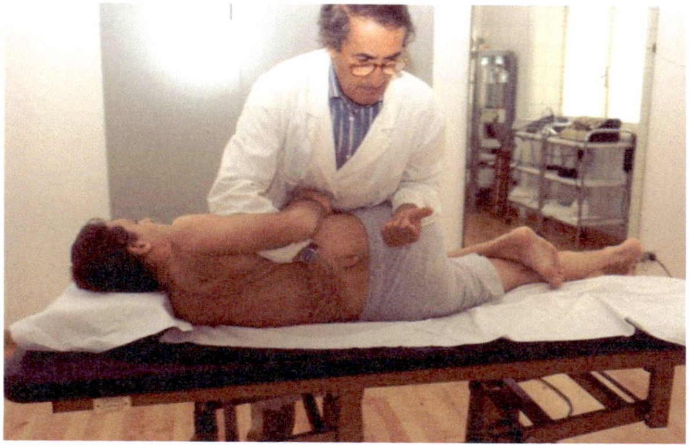

Fig. 9.5 Spinal manipulation of the lumbar region

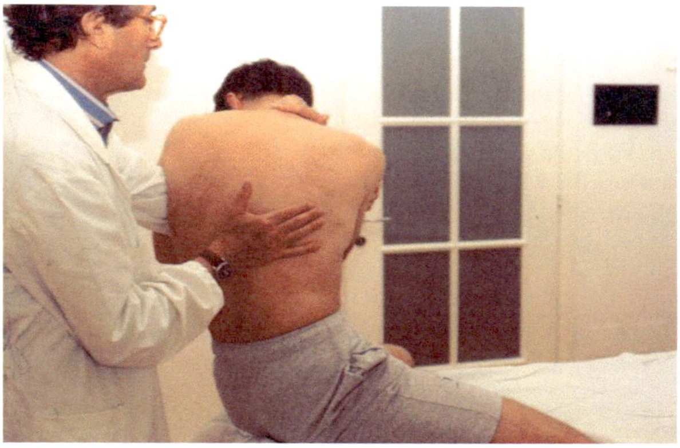

Fig. 9.6 Manipulation of the thoracolumbar passage

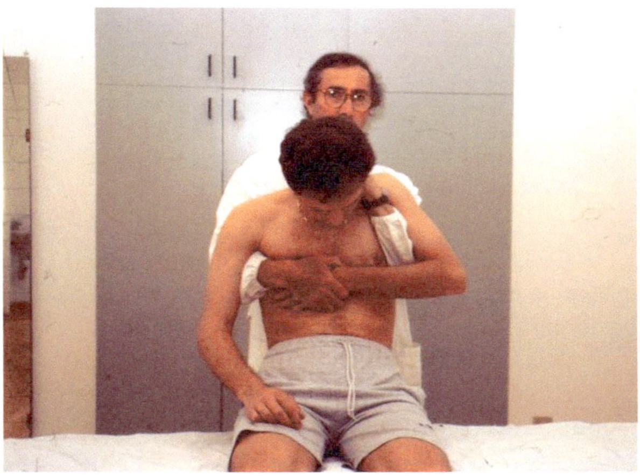

Fig. 9.7 Manipulation of the mid-thoracic passage in extension by means of epigastric support

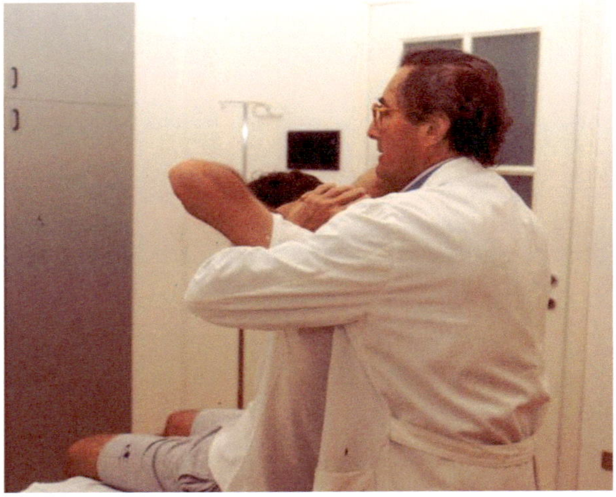

Fig. 9.8 Manipulation in extension by means of sternum support of the cervicothoracic passage

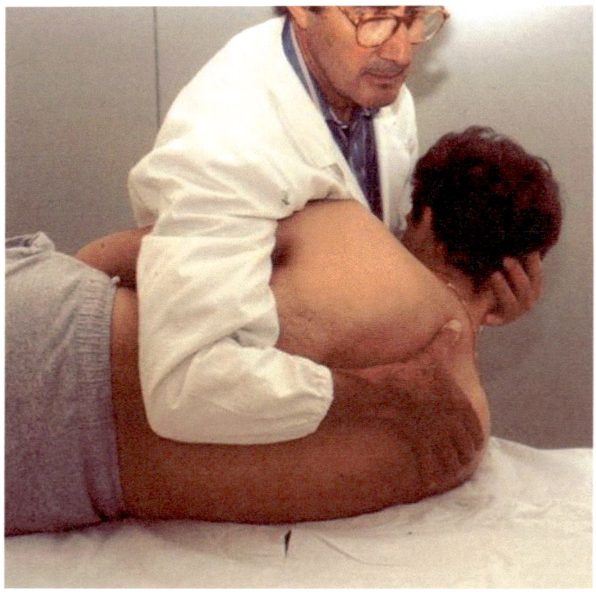

Fig. 9.9 Manipulation of the same spinal region with the patient in the supine position (the so-called Deroullè manipulation)

In CBD the cervicothoracic segment is treated also in the absence of PMID, in extension using a sternum support position (Fig. 9.8) or with the patient in a supine position (Fig. 9.9).

Finally, also the neck is manipulated (Fig. 9.10).

The atlo-occipital segment is the most dangerous to manipulate, and thus gentle mobilization and soft tissues treatment are indicated, with the patient in a supine or sitting position.

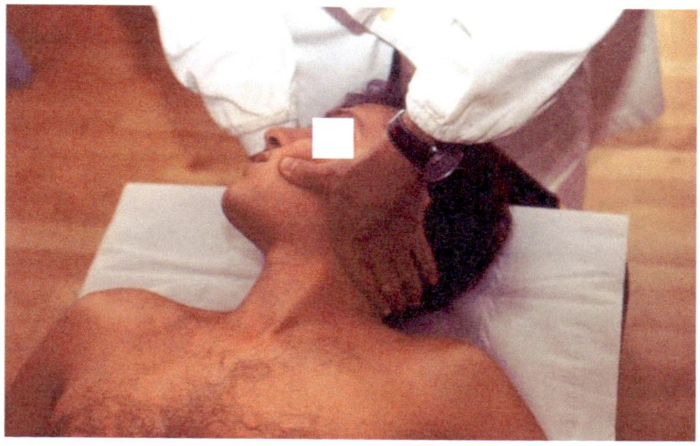

Fig. 9.10 Cervical manipulation

9.4.2 Counselling

It is important to pay attention to lifestyle and to maintain proper postural control during usual daily and working activities.

The main suggestions are:

- Perform regular and constant aerobic physical activity, e.g. rapid walking (not running neither jogging) 30′ daily three times/week.
- Avoid maintaining the same position of the head/neck for more than 30 min.
- Avoid maintaining an incorrect position of the head/neck, in particular check the proper position when watching television or working on a PC.
- Anyway, every 30 min change your head/neck position, and mobilize your head and shoulders.
- Maintain adequate water intake (at least 1.5 l for females and 2 l for males).
- Restrict alcohol intake (less than 120 ml for women and 240 ml for men).
- Restrict smoke and, obviously, avoid drug abuse.
- Sleep using two pillows in order to maintain the head lifted about 20°.

9.5 Physiotherapy

The physiotherapy programme is constituted by ten sessions subdivided into three sessions per week for two weeks followed by two sessions per week for the following two weeks. The first step is to prepare the patient to cooperate in a complex programme involving movement, thinking and learning. Musculoskeletal impairments are often provoked or associated to tension and anxiety, that is why head and neck disorders have to be manually treated before. Furthermore, it is more necessary to begin treatment with simple relaxation exercises to improve patient's tension management.

Simple exercises have to be planned, and they are generally pointed to mobilization of the pelvis, of the cervical rachis and of the thoracolumbar spine.

9.5.1 First week

Supine (All the Exercises Are Performed Having the Patient's Head Comfortably Lying on a Pillow)

1. Relaxation exercises with control of breathing improving consciousness of abdominal or thoracic breathing: deep inhalation followed, after a few seconds, by a forced exhalation pronouncing the word "one". This exercise is repeated 8–10 times.
2. The patient moves the head, first slowly and then faster, in all directions focusing a target straight on the ceiling.
3. The patient holds the right knee against the chest, then extends the leg and takes the left knee against the chest. A gentle traction of the flexed leg is performed by the patient himself/herself when the knee is held against the chest.
4. The patient holds her/his two knees to the chest, with the hands simultaneously helping, gently.
5. The patient lifts her/his pelvis simultaneously extending the arms over the head. Then the patient repositions the arms along the body lowering the pelvis.
6. The patient grasps a stick. Then she/he extends the arms over the head and then returns to the primary position.

In the Quadrupedal Position

7. The patient inhales and arches the back with the head between the arms. Then she/he exhales with a simultaneous retroflexion of the head and rotation of the pelvis in hyperlordosis.
8. The patient simultaneously extends the right arm and the left leg and then repeats the exercise with the left arm and the right leg.
9. In the prone position the patient lifts her/his left arm and the right leg holding the forehead over the bed. She/he then repeats with the right arm and the left leg.

9.5.2 Second Week

Sitting

10. The patient moves the head first slowly and then faster in all directions focusing on a target straight in front of her/him.
11. The patient looks for three targets sited, respectively, in front, at her/his left and at her/his right. Then the patient fixates the front target, then she/he moves the head and fixates the right-sited target. Finally, she/he rotates leftward with the head maintaining the focus on the right-sited target.
12. The patient fixates the frontal target. Then she/he moves the head leftward and fixates the left-sited target. Finally, she/he rotates rightward with the head maintaining the focus on the left-sited target.
13. The patient turns the head rightward and focuses on a target on the lateral wall. Then she/he positions the head straight maintaining focus, through eye counter-rotation, and counts until 10.

14. The patient turns the head leftward and focuses on a target on the lateral wall. Then she/he positions the head straight maintaining focus on the target, through eye counterrotation, and counts until 10.
15. The patient grasps a stick with both hands and takes the stick behind the shoulder positioning the stick at level of the cervico-dorsal junction. In this position she/he rotates to-and-fro the trunk maintaining the head's position still focusing on a target straight in front. Rotation of the trunk has to be harmonic with calm breathing.
16. The patient puts the stick forward on the sternum at the level of the sternoclavicular joint. Then she/he performs rhythmic backward displacements of the shoulders.
17. In this position the patient rotates to-and-fro the trunk maintaining the head's position still fixating on a target straight in front. Rotation of the trunk has to be harmonic with calm breathing.
18. Paying attention to calm breathing, the patient inhales, then, exhaling, she/he bends forward taking the head to the right knee. She/he holds this position for 10 s. Then, inhaling she/he goes back to the sitting position.
19. Paying attention to calm breathing, the patient inhales, then, exhaling, she/he bends forward taking the head to the left knee. She/he holds this position for 10 s. She/he inhales and goes back to the sitting position.
20. The patient inhales. Exhaling she/he bends forward to place an object on the floor. Then she/he inhales and takes it up over the head, and then she/he fixates it for 10 s. Exhaling she/he bends forward and places the object back on the floor.

9.5.3 Third and Fourth Weeks

Standing

21. The patient, in front of a mirror, aligns correctly her/his posture. She/he then maintains equilibrium for 1 min, paying attention to breathing; before she/he maintains equilibrium, she/he opens and closes the eyes visualizing the correct position.
22. The patient remains in this position for at least 1 min paying attention to breathing. Then, she/he oscillates to-and-fro according to the breathing rhythm, hearing the air that enters and then exits from the lungs.
23. The patient in upright position fixates a target on a mirror (a paper square, white or coloured, or a picture approximately cm × 5 cm). In this way the patient has two planes of fixation: the target and her/his reflected image. She/he has to be able to extract the correct fixation information from visual inputs. Then, the patient oscillates to-and-fro according to the breathing rhythm hearing the air that enters and then exits from the lungs.
24. The patient holds a little object and lifts it over the head fixating it. Then, she/he deeply inhales. Exhaling, she/he bends forward placing the object on the floor. Then the patient waits 10 s, and then, inhaling, she/he lifts again the object over the head.

25. The patients take a little object over her/his head. Fixating the object she/he moves it in small circles according to the breathing rhythm hearing the air that enters and then exits from the lungs.

9.6 Home Protocol

Home exercises have to be performed once a day, before sleeping, and at least three times/week twice a day, upon awaking and before sleeping. The sequence is different in the morning with respect to the evening.

Evening Exercises

1. In the sitting position rotate your head to-and-fro, with slow but large movements just until the end of the range of movement (Fig. 9.11).
2. In the sitting position bend your head from side to side, with slow but large movements just until the end of the range of movement (Fig. 9.12).

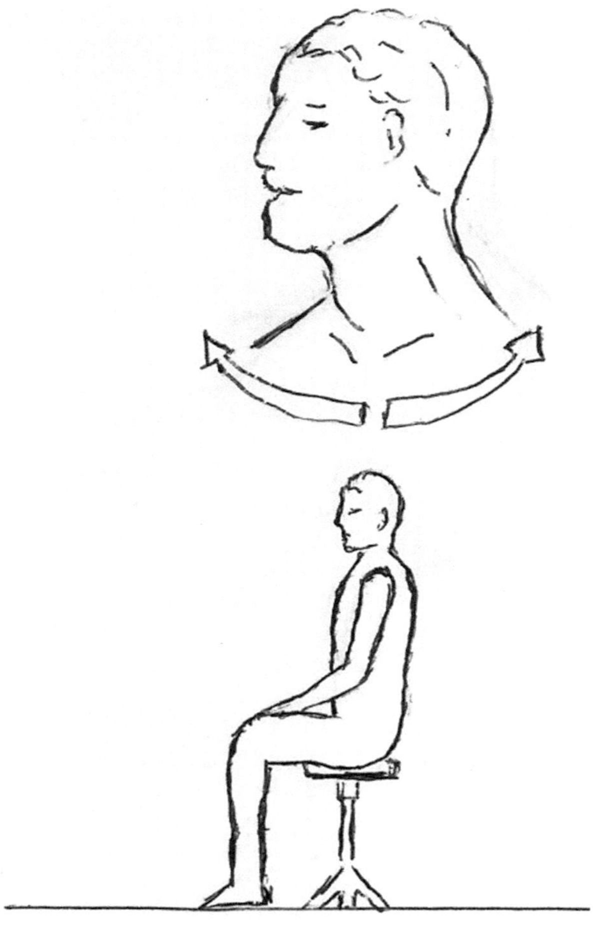

Fig. 9.11 Slow but large rotation of the head, in sitting position

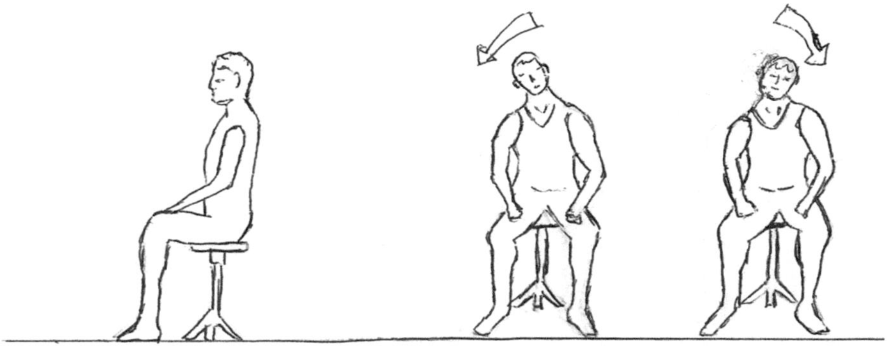

Fig. 9.12 Slow but large lateroflexion of the head, in sitting position

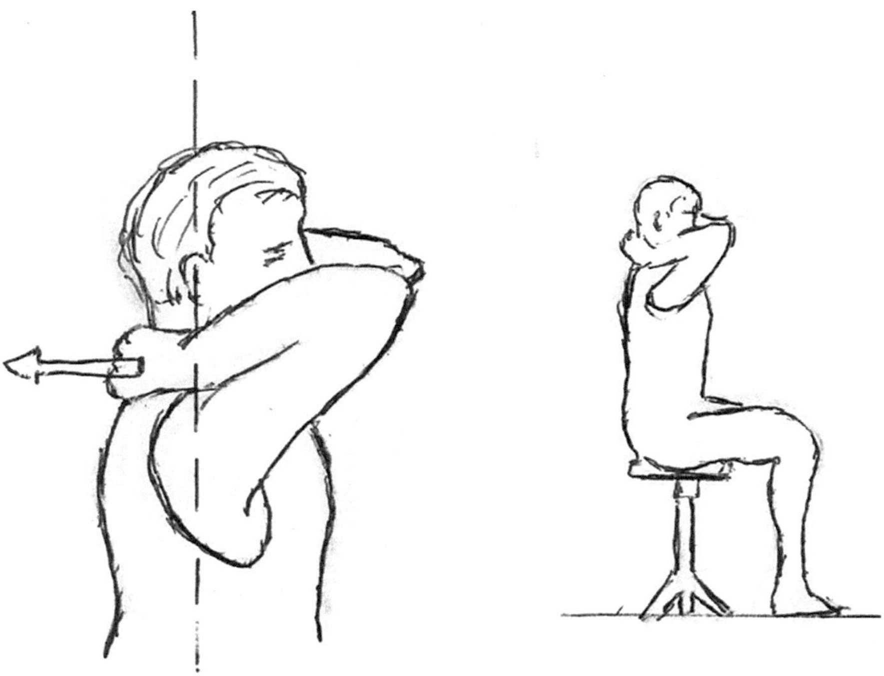

Fig. 9.13 In the sitting position together the hands resist backward pushes of the head

3. In the sitting position put your hands together on your neck. Using the hands together as a resistance, push your head backward in order to obtain isometric contractions of the cervical and dorsal muscles (Fig. 9.13).
4. In the sitting position put your hands together on the occiput. Inhale. Then exhaling bend forward your trunk using the hands together to gently accompany trunk bending. After awhile, inhaling, relax your arms and reposition your head and trunk (Fig. 9.14).

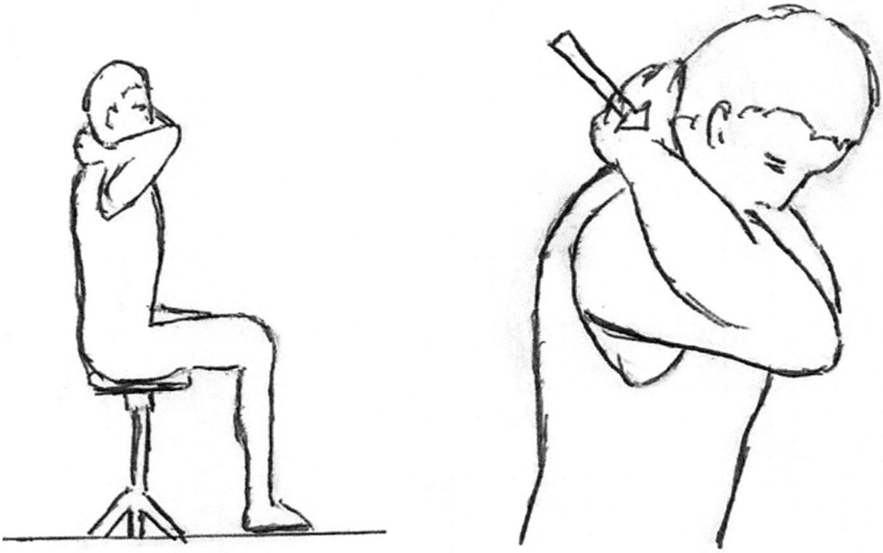

Fig. 9.14 In the sitting position together the hands on the occiput accompany the slow and rhythmic forward bending of the head and the trunk: exhaling the patient bends the trunk; inhaling she/he repositions

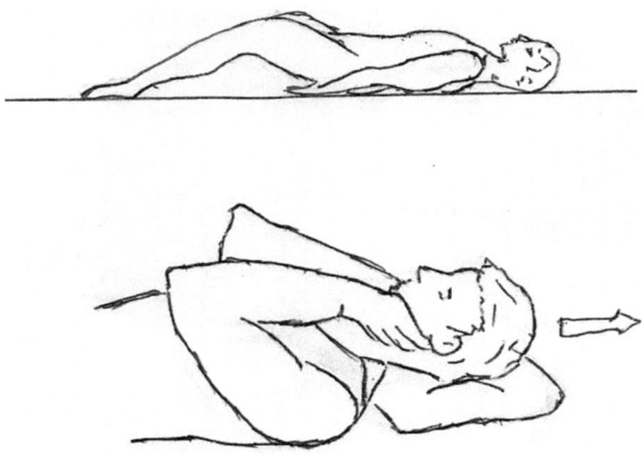

Fig. 9.15 In the supine position put a pillow under both your knees and your head, the hands slowly and gently push the head following the breathing rhythm: the patient pushes when inhaling and stops when exhaling

5. In the supine position with a pillow under the knees and a pillow under the head, with your hands push your head, slowly and gently, several times: when you inhale push your head; when you exhale stop the pushes (Fig. 9.15).
6. In the supine position put your right hand on your left ear and, slowly and gently, pull your head rightward. Follow the breathing rhythm: pull when you inhale; stop when you exhale. Repeat several times and then repeat using your left hand on your right ear (Fig. 9.16).

   In the *morning*, the awaking sequence is 6–5 1–2 3–4.

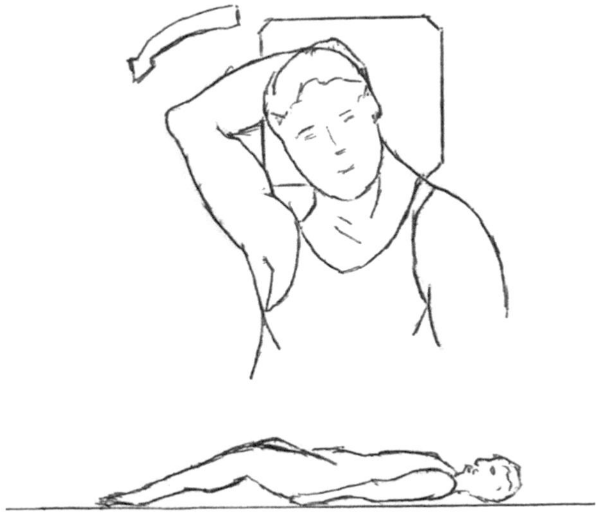

Fig. 9.16 In the supine position put a pillow under both your knees and your head, then the patient uses her/his right hand to pull rightward her/his head, slowly and gently, following the breathing rhythm: the patient pulls when inhaling and stops when exhaling. The patient repeats the same exercise using the opposite hand on the right ear

References

1. Ryan G, Cope S (1955) Cervical vertigo. Lancet 31:1355–1358
2. Lafon H (1990) Les vertiges d'origine proprioceptive par lesion mecanique vertebrocervicale. J Francais d'Oto-Rhino-Laryngologie 39(5):269–278
3. Brandt T, Bronstein AM (2001) Cervical vertigo. Neurol Neurosurg Psychiatry 71(1):8–12
4. Abrahams VC (1977) The physiology of neck muscles; their role in head movement and maintenance of posture. Can J Physiol Pharmacol 55(3):332–338
5. Liu J-X, Thornell L-E, Pedrosa-Domellöf F (2003) Muscle spindles in the deep muscles of the human neck: A morphological and immunocytochemical study. J Histochem Cytochem 51(2):175–186
6. Treleaven J (2008) Sensorimotor disturbances in neck disorders affecting postural stability, head and eye movement control. Man Ther 13(1):2–11
7. Berthoz A, Llinas R (1974) Afferent neck projection to the cat cerebellar cortex. Exp Brain Res 20:385–401
8. Boyle R, Pompeiano O (1981) Convergence and interaction of neck and macular vestibular inputs on vestibulospinal neurons. J Neurophysiol 45:852–866
9. Ghez C (1991) Posture. In: Kandel ER, Schwartz JH, Jessell TM (eds) Principles of neural science, 3rd edn. Elsevier, New York, pp 596–607
10. Brink EE, Suzuki I, Timerick SJB, Wilson VJ (1985) Tonic neck reflex of the decerebrate cat: a role for propriospinal neurons. J Neurophysiol 54:978–987
11. Dumas G, Lion A, Gauchard GC, Herpin G, Magnusson M, Perrin PP (2013) Clinical interest of postural and vestibulo-ocular reflex changes induced by cervical muscles and skull vibration in compensated unilateral vestibular lesion patients. J Vestib Res 23(1):41–49
12. Cohen LA (1961) Role of eye and neck proprioceptive mechanisms in body orientation and motor coordination. J Neurophysiol 24:1–11
13. de Jong PTVM, de Jong JMBV, Cohen B, Jongkees LBW (1977) Ataxia and nystagmus induced by injection of local anesthetics in the neck. Ann Neurol 1(3):240–246
14. Alpini D, Cesarani A, Barozzi S (1992) Non pharmacological treatment of acute vertigo. In: Claussen CF, Kirtane MV, Schneider D (eds) Diagnostic procedures and imagining techniques used in neurotology. Proceedings of the XVI NES CONGRESS. Werner Rudat & Co, Nachf ed m + p, Hamburg, pp 337–340

15. Biguer B, Donaldson IML, Hein A, Jannerod M (1988) Neck muscle vibration modifies the representation of visual motion and direction in man. Brain 11(1):1405–1424
16. Wilson V (1991) Vestibulospinal and neck reflexes: interaction in the vestibular nuclei. Arch Ital Biol 129:43–52
17. Horak F, Hlavacka F (2001) Somatosensory loss increases vestibulospinal sensitivity. J Neurophys 86:575–585
18. Mulavara AP, Ruttley T, Cohen HS, Peters BT, Miller C, Brady R, Merkle L, Bloomberg JJ (2012) Vestibular-somatosensory convergence in head movement control during locomotion after long-duration space flight. J Vestib Res 22:153–166
19. Fitz-Ritson D (1991) Assessment of cervicogenic vertigo. J Manipulative Physiol Ther 14(3):193–198
20. Nakagawa H, Ohashi N, Watanabe Y, Mizukoshi K (1993) The contribution of proprioception in posture control in normal subjects. Acta Otolaryngol Suppl 504:112–116
21. Norré ME (1990) Posture in otoneurotology. Acta ORL Belg 44:183–363
22. Roberts TDM (1973) Reflex balance. Nature 244:158–185
23. Rubin AM, Young JH, Milne AC (1975) Vestibular-neck integration in vestibular nuclei. Brain Res 96:99–102
24. Claussen CF (1999) Cranio-Corpo-Graphy (CCG)- 30 years of equilibriometric measurements of spatial and temporal head, neck and trunk movements. In: Claussen CF, Haid CT, Hofferberth B (eds) Equilibrium in research and equilibriometry in modern treatment. Elsevier, Amsterdam, pp 245–259
25. Alpini D, Ciavarro GL, Zinnato C, Andreoni G, Santambrogio GC (2005) Evaluation of head-to-trunk control in whiplash patients using digital CranioCorpoGraphy during a stepping test. Gait & posture 22:308–316
26. Sjostrom H, Allum JH, Carpenter MG, Adkin AL, Honegger F, Ettlin T (2003) Trunk sway measures of postural stability during clinical balance tests in patients with chronic whiplash injury symptoms. Spine 28(15):1725–1734
27. Tjell C, Rosenhall U (1998) Smooth pursuit neck torsion test: a specific test for cervical dizziness. Am J Otol 19(1):76–81
28. Treleaven J, Gwendolen J, LowChoy N (2005) Smooth pursuit neck torsion test in whiplash-associated disorders: relationship to self-reports of neck pain and disability, dizziness and anxiety. J Rehabil Med 37:219–223
29. Wrisley DM, Sparto PJ, Whitney SL, Furman JM (2000) Cervicogenic dizziness: a review of diagnosis and treatment. J Orthop Sports Phys Ther 30(12):755–766
30. Chou LH, Lenrow DA (2002) Cervicogenic headache. Pain Physician 5(2):215–225
31. Antonaci F, Sjaastad O (2011) Cervicogenic headache: a real headache. Curr Neurol Neurosci Rep 11(2):149–155
32. Dvorak J, Dvorak V, Schneider W (1988) Manual medicine. Springer, Heidelberg
33. Maigne R (2006) Douleurs d'origine vertébrale. Elsevier Masson, Issy-les-Moulineaux
34. Maigne J-Y et al (2009) Interexaminer agreement of clinical examination of the neck in manual medicine. Ann Phys Rehabil Med 52(1):41–48
35. Fankhauser CD, Mutter U, Aghayev E, Mannion AF (2012) Validity and responsiveness of the Core Outcome Measures Index (COMI) for the neck. Eur Spine J 21(1):101–114
36. Stanborough M (2004) Direct release myofascial technique: an illustrated guide for practitioners. Churchill Livingstone, Edinburgh
37. Kessler TJ, Brunner F, Künzer S, Crippa M, Kissling R (2005) Effects of Maitland's manual mobilization on the thoracic spine. Rehabilitation (Stuttg) 6:361–366
38. Goodridge JP (1981) Muscle energy technique: definition, explanation, methods of procedure. J Am Osteopath Assoc 81(4):249–254
39. Ernst E, Canter PH (2006) A systematic review of systematic reviews of spinal manipulation. J R Soc Med 99(4):192–196
40. Gross A, Miller J, D'Sylva J et al (2010) Manipulation or mobilisation for neck pain. In Gross, Anita. Cochrane Database Syst Rev (1):CD004249

10 Ménière's Disease

Ménière's disease (MD) is a chronic illness of the inner ear that affects a substantial number of patients every year worldwide. The disease is characterized by intermittent episodes of vertigo lasting from minutes to hours, with fluctuating sensorineural hearing loss, tinnitus and aural pressure. Attacks of vertigo may come on suddenly or after a short period of tinnitus or muffled hearing. Some people have single attacks of vertigo or dizziness once in a while. Others may have many attacks close together over several days. Some people with Ménière's disease may have very severe attacks to lose their balance and fall.

Ménière's disease may be classified according to different levels of certainty (Table 10.1) [1].

The *key lesion* is the histopathological alteration of the inner ear called endolymphatic hydrops, that is, an excess of fluid in the inner ear. It is thought that endolymphatic fluid bursts from its normal channels in the ear and flows into other areas, causing damage. In some cases the aetiology of hydrops may be considered unknown, but in several patients, causal factors may be identified: post-viral infection [2–5], metabolic disorders like hyperinsulinemia [6–9], vascular disorders [10], autoimmune disorders [11–13] and food intolerances like gluten sensitivity [14, 15].

The *key disabilities* are vertigo or dizziness attacks, intercritical unsteadiness and fear of acute attacks. The main therapy is based on drugs and lifestyle amelioration [16, 17].

Vestibular neurectomy and chemical [18, 19] or surgical [20] labyrinthectomy are the treatment of choice when conservative therapies are unsuccessful.

Rehabilitation [21] may be addressed to:

1. Prepare the patient to imbalance provoked by labyrinthectomy by means of a pre-treatment plan before planned vestibular lesions, so-called *vestibular prehab* [22]
2. Treat the *acute vertigo* seen after vestibular neurectomy or labyrinthectomy [23], as a post-operative plan
3. Amelioration of *intercritical unsteadiness*
4. Manage *fear* of acute attacks
5. Decrease the *frequency* of acute attacks

D.C. Alpini et al., *Vertigo Rehabilitation Protocols*,
DOI 10.1007/978-3-319-05482-7_10, © Springer International Publishing Switzerland 2014

Table 10.1 The American Academy of Otolaryngology—Head and Neck Surgery criteria for diagnosis of Ménière's disease

The definition of the disease requires the combination of: 1. Recurrent spontaneous and episodic vertigo. A definitive spell of vertigo lasting at least 20 min, often prostrating, accompanied by disequilibrium that can last several days; usually nausea or vomiting, or both; no loss of consciousness. Horizontal rotatory nystagmus is always present 2. Hearing loss (not necessarily fluctuating) 3. Either aural fullness or tinnitus, or both
The classification of the disease is graded as follows: Certain Ménière's disease Definite disease with histopathological confirmation Definite Ménière's disease Two or more definitive episodes of vertigo with hearing loss, plus tinnitus, aural fullness, or both Probable Ménière's disease Only one definitive episode of vertigo and the other symptoms and signs Possible Ménière's disease Definitive vertigo with no associated hearing loss or hearing loss with non-definitive disequilibrium

10.1 Vestibular Prehab

Prehab has been proposed for subjects undergoing gentamicin treatment, as in chemical labyrinthectomy. Subjects would perform vestibular exercises for 2 weeks before the first gentamicin installation or surgical operation.

Exercises in the gymnasium to be performed with the therapist three times a week

1. Relaxation exercises such as control of breathing with improving consciousness of abdominal or thoracic breathing. A simple exercise consists in deep inhalation followed, after few seconds, by a forced exhalation pronouncing the word "one". This exercise is repeated 8–10 times.
2. From the supine position, the patient shifts to sitting position, fixating a point straight in front of her/him (Fig. 10.1).
3. In the sitting position, the patient grasps a stick with both hands and takes the stick behind her/his shoulder, positioning the stick at the level of the cervico-dorsal junction. In this position, she/he pushes the stick against her/his back, exhaling and inhaling rhythmically and slowly. She/he then repeats the exercise, moving the stick forward on the sternum at the level of the sterno-clavear joint. The patient grasps the stick with both hands frontally positioned.
4. Standing on a foam mattress.
   (a) The patient fixates her-/himself in a mirror. The therapist helps her/him to align her/his position correctly. She/he must maintain equilibrium for 1 min with eyes open and then close her/his eyes visualizing her/his correct position while remaining in this position for at least 1 min.

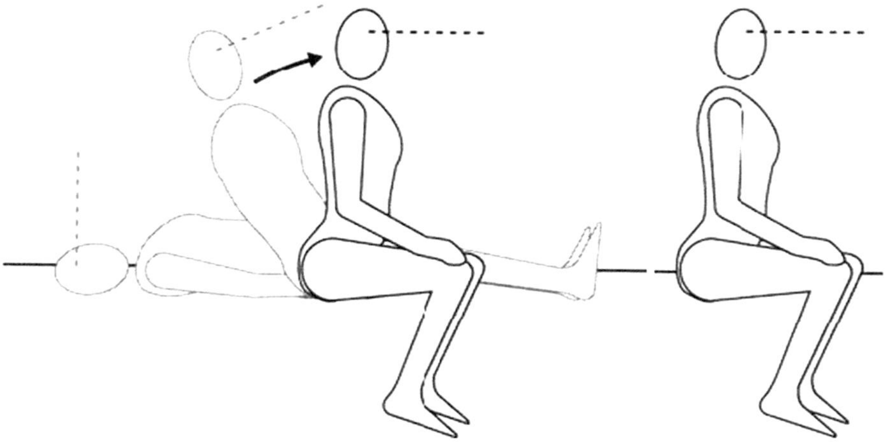

Fig. 10.1 From the supine to sitting position fixating a target (Originally published in Cesarani and Alpini [38] published by Springer © 1999)

(b) The patient fixates her-/himself in a mirror (Fig. 10.2a). Then she/he oscillates right and left (Fig. 10.2b), around her/his pelvis. She/he then resists the therapist's attempts at destabilizations (Fig. 10.2c) and maintains equilibrium, crossing the legs (Fig. 10.2d).
(c) The patient oscillates to and fro around her/his ankles while maintaining fixation in the mirror (Fig. 10.3).
(d) The patient holds a small object and then lifts it over her/his head and fixates it. With his arms extended, she/he moves it in circles of increasing width while maintaining the fixation of the object (Fig. 10.4).

5. Standing on an oscillating platform (so-called Freeman board, or balance board, etc.), looking in the mirror.
   (a) The patient concentrates on a proper posture using a mirror to see her/his reflection and thus she/he tries to maintain equilibrium as longer as possible (no more than 1′)
   (b) The patients transfers her/his weight from one foot to the other with a smooth flowing motion.
   (c) The patient tries to maintain a proper posture while the therapist destabilizes her/him with gentle pushes
   (d) The patient tries to touch some targets (post-its of different colours) placed in different positions on a facing mirror.
   (e) The patient maintains equilibrium on one leg, the leg on the good side and then the leg on the affected side, as long as possible
   (f) Repeat exercises *d* and *e* wearing pinhole glasses.

   Home exercises to be performed once a day (*see* Sect. 10.5)

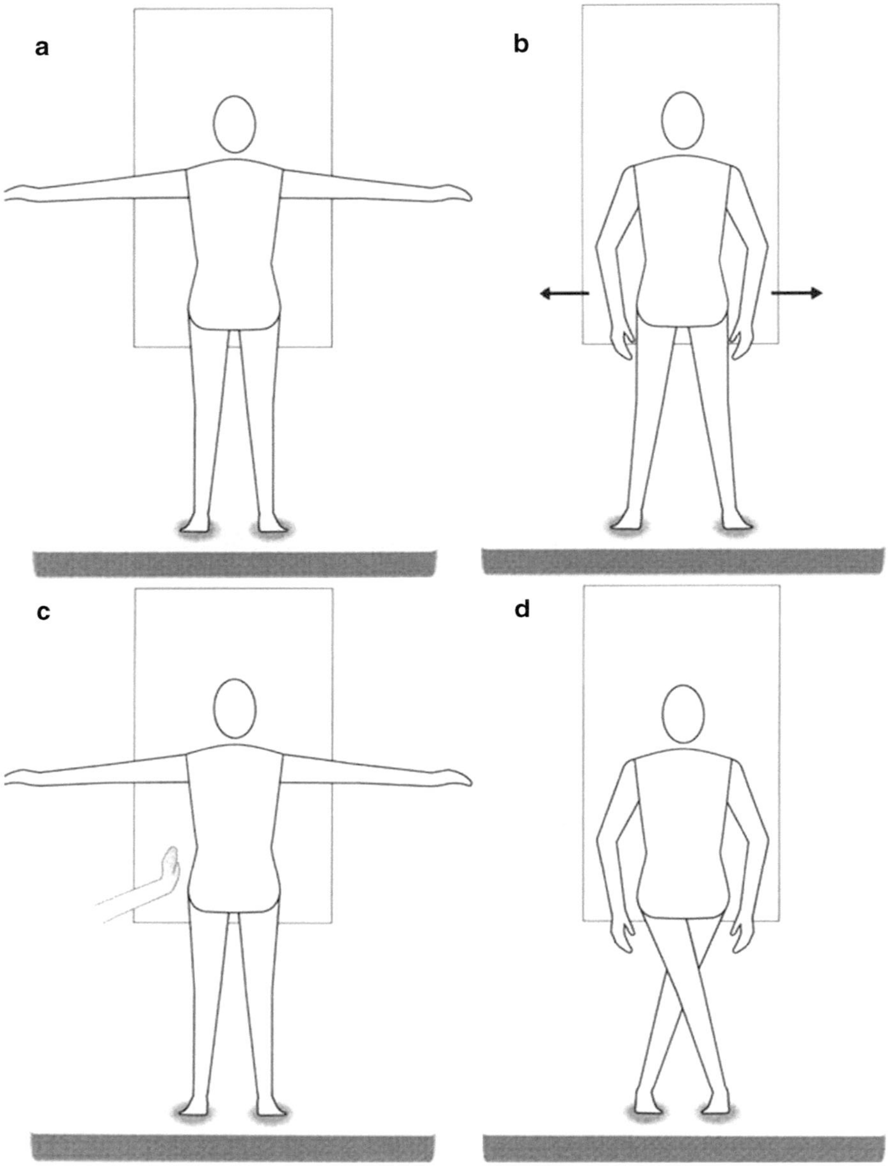

Fig. 10.2 The patient aligns himself looking at a mirror (**a**), then he oscillates (**b**), then resists when the therapist destabilizes him (**c**) or he maintains equilibrium crossing the legs (**d**) (Originally published in Cesarani and Alpini [38] published by Springer © 1999)

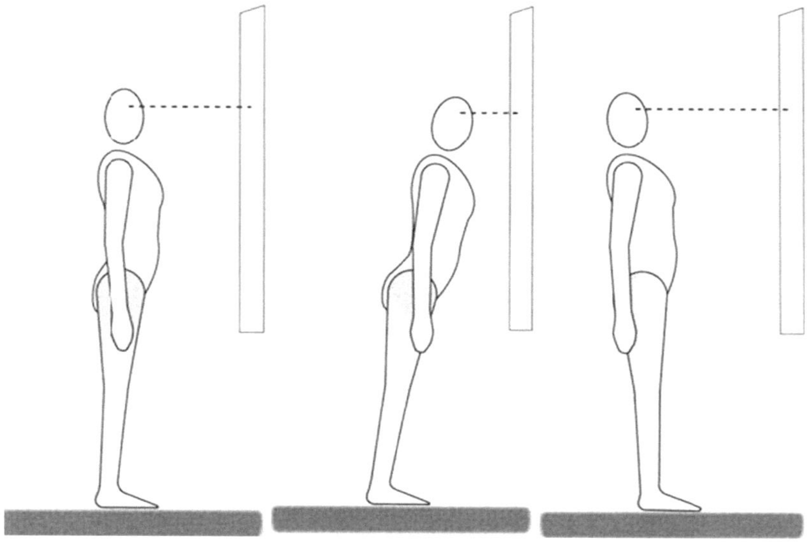

Fig. 10.3 The patient oscillates around his ankles maintaining the pelvis still (Originally published in Cesarani and Alpini [38] published by Springer © 1999)

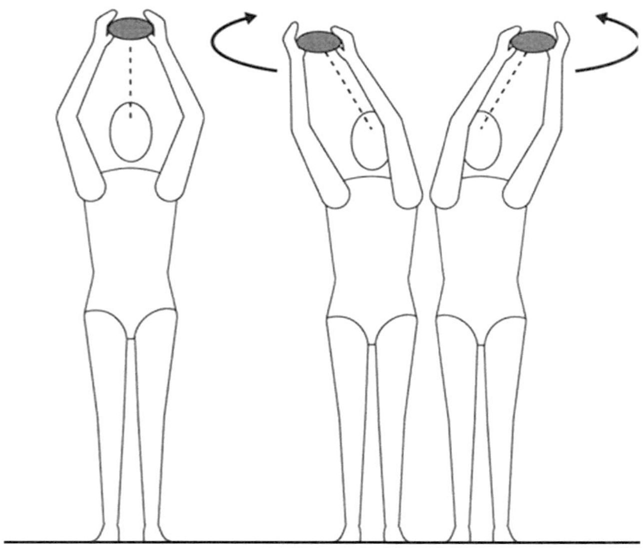

Fig. 10.4 Patient fixates a small object while moving it in circles, standing on a mattress (Originally published in Cesarani and Alpini [38] published by Springer © 1999)

10.2 Post-operative

Post-operative acute vertigo has to be treated as a form of *sudden unilateral vestibular loss* as shown in Chap. 5.

10.3 Intercritical Unsteadiness

Intercritical dizziness has to be treated as a form of *chronic vestibular loss* as shown in Chap. 6.

10.4 Vertigo Attack Fear

Vertigo spells fear has to be treated as a form of *phobic postural vertigo* as shown in Chap. 13.

10.5 Decrease the Frequency of Acute Attacks

The primary histopathological correlate is endolymphatic hydrops. Paparella [24] used the notion of "lake–river–pond" to explain the occurrence of malabsorption of endolymph leading to hydrops. This notion describes the endolymphatic sac as a pond, with the vestibular aqueduct (the river) connecting it to the endolymphatic fluid space that is like a lake. When there is an obstruction near the endolymphatic sac or duct, a backlog of endolymphatic fluid is created, leading to hydrops [25].

This notion has to be implemented to contest the vestibulo-vertebral functional unit as shown in Chap. 1 to explain why the neck and the stomatognathic apparatus are so frequently involved in MD patients.

Franz et al. [26] defined the *cervicogenic oto-ocular (COO) syndrome*, that is to say, vertigo, fluctuating hearing and tinnitus in patients showing a mild Eustachian tube dysfunction, mydriasis on the side of the affected ear and a functional disorder of the upper cervical spine. Bjorne et al. [27] showed that symptoms of cervical spine disorders, such as head and neck/shoulder pain, are significantly more frequent in Ménière patients than in the control group. According to the authors, most of the patients (75 %) reported a strong association between head–neck movements in the atlanto-occipital and atlanto-axial joints and triggered attacks of vertigo. Furthermore, the same AA [28] reported that a coordinated treatment of temporomandibular disorders (TMD) and cervical spine disorders in patients diagnosed with Ménière's disease, after a 3 years follow-up, showed simultaneous decreases in the intensities of vertigo, nonwhirling dizziness, tinnitus, feeling of fullness in the ear, pain in the face and jaws, pain in the neck and shoulders and headache.

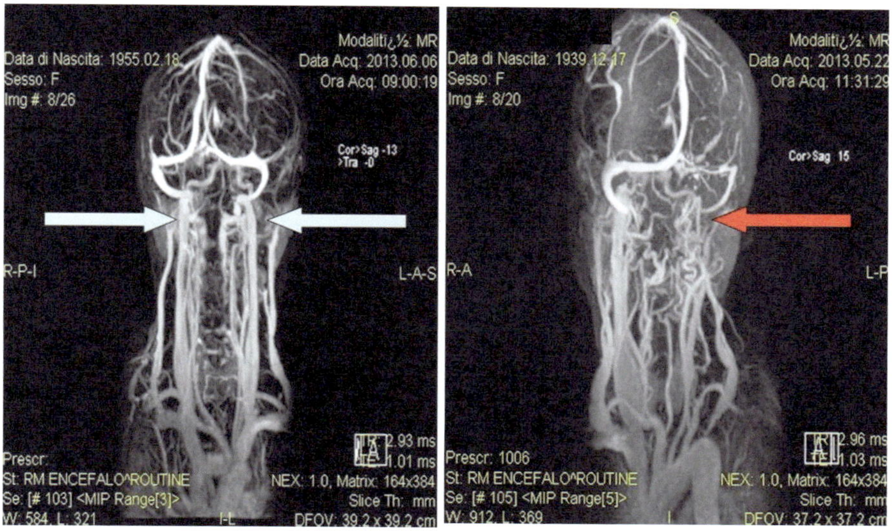

Fig. 10.5 2D time-of-flight MR venography of the upper neck region to visualize the venous vasculature in two vertiginous patients. Venography of the patient affected with Ménière's disease is on the right. *Arrows* indicate internal jugular veins (IJV) that appear normal in the left image (*blue arrows*). The *red arrow* in the right image indicates left IJV stenosis

The role of labyrinth hemodynamic in hydrops is highlighted by the recent investigations about the so-called CCSVI, *Chronic Cerebrospinal Venous Insufficiency*. CCSVI was described by Zamboni [29] as being strongly associated with multiple sclerosis (MS). It is characterized by multiple stenoses of the extracranial venous draining pathways, i.e. the internal jugular veins (IJV) and the azygos veins (AV), which lead to collateral formation, congestion of the vertebral veins (VV) and alteration of the blood-brain barrier. It could be diagnosed by means of MRI digital venography and, especially, duplex examination of the cerebral and cervical vein system.

Abnormalities of the cerebrospinal venous flow have been described also in no-MS patients such as in patients with migraine [30]. Bavera et al. [31] and Alpini et al. [32] showed CCSVI to be present in patients affected with sudden sensorineural hearing loss (SSHL). Furthermore, Alpini et al. [33, 34] performed echo-colour Doppler (ECD) arterial and venous tests in patients affected with cochleo-vestibular disturbances subdivided into three groups: definite unilateral Ménière's disease, no-Ménière subjects affected with unilateral cochleo-vestibular impairment and patients affected with benign paroxysmal positioning vertigo (BPPV) with cochlear hearing loss. The authors found asymmetrical venous flow to be more frequent in Ménière patients than in others as shown. These results suggest that blood outflow could play a pathogenetic role in Ménière's disease and thus may explain the correlation between cervical and TMJ disturbances as reported. CCSVI in MD may be

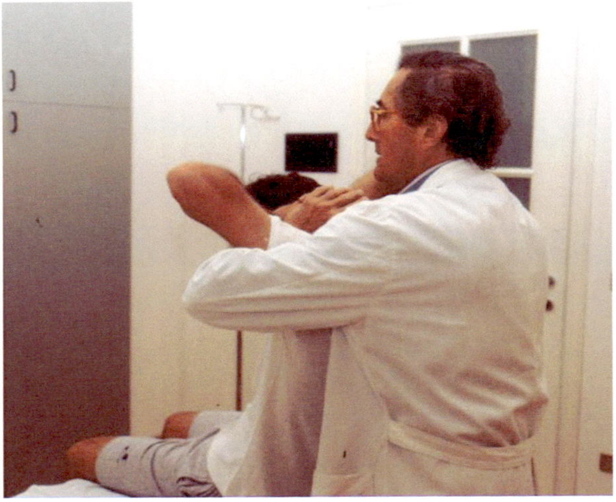

Fig. 10.6 Manipulation in extension by means of sternum support of the cervico-thoracic passage

investigated also by means of 2D time-of-flight MR venography as shown in Fig. 10.5.

In 1999, Brugnoni et al. [35] proposed the manipulation of the cervico-thoracic joint (Fig. 10.6) as an effective treatment in preventing vertigo attacks. The effectiveness of this kind of approach may be understood on the basis of the above-shown research considerations, taking into account the physiology of the *vestibulo-vertebral functional unit* as explained in Chap. 1.

The combination of manual medicine techniques [36] and physiotherapy may be thus used to reduce the frequency of Ménière vertigo crisis. Manual medicine treatment in vertiginous patients is explained in Chap. 9.

Manual treatment of Ménière patient has to be performed during the intercritical period, once a week for 4–5 weeks and it is planned as follows:

1. *Cervico-thoracic spinal manipulation*, a therapeutic intervention performed on spinal articulations that has to be performed only by well-trained doctors.
2. *Soft tissues* treatment, that is to say, delicate massage of superficial and deeper layers of muscles and connective tissues of the shoulders and the neck.
3. Gentle, oscillatory and passive mobilization of the *atlanto-occipital* and *atlanto-axial* joints. The atlanto-occipital segment is the most dangerous to manipulate, and thus gentle mobilization and soft tissue treatment are more indicated, with the patient in a supine or sitting position.

The treatment is to be completed by "Home Exercises", as follows, to be performed three times a week.

1. In the supine position, control of breathing with improving consciousness of abdominal or thoracic breathing. A simple exercise consists in deep inhalation followed, after few seconds, by a forced exhalation pronouncing the word "one". This exercise is repeated 8–10 times.

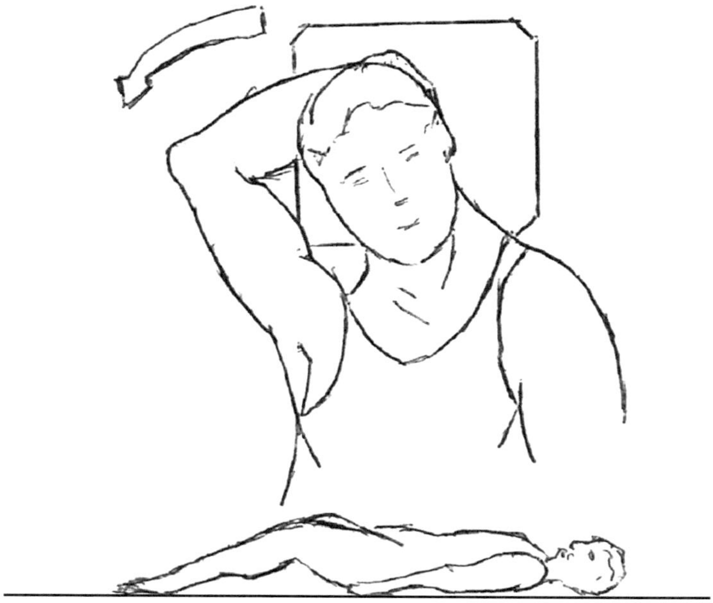

Fig. 10.7 In the supine position with a pillow under both the knees and head, the patient uses her/his right hand to pull rightward her/his head, slowly and gently, following the breathing rhythm: the patient pulls when inhaling and stops when exhaling. The patient repeats the same exercise using the opposite hand on the right ear

2. In the supine position, put your right hand on the left ear and, slowly and gently, pull rightward your head. Follow the breath rhythm: pull when you inhale, stop when you exhale. Repeat some times and then repeat using your left hand on your right ear (Fig. 10.7).
3. In the sitting position, grasp a stick with both hands and take the stick behind your shoulder, positioning the stick at the level of the cervico-dorsal junction. In this position, push the stick against your back, exhaling and inhaling rhythmically and slowly. Then repeat the exercise, moving the stick forward on the sternum at the level of the sterno-clavear joint. Please grasp the stick with the hands frontally positioned.
4. In the sitting position, put your hand together on your neck. Using both hands together as a resistance, push your head backward in order to obtain isometric contractions of the cervical and dorsal muscles (Fig. 10.8).
5. In the sitting position, put your hands together on the occiput. Inhale, then exhaling, bend forward your trunk using the hands together to gently accompany trunk bending. After a while, inhaling, relax your arms and reposition your head and trunk (Fig. 10.9).

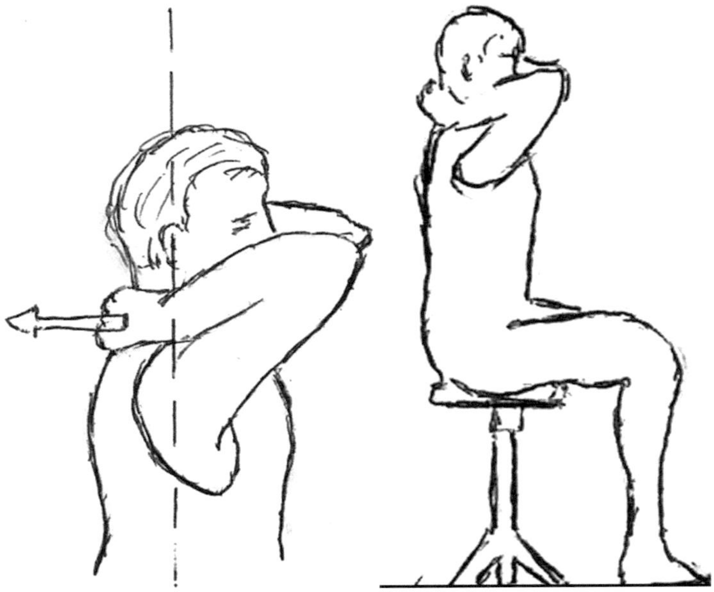

Fig. 10.8 In the sitting position, the patient uses her/his hands together to resist backward pushes of the head

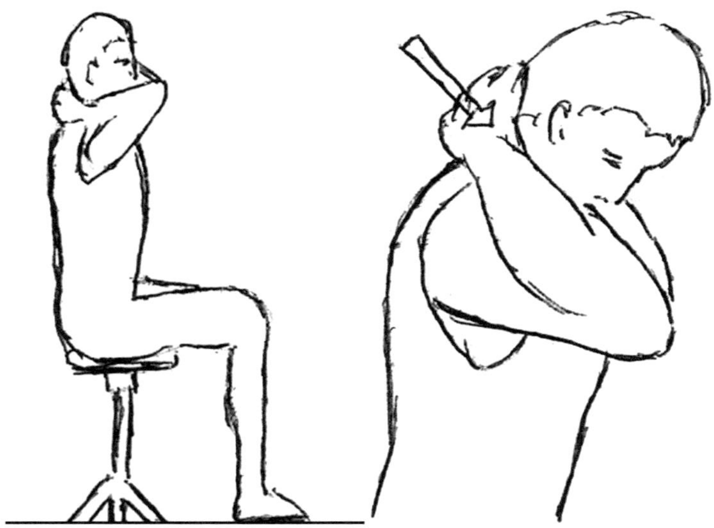

Fig. 10.9 In the sitting position, the patient uses her/his hands together on the occiput to accompany the slow and rhythmic forward bending of the head and the trunk; exhaling, the patient bends the trunk, inhaling she/he repositions

10.6 Counselling

It is important to pay attention to lifestyle and to maintain proper postural control during usual daily and working activities. The main suggestions are:

- Perform regular and constant aerobic physical activity: e.g. rapid walking (not running neither jogging) 30′/day three times/week
- Avoid maintaining the same position of the head/neck for more than 30 min when reading, working on a PC, watching television, etc.
- Avoid maintaining incorrect position of the head/neck, in particular check proper position when watching television or working on a PC.
- In any way, change your head/neck position every 30 min and mobilize your head and shoulders.
- Maintain adequate water intake (at least 1.5 l for females and 2 l for males).
- Maintain a diet rich of fruit and vegetables (five servings/day) especially in autumn and spring.
- Avoid industrial food.
- Avoid hot chilli pepper and generally foods containing capsaicin [37].
- Restrict salt intake in cases of hypertension.
- Restrict gluten intake [15].
- Restrict alcohol intake (less than 120 ml for women and 240 ml for men).
- Restrict smoking and, obviously, avoid drug abuse.
- Sleep using two pillows in order to maintain the head lifted about 20°.
- Maintain proper night-and-day rhythm and at least 6–8 h of sleep (melatonin 5 mg at bedtime may be useful)
- Reduce stress, in general.

References

1. Committee on Hearing and Equilibrium guidelines for the diagnosis and evaluation of therapy in Menière's disease. American Academy of Otolaryngology-Head and Neck Foundation, Inc. Otolaryngol Head Neck Surg. 1995;113(3):181–185
2. Vrabec JT (2003) Herpes simplex virus and Meniere's disease. Laryngoscope 113(9):1431–1438
3. Gartner M, Bossart W, Linder T (2008) Herpes virus and Ménière's disease. ORL J Otorhinolaryngol Relat Spec 70(1):28–31
4. Gacek RR (2009) Ménière's disease is a viral neuropathy. ORL J Otorhinolaryngol Relat Spec 71(2):78–86
5. DiBerardino F, Cesarani A, Hahn A, Alpini D (2007) Viral infection and serum antibodies to heat shock protein 70 in the acute phase of Ménière's disease. Int Tinnitus J 13(2):90–93
6. D'Avila C, Lavinsky L (2005) Glucose and insulin profiles and their correlations in Ménière's disease. Int Tinnitus J 11(2):170–176
7. Brookler KH (2006) Meniere's syndrome, otosclerosis, and insulin resistance syndrome. Ear Nose Throat J 85(2):82–83
8. Lavinsky J, Wolff ML, Trasel AR, Valerio MM, Lavinsky L (2014) Effect of hyperinsulinism on sensorineural hearing impairment in Ménière's disease: a cohort study. Otol Neurotol 35(1):155–161

9. Raponi G, Alpini D, Volontè S, Capobianco S, Cesarani A (2003) The role of free radicals and plasmatic antioxidant in Ménière's syndrome. Int Tinnitus J 2:104–108
10. Foster CA, Breeze RE (2013) The Meniere attack: an ischemia/reperfusion disorder of inner ear sensory tissues. Med Hypotheses 81(6):1108–1115
11. Greco A, Gallo A, Fusconi M, Marinelli C, Macri GF, de Vincentiis M (2012) Meniere's disease might be an autoimmune condition? Autoimmun Rev 11(10):731–738
12. Gazquez I, Soto-Varela A, Aran I, Santos S, Batuecas A, Trinidad G, Perez-Garrigues H, Gonzalez-Oller C, Acosta L, Lopez-Escamez JA (2011) High prevalence of systemic autoimmune diseases in patients with Menière's disease. PLoS One 6(10):e26759. doi:10.1371/journal.pone.0026759
13. Fattori B, Nacci A, Dardano A, Dallan I, Grosso M, Traino C, Mancini V, Ursino F, Monzani F (2008) Possible association between thyroid autoimmunity and Menière's disease. Clin Exp Immunol 152(1):28–32
14. Di Berardino F, Cesarani A (2012) Gluten sensitivity in Meniere's disease. Laryngoscope 122(3):700–702
15. Di Berardino F, Filipponi E, Alpini D, O'Bryan T, Soi D, Cesarani A (2013) Ménière disease and gluten sensitivity: recovery after a gluten-free diet. Am J Otolaryngol 34(4):355–356
16. Djelilovic-Vranic J, Alajbegovic A, Tiric-Campara M, Volic A, Sarajlic Z, Osmanagic E, Todorovic L, Beslagic O (2012) Betahistine or Cinnarizine for treatment of Meniere's disease. Med Arh 66(6):396–398
17. Kentala E, Levo H, Pyykkő I (2013) How one hundred and eighty three people with Menière's disorder relieve their symptoms: a random cohort questionnaire study. Clin Otolaryngol 38(2):170–174
18. Crane BT (2013) Comparison of intratympanic methylprednisolone and gentamicin for Meniere's disease may be misleading. Otolaryngol Head Neck Surg 149(1):175
19. Gabra N, Saliba I (2013) Response to: comparison of intratympanic methylprednisolone and gentamicin for Meniere's disease may be misleading. Otolaryngol Head Neck Surg 149(1):175–176
20. Pullens B, Verschuur HP, van Benthem PP. Surgery for Ménière's disease. Cochrane Database Syst Rev. 2013 Feb 28;2:CD005395. doi: 10.1002/14651858.CD005395.pub3. Review. PubMed PMID: 23450562.
21. Gottshall KR, Topp SG, Hoffer ME (2010) Early vestibular physical therapy rehabilitation for Meniere's disease. Otolaryngol Clin North Am 43(2):1113–1119
22. Magnusson M, Kahlon B, Karlberg M, Lindberg S, Siesjö P, Tjernström F (2009) Vestibular "PREHAB". Ann N Y Acad Sci 1164:257–262
23. Gottshall KR, Hoffer ME, Moore RJ, Balough BJ (2005) The role of vestibular rehabilitation in the treatment of Meniere's disease. Otolaryngol Head Neck Surg 133(3):326–328
24. Paparella MM (1985) The cause (multifactorial inheritance) and pathogenesis (endolymphatic malabsorption) of Meniere's disease and its symptoms (mechanical and chemical). Acta Otolaryngol (Stockh) 99:445–451
25. Sajjadi H, Paparella MM (2008) Meniere's disease. Lancet 372(9636):406–414
26. Franz B, Altidis P, Altidis B, Collis-Brown G (1999) The cervicogenic otoocular syndrome: a suspected forerunner of Ménière's disease. Int Tinnitus J 5(2):125–130
27. Bjorne A, Berven A, Agerberg G (1998) Cervical signs and symptoms in patients with Meniere's disease: a controlled study. Cranio 16(3):194–202
28. Bjorne A, Agerberg G (2003) Symptom relief after treatment of temporomandibular and cervical spine disorders in patients with Meniere's disease: a three-year follow-up. Cranio 21(1):50–60
29. Zamboni P, Galeotti R (2010) The chronic cerebrospinal venous insufficiency syndrome. Phlebology 25(6):269–279
30. Koerte IK, Schankin CJ, Immler S, Lee S, Laubender RP, Grosse C, Eftimov L, Milde-Busch A, Reiser M, Straube A, Heinen F, Alperin N, Ertl-Wagner B (2011) Altered cerebrovenous drainage in patients with migraine as assessed by phase-contrast magnetic resonance imaging. Invest Radiol 46(7):434–440

31. Bavera PM, Agus GB, Alpini D, Cecconi P, Guazzoni A, Tori A, Costantini E, Lupattelli T (2012) Results from 823 consecutive Duplex exams for CCSVI in a Vascular Centre. Acta Phlebologica 13(3):141–146
32. Alpini DC, Bavera PM, Di Berardino F, Barozzi S, Cesarani A (2013) Bilateral sudden sensorineural hearing loss and chronic venous cerebrospinal insufficiency: a case report. Phlebology 28(5):231–233
33. Alpini DC, Bavera PM, Hahn A, Mattei V (2013) Chronic cerebrospinal venous insufficiency (CCSVI) IN Meniere disease. Case or cause? Science Med 4(1):9–15
34. Di Berardino F, Alpini DC, Bavera PM, Cecconi P, Farabola M, Mattei V, Ambrosetti U, Cesarani A. Chronic cerebrospinal venous insufficiency in Meniere disease. Phlebology. 2014 Mar 4. [Epub ahead of print] PubMed PMID: 24594584.
35. Cesarani A, Brugnoni G, Barozzi S (1999) Vertige de la maladie de Meniere Traitement par manipulation vertebrales. Revue de Medicine Orthopedique 59:17–19
36. Dvorak J, Dvorak V, Schneider W (1988) Manual medicine. Springer, Berlin, Heidelberg
37. Vass Z, Dai CF, Steyger PS, Jancsó G, Trune DR, Nuttall AL (2004) Co-localization of the vanilloid capsaicin receptor and substance P in sensory nerve fibers innervating cochlear and vertebro-basilar arteries. Neuroscience 124(4):919–927
38. Cesarani A, Alpini D (1999) Vertigo and dizziness rehabilitation – the MCS method. Springer, Milan, Heidelberg

11 Dizziness and Unsteadiness in the Elderly

Vertigo, dizziness and unsteadiness are common in the aged. They can be caused by distinct vestibular disorders but can also be a symptom in other medical conditions like non-vestibular sensory loss, vascular encephalopathy or anxiety. Anyway, they independently and relevantly contribute to population-attributable disability in the aged. They are not inevitable consequences of aging but arise from distinct disease entities.

In aged people, specific vestibular vertigo may be recognized just as in general population: unilateral sudden vestibular loss, chronic unilateral vestibular loss, vestibular ataxia, benign positioning paroxysmal vertigo and cervical vertigo.

Although the general medical condition of the aged patient has to be taken into account, this kind of vestibular vertigo may be treated as in general population, and the rehab protocol shown in the dedicated chapters may be usually adopted.

Dizziness and unsteadiness in the elderly are particularly important because they decrease social autonomy and are often the cause of falls. In both men and women between 65 and 79 years, vertigo and dizziness are among the strongest contributors to the burden of disability with a prevalence of 10.5 % in men and 9.0 % in women [1]. In men, this effect is stable across all age groups, whereas it decreases with age in women.

Dizziness affects one in five people over the age of 65 years and is associated with substantial healthcare costs. Serious causes of dizziness are found in 20 % of patients over 50 years. The causes of dizziness are always multifactorial [2].

For the vestibular system, aging is associated with degenerated otoconia and loss of hair cells, vestibular afferents and cells in the vestibular nuclei [3]. Although an overall decline in semicircular canal as well as otolith function associated with aging is observed [4], the magnitude of impairment is greater for the semicircular canals than the otoliths. Particularly, the prevalence of semicircular canal dysfunction is highest followed by saccular then utricular impairment, although some individuals may present with isolated otolith deficits [5].

Neurodegenerative processes involve cortical, extrapyramidal motor and cerebellar structures. Furthermore, the elderly is characterized by perturbation at several levels of the sensorimotor system, including decreases in muscle mass, increases in

D.C. Alpini et al., *Vertigo Rehabilitation Protocols*,
DOI 10.1007/978-3-319-05482-7_11,

the threshold of vibratory sensations and the cognitive processes like memory and attention span.

Gait stability, especially in old women, may be compromised by the combination of increased body weight and decreased muscle strength and postural responses. Somatosensation is the primary sense that triggers automatic postural responses when a standing adult experiences a sudden horizontal support surface displacement. The activation of the distal leg muscles has short latency, and it may serve as the primary defence mechanism, with the supplement of the visual and vestibular inputs, to prevent falls when a person encounters an unexpected support surface displacement, such as a slip. With advancing age thresholds of joint position sense, vibration sense and cutaneous sense increase. Older subjects show a higher threshold for detecting movement in the metatarsophalangeal joint [6].

Also, reduced peripheral proprioceptive information plays an important role, especially in developing falls. Single stance instability would appear as a major risk factor in older individuals (75–84 years). The significant decline of stability in the older subjects observed by Riva et al. [7] may be explained by the impairment of proprioceptive control together with the decrease in compensatory visual stabilization and emergency responses. In their experience, younger subjects (65–74 years) exhibit better, but still inadequate, proprioceptive control with compensatory visual stabilization. Gender differences appeared in older subjects: women were significantly less stable than men.

There is a close relationship between increased sway and impaired vibration sense in the legs. Cutaneous and proprioceptive sensation thresholds increase with age. Alterations that develop as a result of the gradual loss of function of the receptors are considered an inevitable concomitant of the aging process. Abnormalities in the reflexogenic functions of the cervical articular mechanoreceptors make a significant contribution to the disorders of posture and gait that afflict old people [8].

The neck plays an important role in presby-dizziness as a possible cause of falls also through the carotid sinus hypersensitivity that has a high prevalence in the elderly. In carotid sinus hypersensitivity, external triggers cause sudden reductions in blood pressure, leading to dizziness or syncope, resulting in falls. Turning of the head is considered an important example of such an external trigger in everyday life, wherein rotation of the neck is thought to manipulate the hypersensitive carotid sinus [9].

Reduced visual acuity is frequent with age. It appears to be accompanied by increased postural sway, particularly in the anteroposterior direction. The following deficits in focal vision have been found in the older adult: decreased visual acuity, restriction of visual field, poor depth perception and losses in contrast sensitivity at the intermediate and high spatial frequencies. Older adults show diminished sensitivity to a moving target with low spatial frequencies, especially when this target moves at a high speed. Older adults not only have difficulty in perceiving a moving object but also have difficulty in perceiving self-motion with reference to the external space. Thus, decline in balance control abilities and consequent falls in older adults may be partially attributable to eye diseases and impaired vision [10].

In older fallers, also the perception of verticality and horizontality is impaired compared to older non-fallers [11] especially in those affected with orthostatic hypotension [12].

In the elderly, a more frequent presence of central components or of central pathology is expected such as typical neurological diseases, the influence of vertebrobasilar insufficiency and cardiovascular and degenerative changes in the CNS. Disturbance in the integrating mechanisms in the brainstem and cerebellum is common as a result of ischemia. Cerebrovascular disease often may have resulted in pre-existing central nervous disease, and compensation of vestibular injuries is frail and may break down if there is subsequent additional damage to any of the mechanisms responsible [13].

Aging is associated with a progressive decline in overall muscle strength. In fact, in aged human, the number of muscle fibres and motor units decreases. The remaining motor units lose their functionality (decrease of the discharge frequency, greater fluctuation of the discharge) particularly those which contain type II fibres. The renewal of intracellular proteins declines which creates a negative balance between the daily protein losses and the capacities to renew them. Besides, the process of activation and proliferation of satellite cells is affected, and the production of anabolic hormones and local factors is decreased. Loss of lower limb strength leads to an increased risk of falls and [14].

In conclusion, dizziness and unsteadiness in the elderly are typically caused by multiple deficits, multiple deficits that can add up to produce disability disproportionate to their individual contributions.

The key disability is the reduced motor and social autonomy with postural instability, falls and fear of falls.

Although hair cell regeneration is a recent field of research [15], rehabilitation is the worldwide specific treatment of dizziness and unsteadiness in the elderly [16–19]. The role of rehab in the prevention of falls is still a matter of discussion [20], but regular physical exercises appear to be the appropriate treatment [21]. Exercise in the elderly needs to be carefully tailored and individualized with the specific objectives of the person or group in mind. The beneficial effects of exercise in two of the main age-related diseases, sarcopenia and Alzheimer's disease, are dealt with at the beginning of this report [22].

Rehabilitative treatment has to be pointed to:

1. Improve ankle, hip and neck mobility
2. Increase antigravity muscle tone
3. Improve balance reactions
4. Ameliorate motor coordination
5. Improve attention to balance phenomena
6. Correct internal representation of posture

Each aged subject presents a personal variety of multiple sensorimotor involvement, some with special regard to sensorial aspects, some with special regard to motor aspects and some with special regard to cognitive aspects. Thus, the treatment protocol has to be strictly personalized adapting each phase to each patient. In some subjects, attention must be paid to motor involvement; in some, sensorimotor involvement will be stressed, while in others, cognitive–motor interaction will be the key of treatment.

11.1 Exercises in the Gymnasium

11.1.1 First Week

1. The patient holds her/his left knee against the chest and then extends her/his leg and holds the right knee against the chest. When she/he holds the knee against the chest, she/he applies gentle traction to the flexed leg with the hands (Fig. 11.1a).
2. The patient holds both knees against the chest simultaneously with the help of her/his hands (Fig. 11.1b).
3. The patient takes her/his left arm extending over her/his head and simultaneously holds the right flexed leg to the chest, with her/his hand. She/he maintains this position for 10 s and then repeats the exercise with the opposite arm and leg (Fig. 11.2).
4. With the legs flexed and the feet on the bed, the patient rotates her/his pelvis rightward and leftward keeping the knees flexed and the legs together (Fig. 11.3).
5. The patient lifts her/his pelvis simultaneously extending the arms over her/his head. She/he repositions the arms along the body, lowering the pelvis (Fig. 11.4).

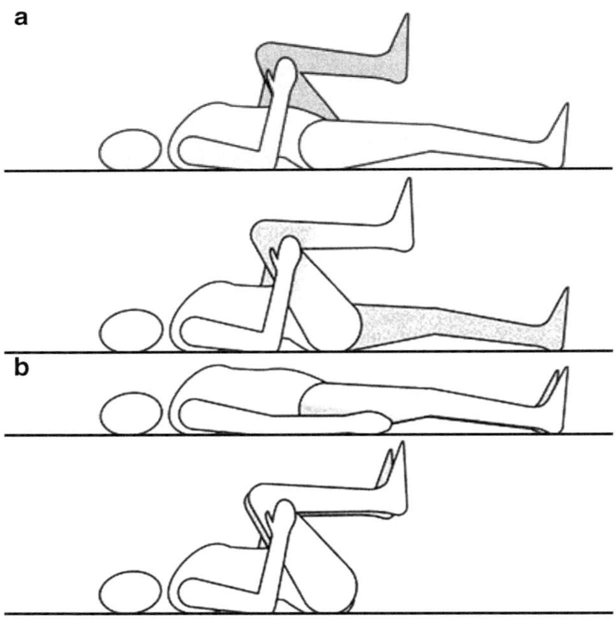

Fig. 11.1 (**a**, **b**) Flexions of the knees (Originally published in Cesarani and Alpini [37] published by Springer © 1999)

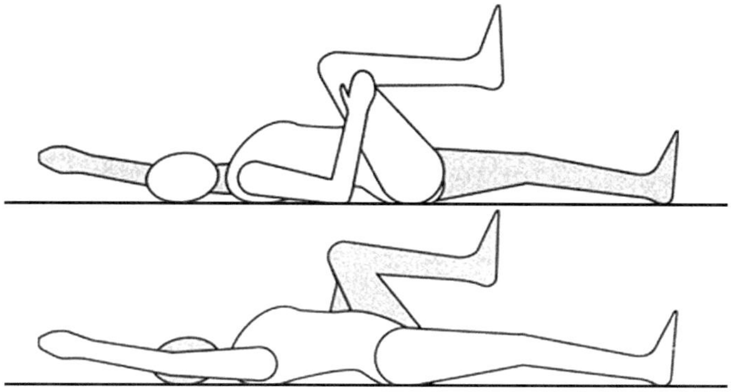

Fig. 11.2 Flexion of the knee and extension of the opposite arm (Originally published in Cesarani and Alpini [37] published by Springer © 1999)

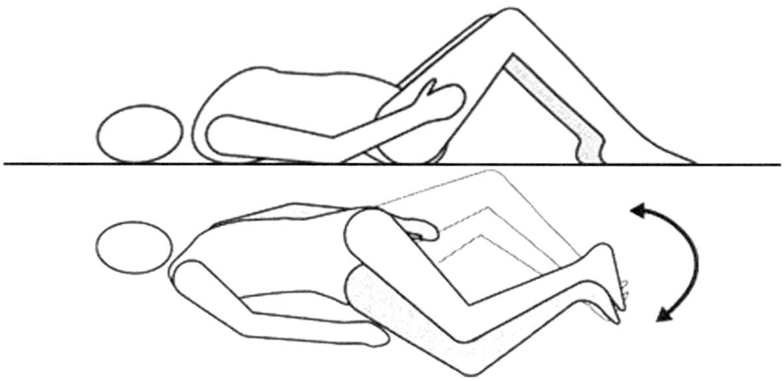

Fig. 11.3 Rotation of the pelvis (Originally published in Cesarani and Alpini [37] published by Springer © 1999)

6. The patient grasps a stick and extends the arms over her/his head and then returns to the resting position.
7. In the quadrupedal position, the patient simultaneously extends the right arm and the left leg. She/he repeats the exercise with the left arm and the right leg (Fig. 11.5).
8. In the quadrupedal position, the patient arches her/his back for hyperkyphosis of the thoraco-lumbar spine (Fig. 11.6).
9. The patient moves her/his head first slowly and then more rapidly in all directions, fixating a target straight in front of her/him.

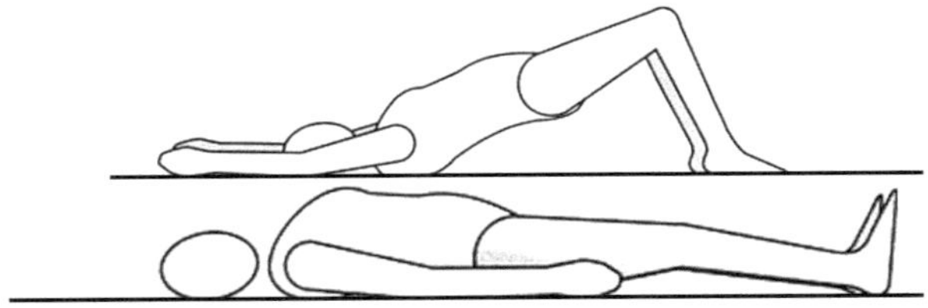

Fig. 11.4 Lifting the pelvis (Originally published in Cesarani and Alpini [37] published by Springer © 1999)

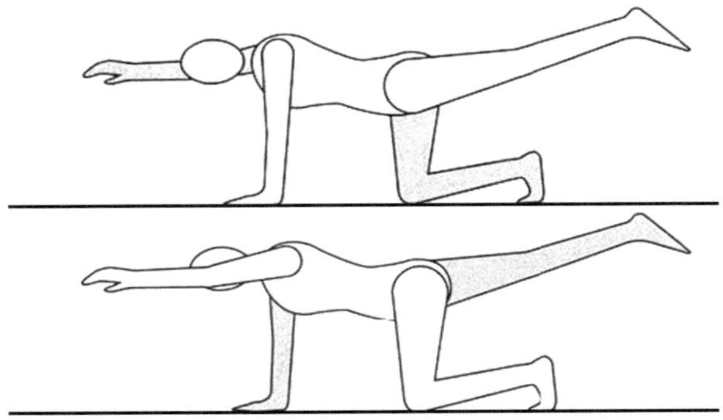

Fig. 11.5 Synchronization of arm–leg extension (Originally published in Cesarani and Alpini [37] published by Springer © 1999)

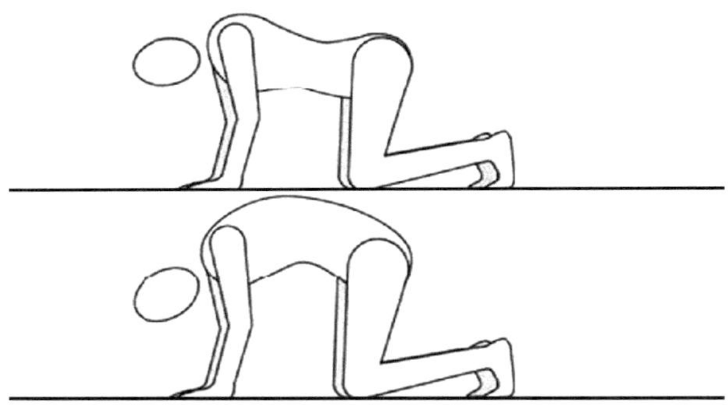

Fig. 11.6 In the quadrupedal position, the patient arches the trunk (Originally published in Cesarani and Alpini [37] published by Springer © 1999)

10. The patient inhales, and then, exhaling, she/he bends forward to pick an object on the floor. She/he then inhales and takes it up over her/his head fixating it for 10 s. The patient inhales and then, exhaling, she/he bends forward and places the object back on the floor (Fig. 11.7).
11. With the hands on a chair, the patient lifts her-/himself on tiptoes and maintains this position for 30 s (Fig. 11.8a).
12. With the hands on a table, the patient lifts her-/himself on your heels and maintains this position for 30 s (Fig. 11.8b).
13. The patient walks on the floor with eyes open (Fig. 11.9).

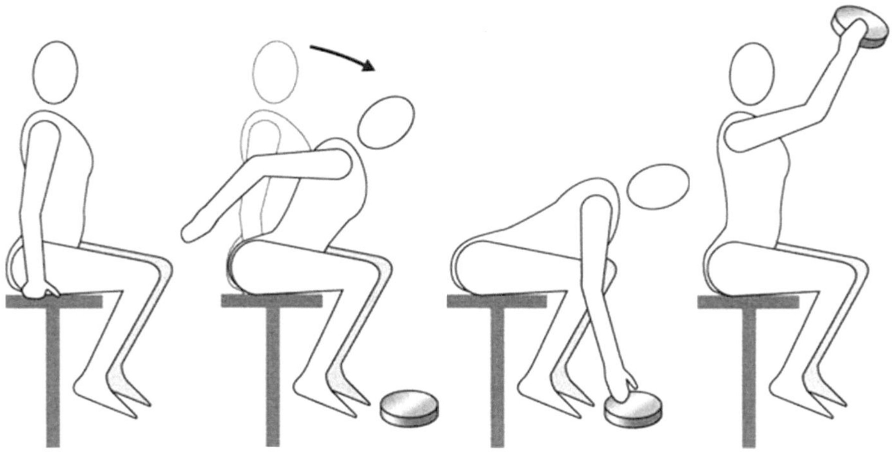

Fig. 11.7 Picking up and lifting an object from the floor (Originally published in Cesarani and Alpini [37] published by Springer © 1999)

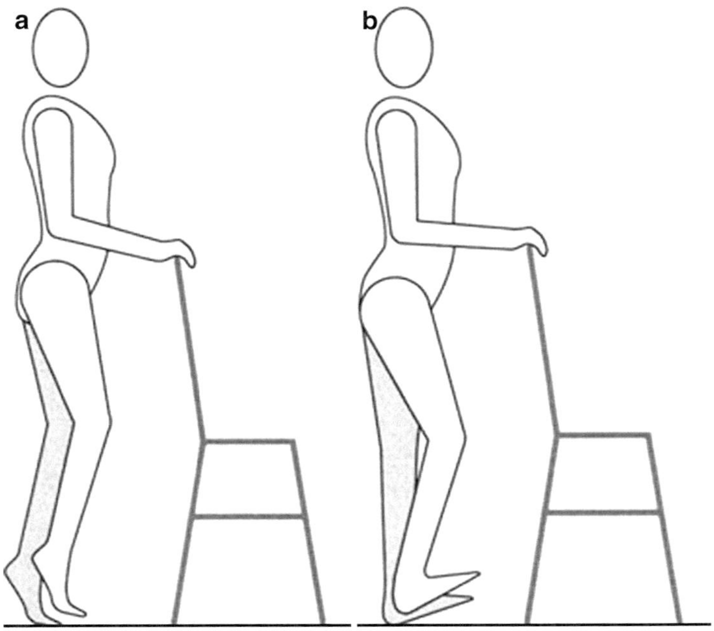

Fig. 11.8 Rising in tiptoes (**a**) and heels (**b**) (Originally published in Cesarani and Alpini [37] published by Springer © 1999)

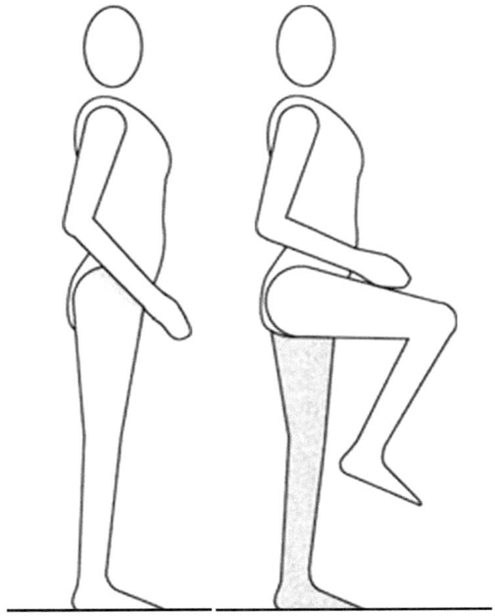

Fig. 11.9 Stepping (Originally published in Cesarani and Alpini [37] published by Springer © 1999)

11.1.2 Second Week

14. The patient turns her/his head rightward and fixates a target on the lateral wall. Then she/he straightens her/his head, maintaining the visual fixation and counting from one up to ten; then she/he turns her/his head (Fig. 11.10a).
15. The patient turns her/his head leftward and fixates a target on the lateral wall. Then she/he straightens her/his head, maintaining the visual fixation and counting from one up to ten; then she/he turns her/his head (Fig. 11.10b).
16. The patient looks for three targets sited, respectively, in front of her/him, on her/his left and on her/his right. She/he fixates the front target; then rapidly she/he moves her/his head fixating the right-hand target. She/he then turns her/his head leftward maintaining the fixation of the right-hand target. The patient fixates the front target and then moves her/his head rapidly leftward and fixates the left-hand target. She/he then turns her/his head rightward maintaining the fixation of the left-hand target.
17. The patient fixates herself/himself in a mirror and aligns correctly her/his posture (Fig. 11.11a). She/he maintains equilibrium for 1 min, and then she/he closes her/his eyes visualizing her/his correct position, remaining in this position for at least 1 min. She/he then lifts her-/himself on tiptoes maintaining equilibrium first with the eyes open fixating a mirror and then with the eyes closed

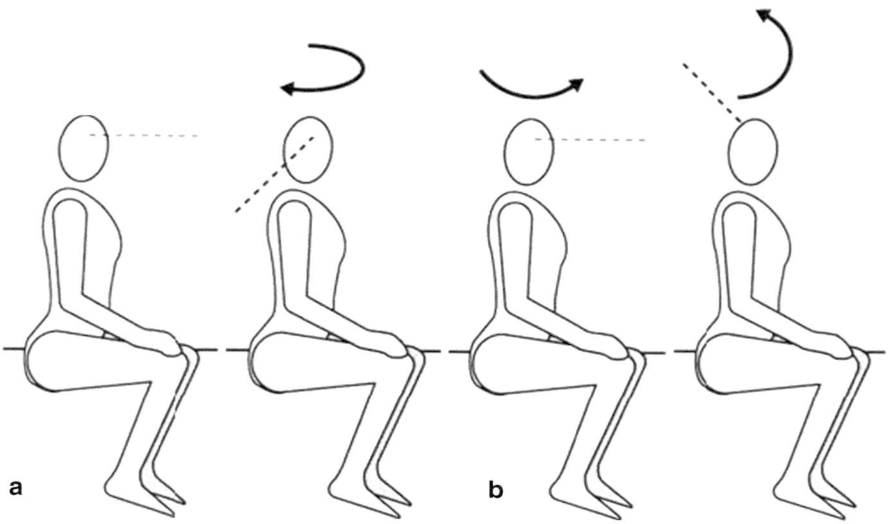

Fig. 11.10 (**a**, **b**) Turning the head fixating a target (Originally published in Cesarani and Alpini [37] published by Springer © 1999)

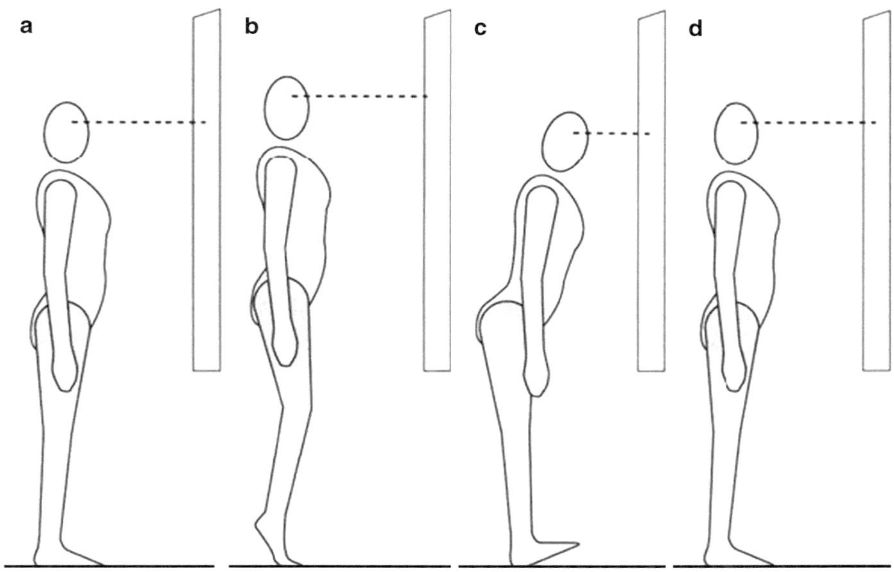

Fig. 11.11 Correct alignment in front of a mirror in normal stance (**a**–**d**), on tiptoes (**b**) and on heels (**c**) (Originally published in Cesarani and Alpini [37] published by Springer © 1999)

(Fig. 11.11b). Then she/he lifts her-/himself on her/his heels maintaining equilibrium first with the eyes open fixating a mirror and then with the eyes closed (Fig. 11.11c). Finally, she/he returns to the resting position standing quietly in front of the mirror (Fig. 11.11d).

18. The patient steps up and down, fixating a target according to the following sequence:

Right foot up	Left foot up
Right foot down	Left foot down
Left foot up	Right foot up
Left foot down	Right foot down

She/he then repeats the exercise with the eyes closed.

19. On a soft mattress:
    (a) The patient fixates herself/himself in a mirror and correctly aligns her/his posture. She/he maintains equilibrium for 1 min, and then she/he closes her/his eyes visualizing the correct position and remains in this position for at least 1 min (Fig. 11.12a). Then she/he oscillates rhythmically laterally (Fig. 11.12b). In succession, she/he resists the attempts of the therapist to push her/him (Fig. 11.12c), and she/he maintains equilibrium crossing the legs (Fig. 11.12d).
    (b) The patient fixates her-/himself in a mirror and then oscillates to and fro and right and left, around the ankles keeping her/his pelvis still (ankle strategy) (Fig. 11.13a).
    (c) The patient fixates her-/himself in a mirror; keeping the feet still, she/he bends her/his trunk to and fro and right and left (hip strategy) (Fig. 11.13b).
    (d) The patient grasps a stick (Fig. 11.14a), and then she/he lifts it over her/his head fixating it (Fig. 11.14b).
    (e) The patient holds a small object and lifts it over her/his head fixating it. Then she/he inhales. Exhaling, she/he bends her-/himself forward placing the object on the floor. She/he waits for 10 s, and then, inhaling, she/he lifts the object again over her/his head (Fig. 11.15).
    (f) The patient walks in place with the eyes open, fixating a target.
20. The patient stands comfortably and stable on the board with the feet apart on a balance board:
    (a) The patient concentrates on proper posture using a mirror to see her/his reflection and transfers her/his weight from one foot to the other with a smooth flowing motion. During this smooth and rhythmic weight transfer, the therapist accompanies and directs the patient's movements.

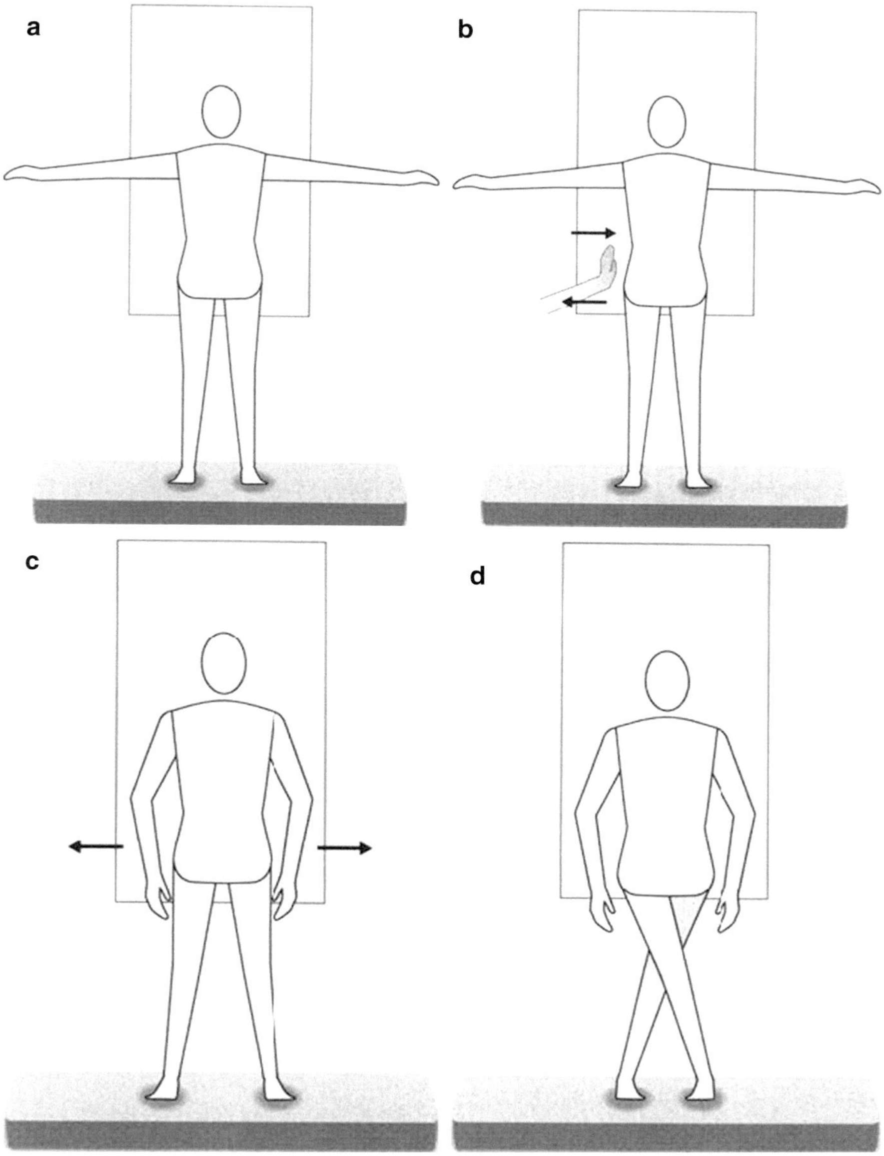

Fig. 11.12 (**a–d**) Standing on a mattress, the patient controls his or her posture (Originally published in Cesarani and Alpini [37] published by Springer © 1999)

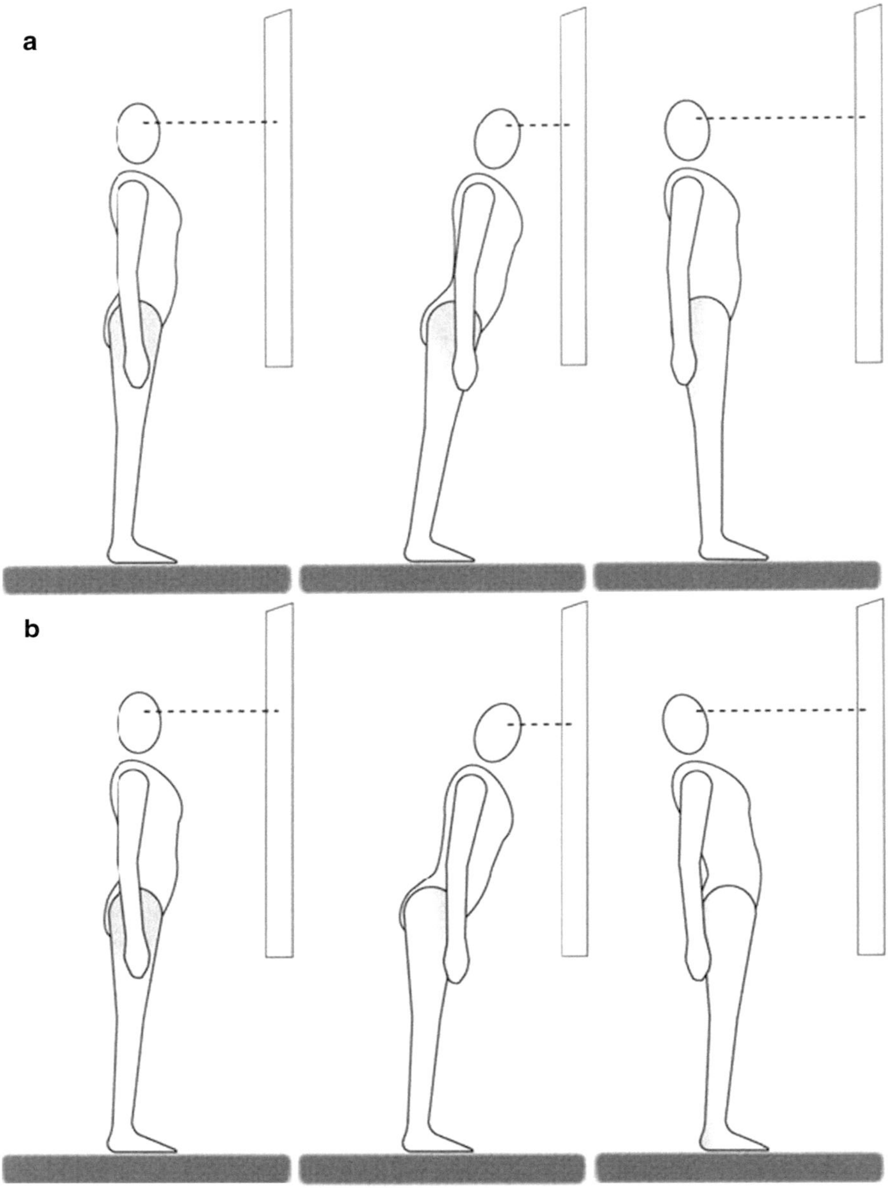

Fig. 11.13 (**a**) Ankle oscillations and (**b**) hip oscillations, standing on a mattress (Originally published in Cesarani and Alpini [37] published by Springer © 1999)

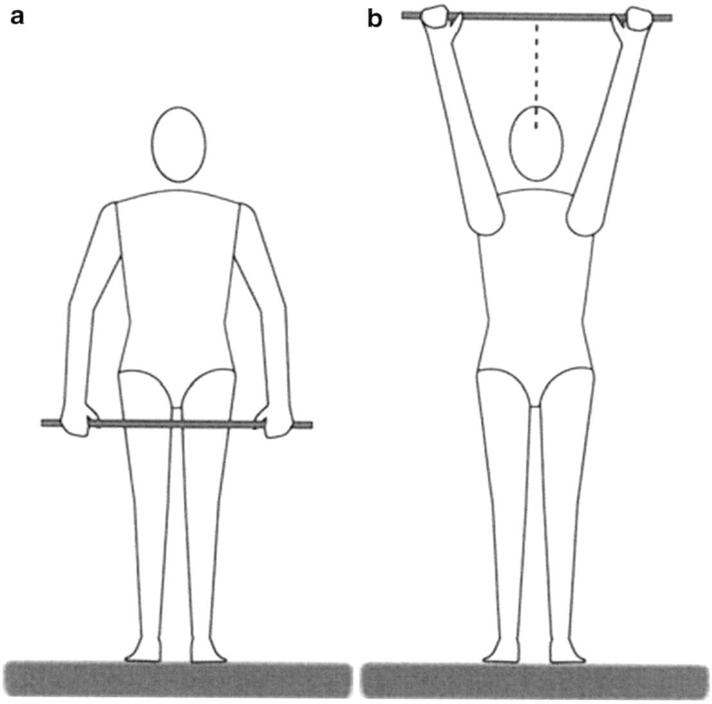

Fig. 11.14 (**a**, **b**) Grasping and lifting a stick, standing on a mattress (Originally published in Cesarani and Alpini [37] published by Springer © 1999)

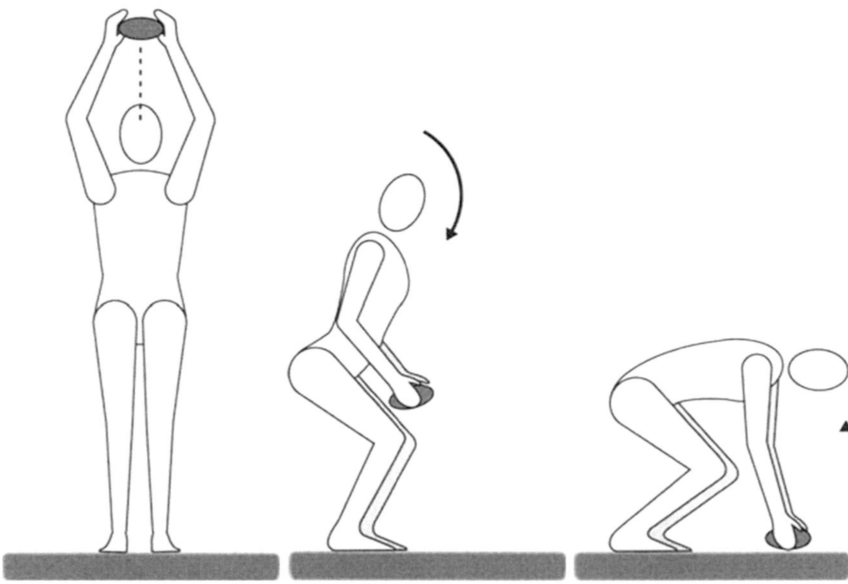

Fig. 11.15 Fixating an object and then placing it on the floor and standing on a mattress (Originally published in Cesarani and Alpini [37] published by Springer © 1999)

(b) A small target is placed on the wall in front of the patient, and a small laser pointer is fixed on her/his head (e.g. on cap). The patient is required to maintain the laser pointed on the target. The same exercise may be repeated placing the target on a mirror.
(c) Targets of different colours are placed on the wall in front of the patient that keeps the laser pointer with her/his hand. The patient is required to point the laser on a target according to the therapist's commands (e.g. "touch the red target, now the yellow one, etc."). The same exercise may be repeated placing the targets on a front mirror.
(d) The patient with her/his limbs extended tries to touch some visual targets of different colours placed on a front mirror according to the therapist's commands (e.g. "touch the red target, now the yellow one, etc.").

11.1.3 Third Week

In this phase, exercises have to be performed during TENS [23]. If vestibular hypofunction has been documented, electrodes need to be placed according to the side of hypofunction. In the other cases, electrodes need to be placed symmetrically on both sides of the neck:

21. The patient is sitting and extends the right arm and lifts her/his thumb. She/he moves the arm to and fro slowly first in a horizontal direction and then in a vertical direction. She/he follows the thumb with the eyes only, first slowly and then increasing progressively the velocity of thumb displacement.
22. Repeat as above but simultaneously moving also the head while trying to keep the eyes still.
23. Exercises 21 and 22 are repeated while standing on the floor.
24. Exercises 21 and 22 are repeated while standing on a foam mattress.
25. The patient walks for five steps forward and backward moving her/his head to and fro.
26. The patient walks for five steps forward and backward reading a book aloud.
27. The patient stands on a soft mattress:
    (a) She/he opens a book in front of her/him. She/he reads it aloud while at the same time moving the book right and left and then to and fro.
    (b) The patient opens a book in front of her/him and then moves it away from her/him extending her/his arms. She/he reads it aloud. Then, he/she brings it near to her/him, slowly, trying to read it. Then she/he moves it away again and repeats the exercise several times to and fro.
    (c) The patient walks on place moving her/his head to and fro.
    (d) The patient walks on place reading a book aloud.
28. Posturographic visual feedback.

    Position of the target generally reproduces the perimeter of the limits of stability. To induce hip strategies, the targets are placed in a small circle with fast pacing (5 s or less) (Fig. 11.16); to improve ankle strategy, they have to be placed in a larger circle (Fig. 11.17) with a slow pacing (10 s). Based on the previous evaluation of the patient, the targets may be placed especially in the anterior or posterior and lateral positions.

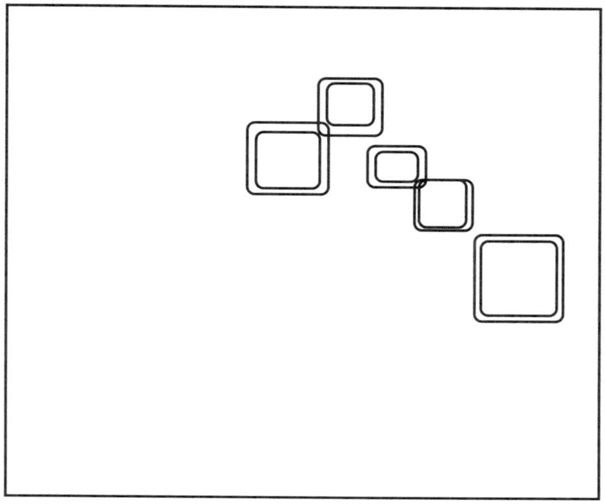

Fig. 11.16 Close arrangement of different-sized targets (Balance Master, reproduced by courtesy of NeuroCom International, Inc., Clackamas, Oregon, USA. Originally published in Cesarani and Alpini [37] published by Springer © 1999)

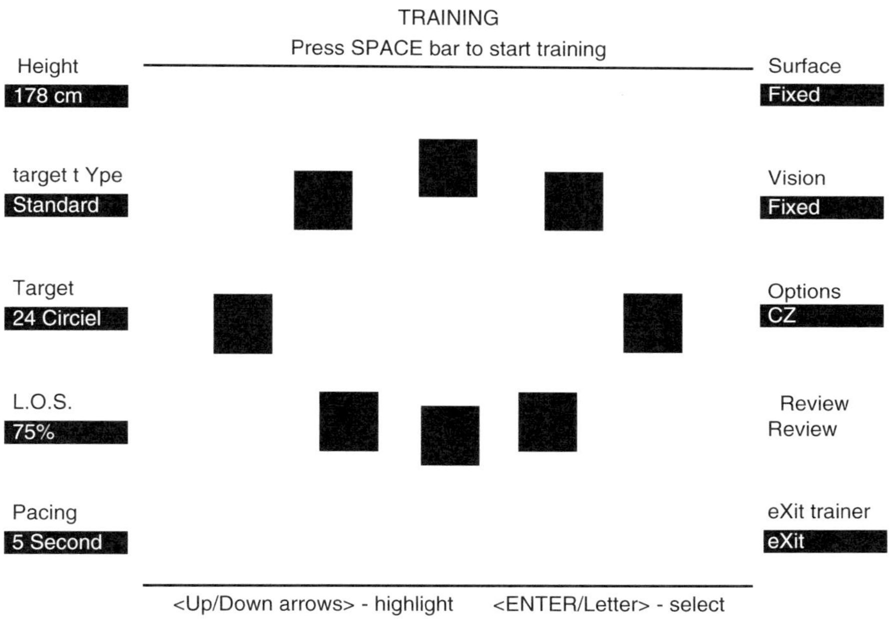

Fig. 11.17 Wide arrangement of targets along the perimeter of stability (Balance Master, reproduced by courtesy of NeuroCom International, Inc., Clackamas, Oregon, USA. Originally published in Cesarani and Alpini [37] published by Springer © 1999)

29. Virtual reality.

    We have experienced virtual reality (VR) in cognitive and motor rehab also in the elderly [24–26]. This kind of technology (VR) can be used to train realistic everyday tasks in the clinic and to combine complex abilities to fulfil complicated tasks without the dangers of the real word. Immersion and a high sense of presence are necessary to obtain enduring results. We propose the self-experienced virtual reality as explained in Chap. 7. VR training is adopted especially to improve unsteadiness and vestibular ataxia. Alternating objective and subjective views of each video are projected.

Static Balance

1. The patient stands on the floor in front of the screen, and she/he has to maintain equilibrium despite the visual stimulation.
2. A laser pointer is mounted on the head. The patient is required to point the laser spot on a target placed on the upper edge of the screen and to maintain steady the laser spot while standing on both legs for at least 30 s.
3. The patient is required to repeat the exercises standing on a foam mattress.

Dynamic Balance

The patient stands upright on a balance board in front of the screen.

1. The patient is required to maintain balance. The therapist helps the patient to avoid falls.
2. When the patient is able to maintain balance for at least 30 s during video projection, a laser pointer will be mounted on the patient's head, and stabilization of the laser spot on a target placed on the upper edge of the screen will be required.

11.2 Home Protocol

Exercises have been subdivided according to different phases of equilibrium, from supine to standing to moving. In each phase, there is a progression from mechanic to synergetic exercises. The exercises must be as simple as effective to ensure both continuous daily repetition and maintenance of the results obtained with the therapist in the gymnasium.

Home exercises can never be substituted for the therapeutic programmes shown in the previous section, performed with the therapist. Home exercises are used to complete the therapy. All the protocols have to be performed for 2 weeks, possibly twice a day. After 2 weeks, it can be reduced to the following exercises: 4, 6–9, 13–14–15, 19–20 and 25–30.

Supine

1. Hold your right knee against the chest and then extend your leg and take your left knee against the chest. When you hold the knee against the chest, softly apply traction to the flexed leg with the hands.
2. Extend your left arm over your head and simultaneously hold the right flexed leg to the chest with your hand. Maintain this position for 10 s and then repeat using the opposite arm and leg.
3. Lift your left leg with the extended knee and then repeat with your right leg.
4. Grasp a stick. Take your extended arms over your head and then return to the starting position.

5. Fixate a target on the ceiling and slowly move your head rightward and leftward.
6. Look for two equidistant targets on the ceiling and then fixate them alternately first moving only the eyes and then moving only the head.
7. Turn your head rightward and fixate a target on the lateral wall. Then straighten your head maintaining the visual fixation. Count from one up to ten and then turn your head.
8. Turn your head leftward and fix a target on the lateral wall. Then straighten your head, maintaining the visual fixation. Count from one up to ten and then turn your head.
9. From the supine position, shift to sitting position fixating a point straight in front of you.
10. In the prone position, lift your left arm and the right leg maintaining your forehead over the bed. Then repeat with the right arm and the left leg.
11. Repeat as above but at the same time also lifting the head.

Sitting

12. Extend your arms and lift your thumbs. Move your arms along a horizontal plane at about 50 cm from your eyes and then fixate your thumbs alternately. Begin slowly and then increase progressively the velocity of alternating the fixation.
13. Extend your arms and lift your thumbs. Move your arms along a vertical plane at about 50 cm from your eyes and then fixate your thumbs alternately. Begin slowly and then increase progressively the velocity of alternating the fixation.
14. Extend your right arm and lift your thumb. Move your arm slowly to and fro first along in a horizontal direction and then in a vertical direction. Follow your thumb with eyes only, first slowly and then increasing progressively the velocity of thumb displacement.
15. Repeat as above but simultaneously moving also the head while trying to keep the eyes still.
16. Move your head first slowly and then more rapidly in all directions fixating a target straight in front of you.
17. Look for three targets sited, respectively, in front of you, at your left and at your right. Fixate the front target and then move your head rapidly fixating the right-hand target. Now rotate your head leftward maintaining the fixation of the right-hand target. Fixate the front target. Now move your head rapidly leftward and fixate the left-hand target. Then rotate your head rightward maintaining the fixation of the left-hand target.
18. Open a book in front of you. Move it away from you extending your arms. Read it aloud. Then move it closer to you, slowly, trying to read it. Then move it away. Repeat several times to and fro.

Standing

19. With your hands on a table, lift yourself on tiptoes and maintain this position for 30 s.
20. With your hands on a table, lift yourself on your heels and maintain this position for 30 s.

21. Fixate yourself in a mirror. Align correctly your position. Maintain equilibrium for 1 min and then close your eyes visualizing your correct position and remain in this position for at least 1 min.
22. Fixate yourself on a mirror. Then oscillate to and fro and right and left, around your ankles keeping your pelvis still.
23. Fixate yourself in a mirror; keeping your feet still, bend your trunk to and fro and right and left.
24. Hold a small object and then lift it over your head and fixate it. With your arms extended, move it in circles of increasing width, maintaining the fixation of the object.
25. Open a book in front of you. Move it away from you extending your arms. Read it aloud. Then move it near to you, slowly, trying to read it. Then move it away. Repeat several times to and fro.

Moving

26. Step on the floor with eyes open fixating a target straight in front of you.
27. Support yourself on a chair and then walk on tiptoes.
28. Support yourself on a chair and then walk on heels.
29. Walk for five steps along a corridor forward and backward fixating a target.
30. Walk for five steps along a corridor forward and backward moving your head to and fro.
31. Walk for five steps along a corridor forward and backward reading a book aloud.
32. During video "objective" projection:
    (a) Maintain equilibrium while standing, first on the floor and then on a soft mattress.
    (b) Maintain equilibrium while stepping, first on the floor and then on a soft mattress.

11.2.1 Counselling

Rehabilitation is an important step in the treatment of dizziness and unsteadiness in the elderly, but it has to be usually accomplished with modifications of lifestyle and home environment and pharmacotherapy. The general suggestions are the following:

- Maintain adequate water intake (at least 1.5 l for females and 2 l for males).
- Restrict alcohol intake (less than 120 ml for women and 240 ml for men).
- Restrict smoking and, obviously, avoid drug abuse.
- Sleep using two pillows in order to maintain the head lifted about 20° in order to relax neck muscles and to ameliorate breathing and digestion avoiding gastro-oesophageal reflux.
- Avoid maintaining the same position of the head/neck for more than 30 min.
- Avoid maintaining incorrect position of the head/neck; in particular, check the proper position when watching television.
- In any way, every 30 min, change your head/neck position and mobilize your head and shoulders.
- Perform regular and constant aerobic physical activity like quiet walking at least 30′/day three times/week.

The most specific considerations linked to the specific aspects of aged biology are the following:

1. Sedative drugs have to be generally avoided, while drugs improving cognitive and motor skills have to be preferred (the so-called nootropic drugs).
2. There is emerging evidence [27] that mild chronic hyponatraemia, highly prevalent in the elderly and once considered asymptomatic, is a major independent risk factor for falls and fall-related fractures.
3. Vitamin D deficiency, very common in the general population and especially in the aged, is associated with reduced functional mobility [28], and it may be relevant for physical and cognitive performance in the older population [29, 30].
4. Combination of physical exercise and protein supplementation, especially leucine, the only dietary amino acid that has the capacity to stimulate muscle protein synthesis, may be useful to improve muscle strength and thus antigravity control [31, 32]. Protein intake has to be at least 1.5 g/kg/day.
5. Sleep disorders are frequent in aged people, and they are frequently due to an alteration of melatonin rhythm [33]. Melatonin supplementation (3 or 5 mg) 30 min before sleeping may be useful.
6. Footwear intervention, including shoe insoles and foot orthoses, may enhance balance control and gait in older people [34].
7. Motor activity has to be stimulated even through playful activities like dance [35] or sport disciplines [36].

11.2.2 Some Suggestions to Ameliorate Lifestyle

(a) *How to get up from a chair:*
   1. Place your hands on the chair's arms (Fig. 11.18a).
   2. Bend forward your trunk and lift yourself pushing on the chair's arms (Fig. 11.18b).
   3. Now get up fixating in front of you (Fig. 11.18c).
   4. Wait for a few seconds before walking and continue to fixate in front of you (Fig. 11.18d).

(b) *How to keep an object from the floor:*
   1. Push the object near a table or something like it (Fig. 11.19a).
   2. Using the table for support, bend your knees and keep the object (Fig. 11.19b).
   3. Lift yourself using the table for support (Fig. 11.19c).

(c) *How to get out of bed:*
   1. Turn yourself to one side (Fig. 11.20b).
   2. Move your legs over the side of the bed (Fig. 11.20c).
   3. Lift your trunk slowly (Fig. 11.20d).
   4. Sit fixating in front of you, remaining still for a few seconds before standing up (Fig. 11.20e).

Note. The contents of this chapter are partially based on *Dizziness in the Elderly* (A. Cesarani, D. Alpini) in A. Cesarani, D. Alpini (1999) Vertigo and Dizziness Rehabilitation – The MCS Method. Springer, p 188.

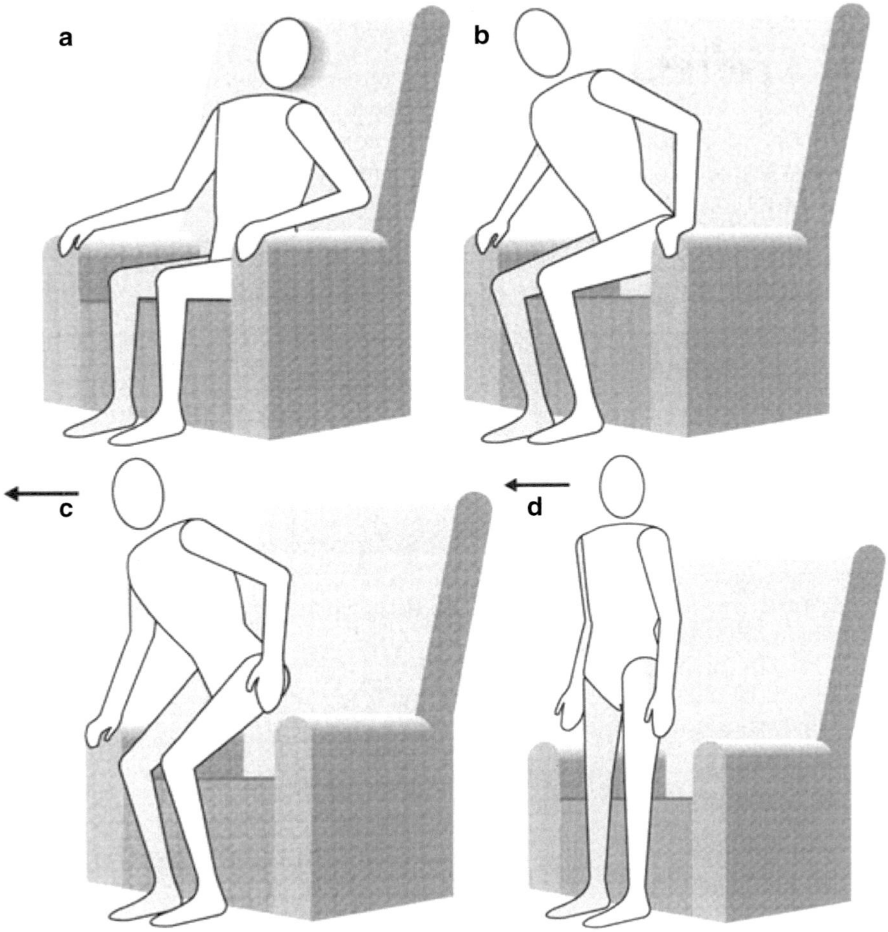

Fig. 11.18 (**a–d**) How to get up from a chair (Originally published in Cesarani and Alpini [37] published by Springer © 1999)

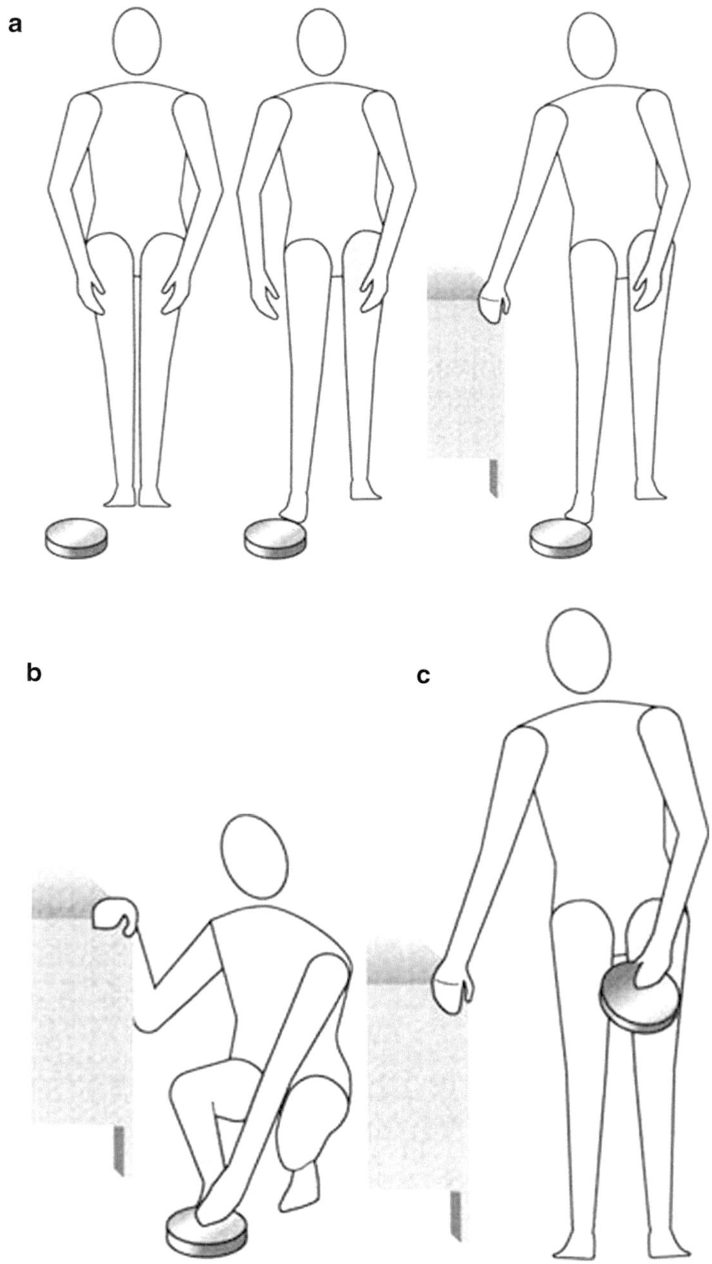

Fig. 11.19 (**a–c**) How to pick up an object (Originally published in Cesarani and Alpini [37] published by Springer © 1999)

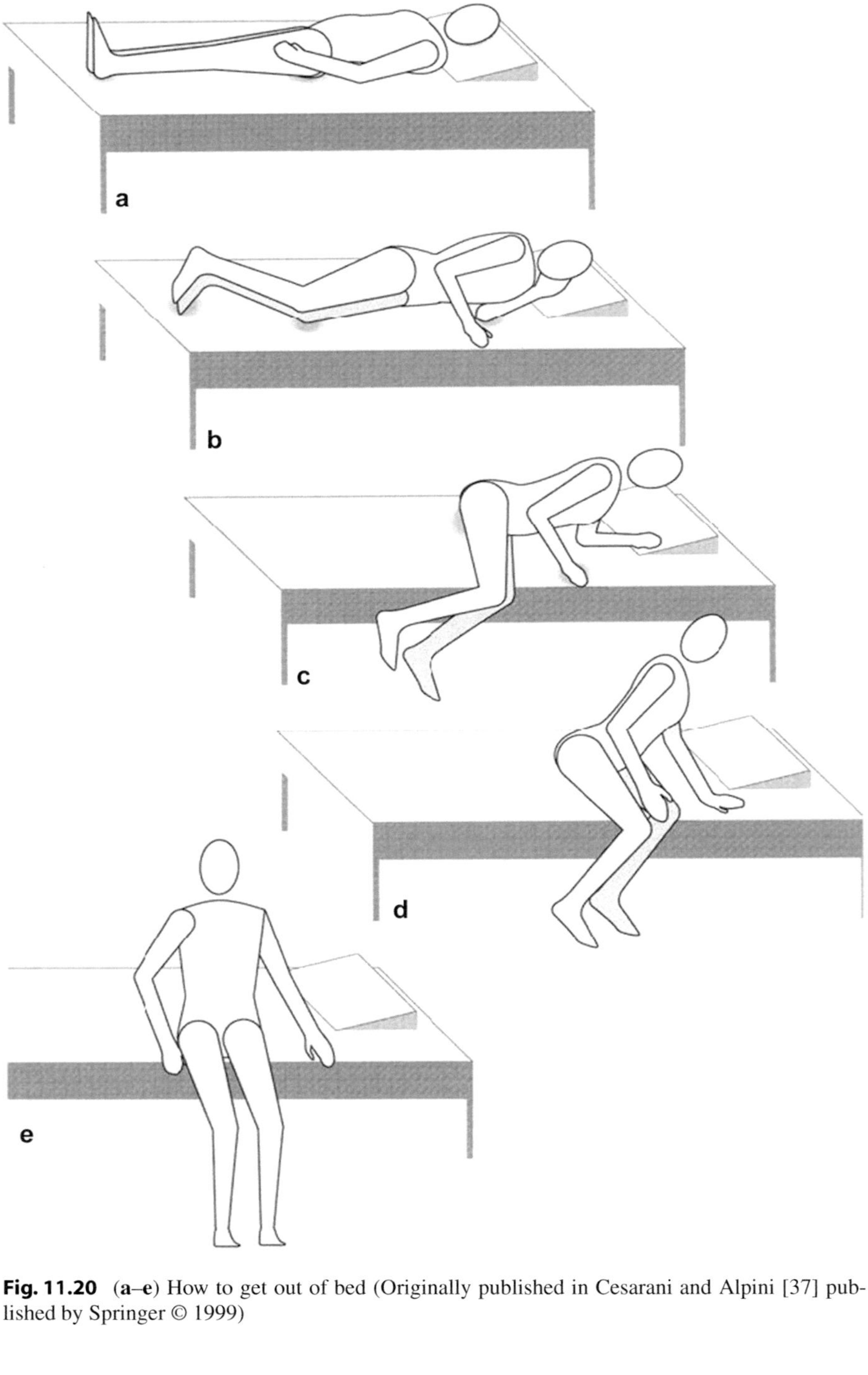

Fig. 11.20 (**a**–**e**) How to get out of bed (Originally published in Cesarani and Alpini [37] published by Springer © 1999)

References

1. Mueller M, Strobl R, Jahn K, Linkohr B, Peters A, Grill E. Burden of disability attributable to vertigo and dizziness in the aged: results from the KORA-Age study. Eur J Public Health. 2013 Nov 19
2. Lo AX, Harada CN (2013) Geriatric dizziness: evolving diagnostic and therapeutic approaches for the emergency department. Clin Geriatr Med 29(1):181–204
3. Ishiyama G (2009) Imbalance and vertigo: the aging human vestibular periphery. Semin Neurol 29(5):491–499
4. Walther LE, Westhofen M (2007) Presbyvertigo-aging of otoconia and vestibular sensory cells. J Vestib Res 17(2–3):89–92
5. Agrawal Y, Zuniga MG, Davalos-Bichara M, Schubert MC, Walston JD, Hughes J, Carey JP (2012) Decline in semicircular canal and otolith function with age. Otol Neurotol 33(5):832–839
6. Alpini D, Kohen-Ratz R, Braun R, Burstin A, Tesio L, Pugnetti L, Mendozzi L, Sambataro G, Cesarani A, Giuliano DA (2001) Falls in the elderly: the development of a risk questionnaire and posturographic findings. Int Tinnitus J 7(2):105–108
7. Riva D, Mamo C, Fanì M, Saccavino P, Rocca F, Momenté M, Fratta M (2013) Single stance stability and proprioceptive control in older adults living at home: gender and age differences. J Aging Res 2013:561695. doi:10.1155/2013/561695. Epub 2013 Jul 28
8. Panel on Prevention of Falls in Older Persons, American Geriatrics Society and British Geriatrics Society (2011) Summary of the Updated American Geriatrics Society/British Geriatrics Society clinical practice guideline for prevention of falls in older persons. J Am Geriatr Soc 59:148–157
9. Schoon Y, Olde Rikkert MG, Rongen S, Lagro J, Schalk B, Claassen JA (2013) Head turning-induced hypotension in elderly people. PLoS One 8(8):e72837. doi:10.1371/journal.pone.0072837
10. Salonen L, Kivelä SL (2012) Eye diseases and impaired vision as possible risk factors for recurrent falls in the aged: a systematic review. Curr Gerontol Geriatr Res 2012:271481. doi:10.1155/2012/271481, Epub 2012 Aug 15
11. Tobis JS, Nayak L, Hoehler F (1981) Visual perception of verticality and horizontality among elderly fallers. Arch Phys Med Rehabil 62(12):619–622
12. Aoki M, Tanaka K, Wakaoka T, Kuze B, Hayashi H, Mizuta K, Ito Y (2013) The association between impaired perception of verticality and cerebral white matter lesions in the elderly patients with orthostatic hypotension. J Vestib Res 23(2):85–93
13. Horak FB (2006) Postural orientation and equilibrium: what do we need to know about neural control of balance to prevent falls? Age Ageing 35(S2):ii7–ii11
14. Paillard T (2013) Neuromuscular system and aging: involutions and implications. Geriatr Psychol Neuropsychiatr Vieil 11(4):379–387
15. Matsui JI, Ryals BM (2005) Hair cell regeneration: an exciting phenomenon…but will restoring hearing and balance be possible? J Rehabil Res Dev 42(4 Suppl 2):187–198
16. Jung JY, Kim JS, Chung PS, Woo SH, Rhee CK (2009) Effect of vestibular rehabilitation on dizziness in the elderly. Am J Otolaryngol 30(5):295–299
17. Marioni G, Fermo S, Lionello M, Fasanaro E, Giacomelli L, Zanon S, Staffieri C, Dall'Igna F, Manzato E, Staffieri A (2013) Vestibular rehabilitation in elderly patients with central vestibular dysfunction: a prospective, randomized pilot study. Age (Dordr) 35(6):2315–2327
18. Costa de Araujo P, Demanez L, Lechien J, Bauvir P, Petermans J (2011) Presbyastasis and application of vestibular rehabilitation in geriatrics. Rev Med Liege 66(3):130–134
19. Peres M, da Silveira E (2010) Effect of vestibular rehabilitation in elder people: regarding balance, quality of life and perception. Cien Saude Colet 15(6):2805–2814

20. Fairhall N, Sherrington C, Lord SR, Kurrle SE, Langron C, Lockwood K, MonaghanN, Aggar C, Cameron ID (2013) Effect of a multifactorial, interdisciplinary intervention on risk factors for falls and fall rate in frail older people: a randomised controlled trial. Age Ageing
21. Lee IH, Park SY (2013) Balance improvement by strength training for the elderly. J Phys Ther Sci 25(12):1591–1593. doi:10.1589/jpts.25.1591, Epub 2014 Jan 8
22. Viña J, Borras C, Sanchis-Gomar F, Martinez-Bello VE, Olaso-Gonzalez G, Gambini J, Ingles M, Gomez-Cabrera MC (2013) Pharmacological properties of physical exercise in the elderly. Curr Pharm Des
23. Osio M Dezuanni E. Alpini D Cesarani A. Mangoni A (1995) Low intensity electrical stimulation of neck muscles modifies motor neuron excitability of the soleus muscles in man. Electroencephalography and Clinical Neurophysiology 95(3):68–69
24. Alpini D Pugnetti L Mendozzi L Barbier E, Monti B, Cesarani A. (1998) Virtual reality in vestibular diagnosis and rehabilitation. In: Proceedings of the 2nd European conference on disability, virtual reality & associated technologies, Skövde, pp 221–227; ECDVRAT and University of Reading; ISBN 0 7049 1 1 41 8 79
25. Pugnetti L Mendozzi L, Barbieri E, Motta A, Alpini D, Attree EA, Brooks BM, Rose FD(1998) Developments of a collaborative research on VR applications for mental health. In: Proceedings of the 2nd European conference on disability, virtual reality & associated technologies, Skövde, pp 77–81; ECDVRAT and University of Reading; ISBN 0 7049 1 1 41 8 79
26. Riva G, Rizzo A, Alpini D, Attree EA, Barbieri E, Bertella L, Buckwalter JG, Davies RC, Gamberini L, Johansson G, Katz N, Marchi S, Mendozzi L, Molinari E, Pugnetti L, Rose FD, Weiss PL (1999) Virtual environments in the diagnosis, prevention, and intervention of age-related diseases: a review of VR scenarios proposed in the EC VETERAN Project. Cyberpsychol Behav 2(6):577–591
27. Zaino CJ, Maheshwari AV, Goldfarb DS (2013) Impact of mild chronic hyponatremia on falls, fractures, osteoporosis, and death. Am J Orthop (Belle Mead NJ) 42(11):522–527
28. Gschwind YJ, Bischoff-Ferrari HA, Bridenbaugh SA, Härdi I, Kressig RW (2014) Association between serum vitamin D status and functional mobility in memory clinic patients aged 65 years and older. Gerontology 60:123–129
29. Boyé ND, Oudshoorn C, van der Velde N, van Lieshout EM, de Vries OJ, Lips P, van Beeck EF, Patka P, van der Cammen TJ (2013) Vitamin D and physical performance in older men and women visiting the emergency department because of a fall: data from the improving medication prescribing to reduce risk of falls (IMPROveFALL) study. J Am Geriatr Soc 61(11):1948–1952. doi:10.1111/jgs.12499, Epub 2013 Oct 1
30. Park S, Ham JO, Lee BK (2013) A positive association of vitamin D deficiency and sarcopenia in 50 year old women, but not men. Clin Nutr pii: S0261-5614(13)00256-2
31. Churchward-Venne TA, Breen L, Phillips SM (2013) Alterations in human muscle protein metabolism with aging: protein and exercise as countermeasures to offset sarcopenia. Biofactors. doi:10.1002/biof.1138
32. Shahar S, Kamaruddin NS, Badrasawi M, Sakian NI, Abd Manaf Z, Yassin Z, Joseph L (2013) Effectiveness of exercise and protein supplementation intervention on body composition, functional fitness, and oxidative stress among elderly Malays with sarcopenia. Clin Interv Aging 8:1365–1375. doi:10.2147/CIA.S46826, Epub 2013 Oct 9
33. Alpini D, Cesarani A, Fraschini F Kohen-Raz F, Capobianco S, Cornelio F (2004) Aging and vestibular system: specific tests and role of melatonin in cognitive involvement. Arch Gerontol Geriatr Suppl (9):13–25
34. Hatton AL, Rome K, Dixon J, Martin DJ, McKeon PO (2013) Footwear interventions: a review of their sensorimotor and mechanical effects on balance performance and gait in older adults. J Am Podiatr Med Assoc 103(6):516–533

35. Kattenstroth JC, Kalisch T, Holt S, Tegenthoff M, Dinse HR (2013). Six months of dance intervention enhances postural, sensorimotor, and cognitive performance in elderly without affecting cardio-respiratory functions. Front Aging Neurosci. 26(5):5. doi: 10.3389/fnagi.2013.00005
36. Nguyen MH, Kruse A (2012) A randomized controlled trial of Tai chi for balance, sleep quality and cognitive performance in elderly Vietnamese. Clin Interv Aging 7:185–190
37. Cesarani A, Alpini D (1999) Vertigo and dizziness rehabilitation – the MCS method. Springer, Milan, Heidelberg

12 Whiplash-Associated Balance Disorders

The term "whiplash" has been used to describe a mechanism of injury and the various clinical manifestations as a consequence of the injury [1]. In 1995, the Quebec Task Force (QTF) on whiplash-associated disorders (WADs) adopted the following definition of whiplash: "whiplash is an acceleration-deceleration mechanism of energy transfer to the neck. It may result from rear-end or side-impact motor vehicle collisions, but can also occur during diving or other mishaps. The impact may result in bony or soft-tissue injuries (whiplash-injury), which in turn may lead to a variety of clinical manifestations called Whiplash-Associated Disorders" [2].

Whiplash injury can be defined, in a most wide interpretation, as a noncontact quick (50 ms) acceleration–deceleration head–neck trauma [3, 4] with involvement of the spine as a whole. This interpretation explains how the WADs comprehend symptoms variably combined:

- Orthopaedic, such as neck pain and functional limitation of cervical and lumbar movements
- Neurological, such as paraesthesias
- Audiological, such as tinnitus and hypoacusia
- Otorhinolaringological, such as dysphagia and disphonias
- Equilibriometric, such as vertigo and dizziness
- Odontoiatric, such as temporomandibular joint disorders

Whiplash injuries vary from minor to severe, and, generally, the evolution of the whiplash is divided into three phases:

- The onset phase, involving local reactions with release of neuromediators, such as serotonin, histamine, bradykinin and classical inflammation
- The recovery phase, locally characterized by synthesis of new collagenous fibres
- The remodelling phase in which the body as a whole modifies its posture and movement strategies in order to restore normal daily life activities

Whiplash patients can be classified according to the severity of signs and symptoms. The QTF-WAD classification system consists of five levels:

0, no complaints or physical signs

I, neck complaints but no physical signs

D.C. Alpini et al., *Vertigo Rehabilitation Protocols*,
DOI 10.1007/978-3-319-05482-7_12,

II, neck complaints and musculoskeletal signs (such as a decreased range of motion or muscle tenderness)
III, neck complaints and neurological signs
IV, neck complaints and fracture/dislocation

The most common presenting symptoms following an acute motor vehicle collision are neck pain (88–100 %) and headache (54–66 %). Other symptoms are neck stiffness, shoulder pain, arm pain/numbness, paraesthesia, weakness, dysphagia, visual and auditory symptoms and dizziness. In most cases, WAD resolves quickly; 47 % of injured people return to normal activities within 4 weeks, and only 2 % continue to be absent from pre-accident activities 1 year after injury [5].

Whiplash injury sometimes causes a labyrinth concussion with a consequent otoconia displacement. In these cases, a benign paroxysmal positioning vertigo (BPPV) is provoked: whiplash-associated BPPV (WA-BPPV).

Most cases of WA-BPPV can be treated using physical therapy (see Chap. 8), by means of Epley's [6] canalith-repositioning procedure (CRP) in the case of canalolithiasis and Semont's [7] liberatory manoeuvre in the case of cupulolithiasis.

Although both manoeuvres have been shown to have therapeutic benefits, they require sequential procedures involving moving the patient's head and body into unnatural positions, making them sometime unsuitable for WAD patients with cervical or back disorders, especially for older patients.

In WA-BPPV patients, it is thus better to use more conservative procedures like the supine to prolonged lateral position (SPLP) [8] or the rolling over manoeuvre (ROM) [9].

The pathogenesis of whiplash-associated balance disorders (WABD) not due to a recognizable BPPV is still debated:

- Mechanical compression with dynamic stenosis of the vertebral arteria or arteriae
- Sympathetic abnormal stimulation
- Proprioceptive disorder especially from cervical and lumbar regions
- Central vestibular system disorder

Probably, WABD derive from different combinations of different mechanisms. The kinematics of the acceleration–deceleration is different, for example, for the driver who is usually opposite to the trauma by means of her/his arms being on the wheel and the passenger who usually receives completely and passively the impact forces. Differences can be observed if the patient wore or not the safety belts during the impact: with safety belts, the movement of the head and the neck is not sagittal but torsional with a torsion having the mid-thoracic vertebrae (T7–8) as fulcrum. The direction of torsional component is different: counterclockwise for the passenger and clockwise for the driver. Furthermore, rarely the impact is caused by a straight rear-end collision, while, very often, the impact causes a rotational acceleration of the vehicle. Torsional and angular accelerations cause brain microlesions in different parts, and this can lead to different combinations of signs and symptoms [10, 11].

Following whiplash, either for mechanical lesions on cervical dynamic or for central dysfunctions, some modifications of patient posture are usually observed:

- The head modifies its position according to an antalgic flexion.
- The head reduces its rotational and lateroflexion movements.

- During normal movements, rotation of the body is along the trunk and not the neck.
- The trunk is ipsilaterally rotated with respect to the side of lesion.
- The pelvis is rotated according to head antalgic position.
- The position of centre of gravity (CoG) is modified.

Generally speaking, WABD may be considered as the result of desynchronization of the proprioceptive interaction between the so-called special proprioception (from the labyrinths) and general proprioceptions (from spine muscles, ligaments, joints, etc.) [12, 13].

Pathogenesis may be interpreted also under a phylogenetic point of view. The specific posture of the human being is the bipedal upright position with a maintenance of dynamic equilibrium as an inverse pendulum on a relatively restricted support surface area. This kind of posture represents a biomechanical evolution strictly correlated to the evolution of high-level cognitive processes specific for the human beings [14]. In adulthood, maintaining stance is perceived as an easy action to be performed, at least in normal conditions on steady surfaces, but it requires a very high level of sensorimotor control in order to allow a low-effort antigravity alignment of the different body segments [15].

The possibility to increase the perception of the environment is the main positive aspects of a bipedal upright posture: in the horizontal plane, the atlo-occipital joint allows the head to extend the exploration possibilities of the eyes [16]; furthermore, the relatively strict base of support allows rapid turns of the body in order to control also the environment at our back; in the vertical plane, the evolution of the lumbosacral spine allows the extension of the head and the trunk in order to explore, also for a long time, the environment over our head [17]. Thus, we can state that human posture is an evolution of the quadrupedal motion with very high possibilities of exploration of the environment all along the three-space axis.

The implementation of bipedal posture on quadrupedal motor control is relatively recent in the phylogenesis, and it can be retraced observing how the child fights against gravity force in her/his early months of life [15].

This concept may explain the pathogenesis of whiplash-associated disorders (WADs) that very frequently cause impairments not proportionate to the intensity of the impact. The relatively low energy transferred to the body during the accident acts specifically at the two most innovative parts of the humans: the atlo-occipital joint and the lumbosacral spine. In this way, whiplash immediately decreases the ability of the subjects to rotate the head and to extend the head and the trunk; in other words, whiplash brings backs the humans to a primate.

Thus, the *key impairment* is the biomechanic disruption of head-to-trunk and lumbar-to-gait coordination.

Treatment must be pointed to restore spine mobility as a whole with special regard to atlo-occipital joint and lumbosacral region and thus to:

- Reorganize self-perception of posture
- Reorganize proprioceptive information from the neck and the pelvis
- Restore visual field stabilization during gait and movement

12.1 Exercises in the Gymnasium

12.1.1 First Week

1. The patient holds her/his knees to the chest simultaneously, gently with the help of her/his hands (Fig. 12.1).
2. With the flexed legs and the feet on the bed, the patient rotates her/his pelvis rightward and leftward keeping his knees flexed and legs together (Fig. 12.2).
3. The patient lifts her/his pelvis simultaneously extending the arms over her/his head. She/he then repositions the arms along the body lowering her/his pelvis (Fig. 12.3).

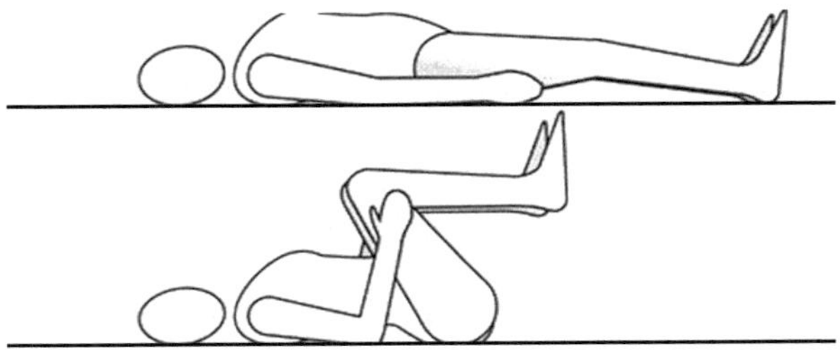

Fig. 12.1 Patient holds both knees against the chest (Originally published in Cesarani and Alpini [21] published by Springer © 1999)

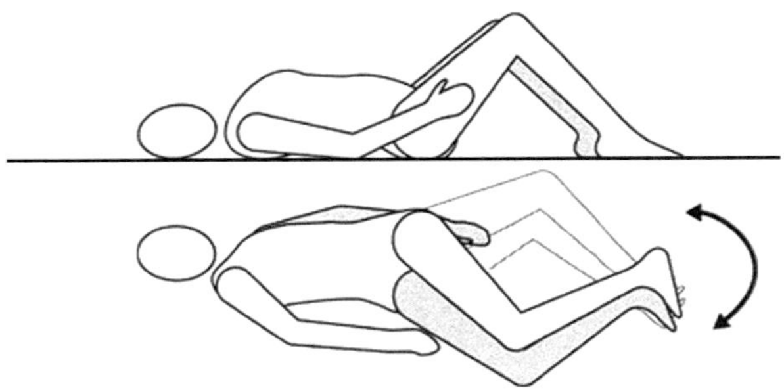

Fig. 12.2 Rotation of the pelvis (Originally published in Cesarani and Alpini [21] published by Springer © 1999)

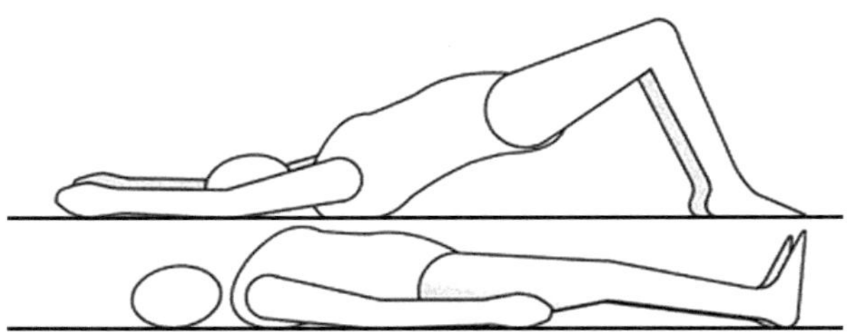

Fig. 12.3 Patient lifts the pelvis and extends the arms. He then returns to the resting position (Originally published in Cesarani and Alpini [21] published by Springer © 1999)

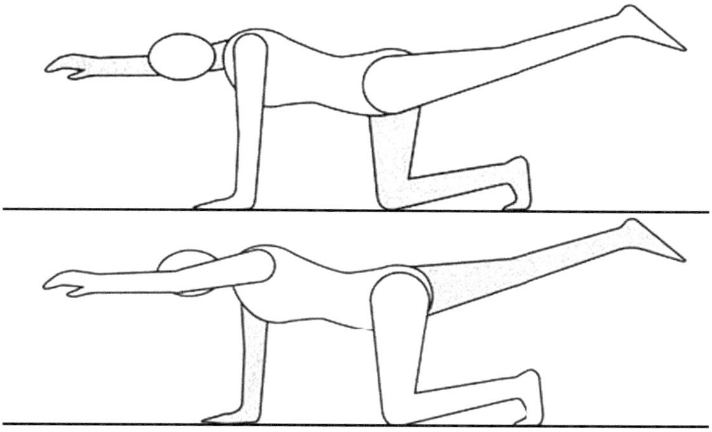

Fig. 12.4 Alternating extension of one arm and the opposite leg (Originally published in Cesarani and Alpini [21] published by Springer © 1999)

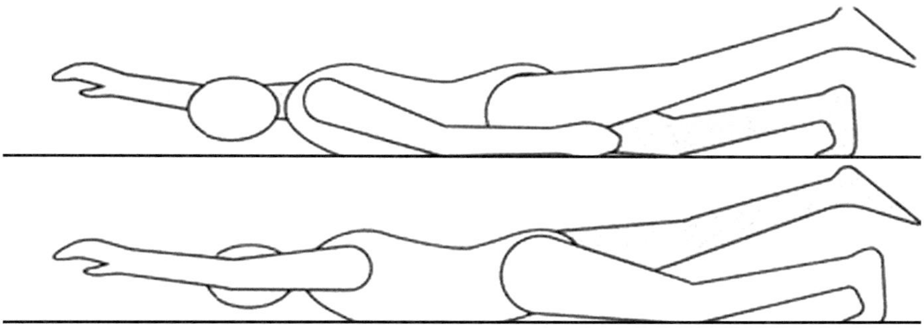

Fig. 12.5 In the prone position, simultaneous extension of one arm and the opposite leg (Originally published in Cesarani and Alpini [21] published by Springer © 1999)

4. In the quadrupedal position, the patient simultaneously extends the right arm and the left leg and then repeats the exercise with the left arm and the right leg (Fig. 12.4).
5. In the prone position, the patient lifts her/his left arm and the right leg, holding the forehead over the bed. She/he then repeats with the right arm and the left leg (Fig. 12.5).
6. The patient repeats the exercise as above but simultaneously also lifting her/his head.
7. The patient inhales. Exhaling, she/he bends forward holding her/his head on the right knee. She/he waits 10 s. Inhaling, she/he returns to sitting position. Exhaling,

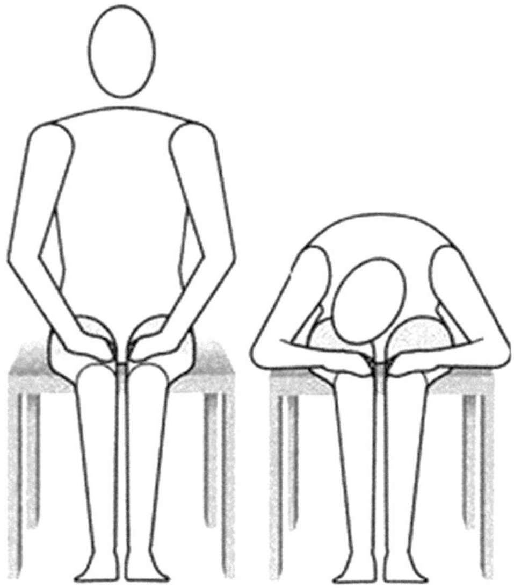

Fig. 12.6 Bending the trunk (Originally published in Cesarani and Alpini [21] published by Springer © 1999)

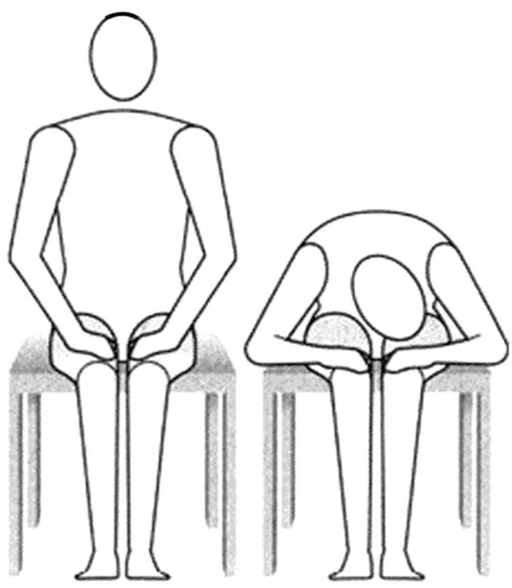

Fig. 12.7 Bending the trunk (Originally published in Cesarani and Alpini [21] published by Springer © 1999)

she/he bends forward taking her/his head on the left knee. She/he waits 10 s, and then inhaling, she/he returns to sitting position (Figs. 12.6 and 12.7).

8. On a balance board:
   (a) The patient steps on the board with the feet centrally positioned and concentrates on a proper posture using a mirror to see her/his reflection. With eyes open, she/he transfers her/his weight from one foot to the other with a smooth flowing motion maintaining a correct postural alignment of the

head and the trunk. In this case, feedback is visual, provided by the mirror.

(b) The patient repeats the exercise but with eyes closed. The therapist controls the patient's movements in order to avoid falls. The therapist is behind the patient helping her/him to maintain correct postural alignment of the trunk. In this case, feedback is somatosensorial, provided by the hands of the therapist.

(c) The patient steps on the board on one leg with the flexed knee and concentrates on a proper posture using a mirror to see her/his reflection. The patient has to maintain equilibrium for at least 10 s. The therapist is behind the patient helping her/him to maintain correct postural alignment of the trunk. In this case, feedback is both visual and somatosensorial.

(d) The patient repeats the exercise with the other leg.

12.1.2 Second Week

9. The patient is supine and fixates a target on the ceiling and slowly moves her/his head rightward and leftward.
10. The patient is supine and looks for two equidistant targets on the ceiling, and then she/he fixates them alternately first moving only the eyes and then moving only her/his head.
11. The patient in supine position shifts to sitting position, fixating a point straight in front of her/him (Fig.12.8).
12. From supine position, the patient shifts to sitting position, fixating a point sited on her/his right.
13. From supine position, the patient shifts to sitting position, fixating a point sited on her/his left.
14. The patient steps up and down, fixating a target according to the following sequence:

Right foot up	Left foot up	Right foot down
Left foot down	Left foot up	Right foot up
Left foot down	Right foot down	

She/he then repeats with the eyes closed.

15. On a soft mattress:
    (a) The patient moves her/his head first slowly and then faster in all directions, fixating a target straight in front of her/him (Fig. 12.9).
    (b) The patient fixates her-/himself in a mirror and aligns her/his position correctly. She/he then maintains equilibrium for 1 min and then closes her/his eyes visualizing her/his correct position while remaining still in the same position for at least 1 min (Fig. 12.10).
    (c) The patient fixates herself/himself in a mirror. She/he then oscillates to and fro and from side to side, around the ankles keeping the pelvis still (ankle strategy) (Fig. 12.11).

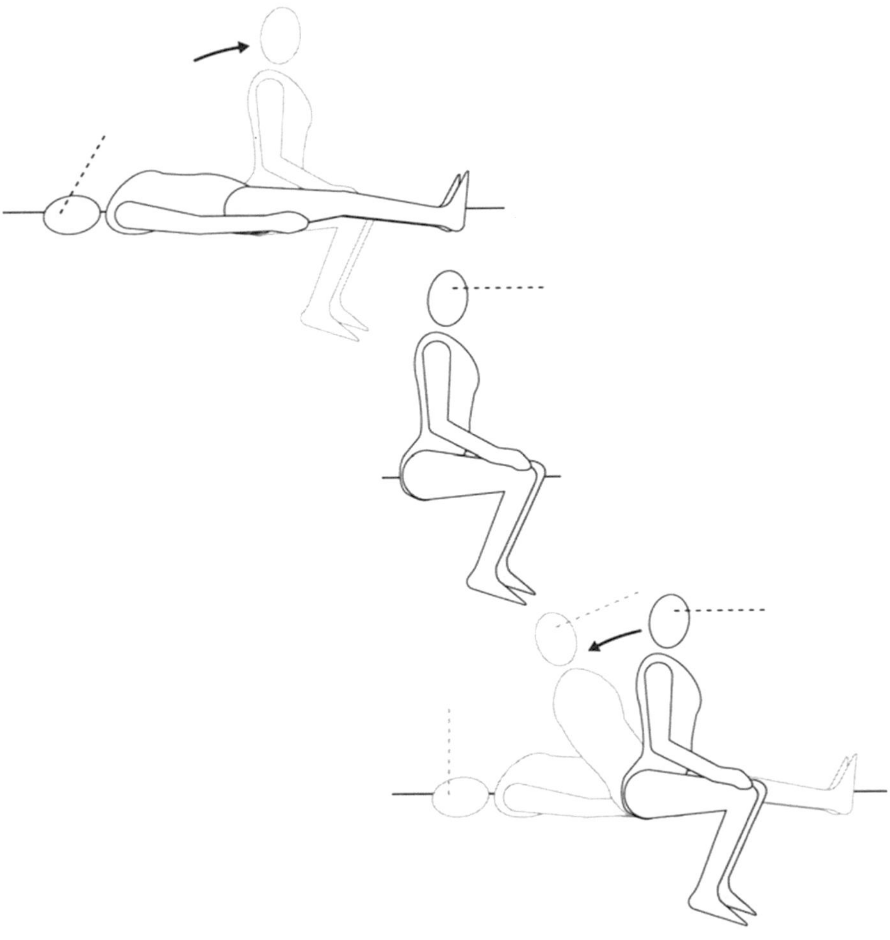

Fig. 12.8 From the supine to sitting position and vice versa (Originally published in Cesarani and Alpini [21] published by Springer © 1999)

(d) The patient fixates her-/himself in a mirror; keeping her/his feet still, she/he bends the trunk to and fro and from side to side (hip strategy) (Fig. 12.12).
(e) The patient holds a small object and lifts it over her/his head while fixating it. She/he lifts it over the head, and then, with arms straight, she/he moves the object in circles of increasing width (Fig. 12.13); then, simultaneously bending the trunk and the knees, she/he places it on the floor (Fig. 12.14).
(f) The patient walks, fixating a target in front of her/him (Fig. 12.15).
(g) In the quadrupedal position on a double mattress, the patient performs synchronization exercises of the arm and leg (Fig. 12.16).

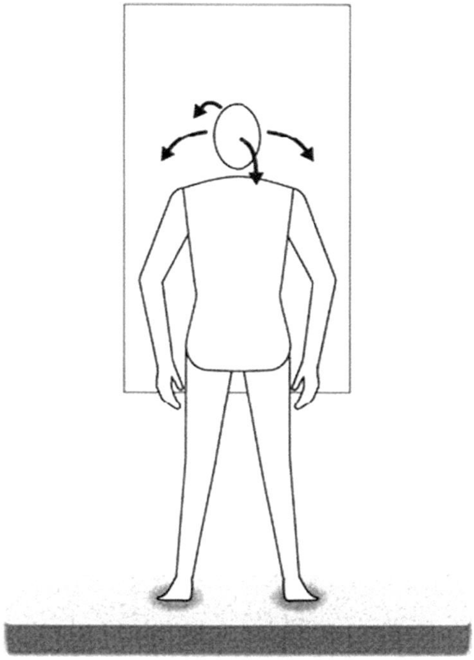

Fig. 12.9 Movements of the head in all directions standing on the mattress (Originally published in Cesarani and Alpini [21] published by Springer © 1999)

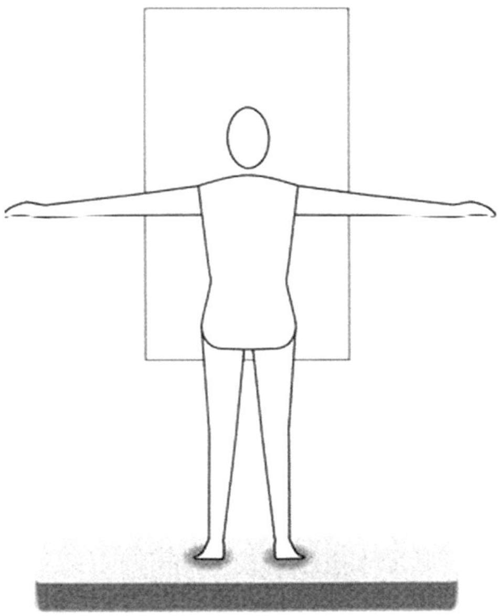

Fig. 12.10 Correct alignment of posture standing on the mattress (Originally published in Cesarani and Alpini [21] published by Springer © 1999)

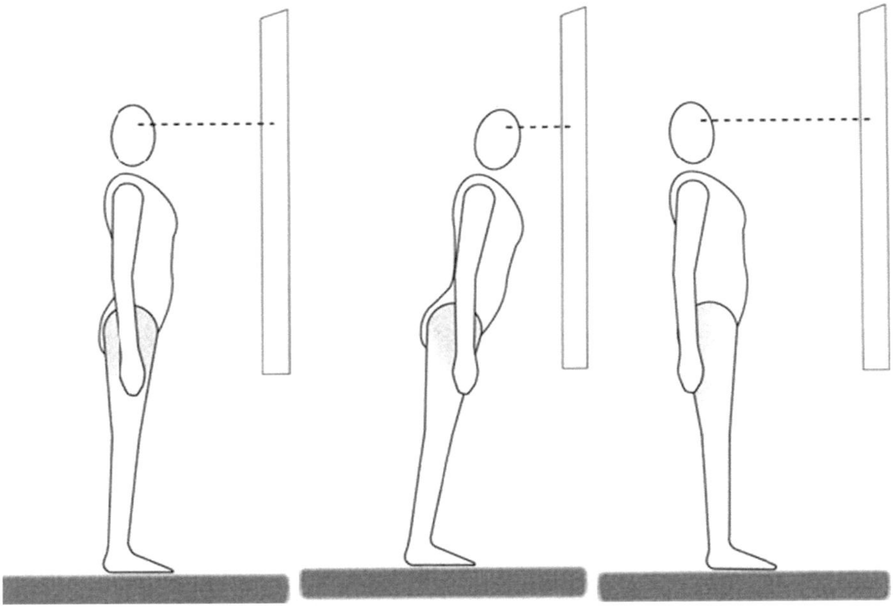

Fig. 12.11 Ankle oscillations (Originally published in Cesarani and Alpini [21] published by Springer © 1999)

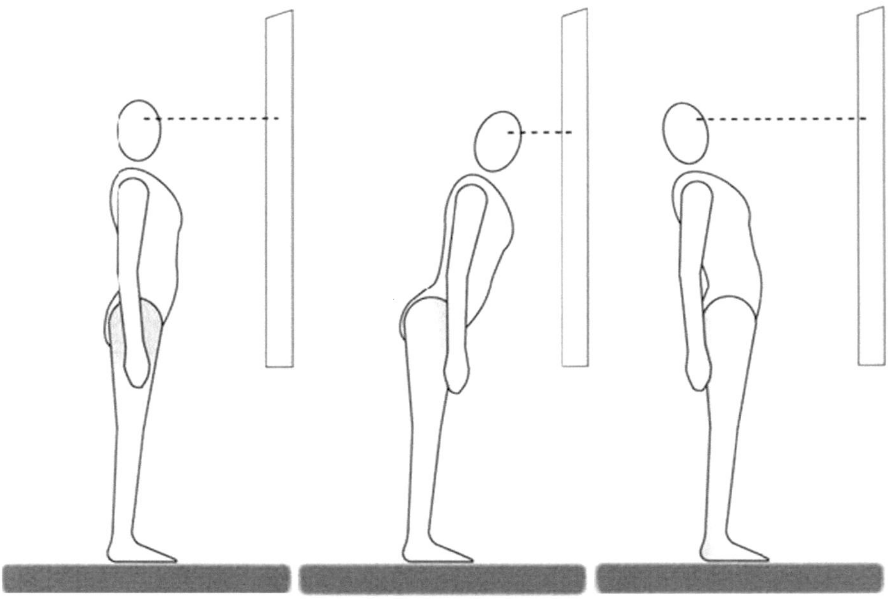

Fig. 12.12 Hip oscillations (Originally published in Cesarani and Alpini [21] published by Springer © 1999)

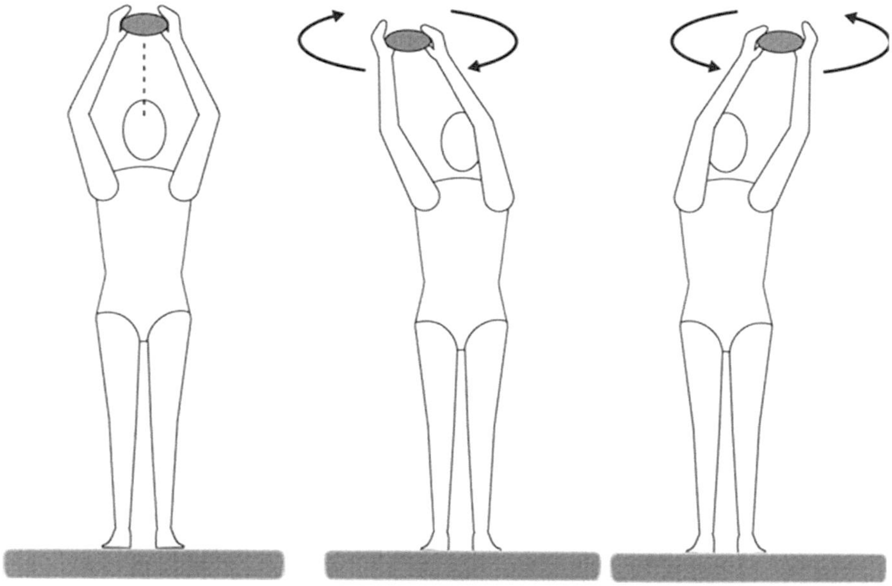

Fig. 12.13 Circular movements of a small object over the head (Originally published in Cesarani and Alpini [21] published by Springer © 1999)

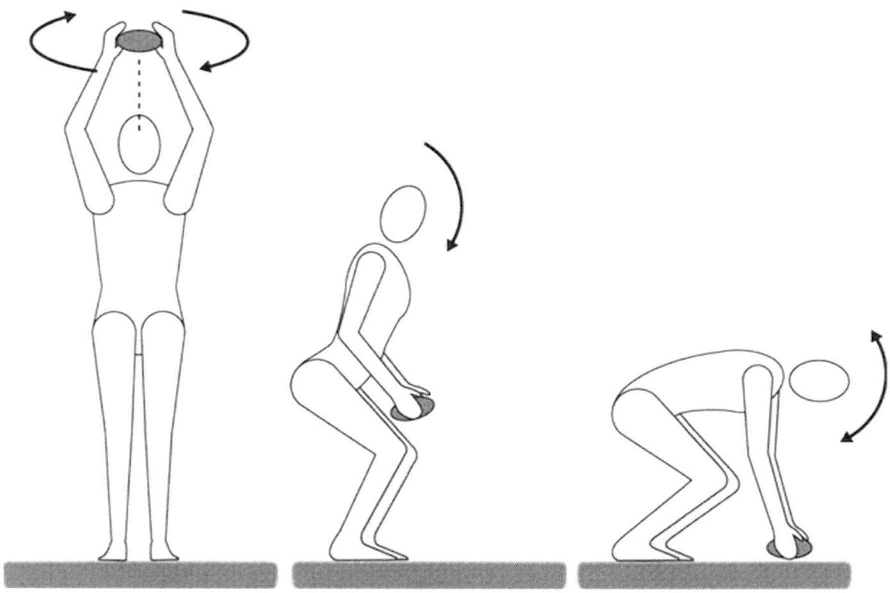

Fig. 12.14 Circular movements of a small object, bending the trunk and placing the object on the floor (Originally published in Cesarani and Alpini [21] published by Springer © 1999)

Fig. 12.15 Stepping on the mattress (Originally published in Cesarani and Alpini [21] published by Springer © 1999)

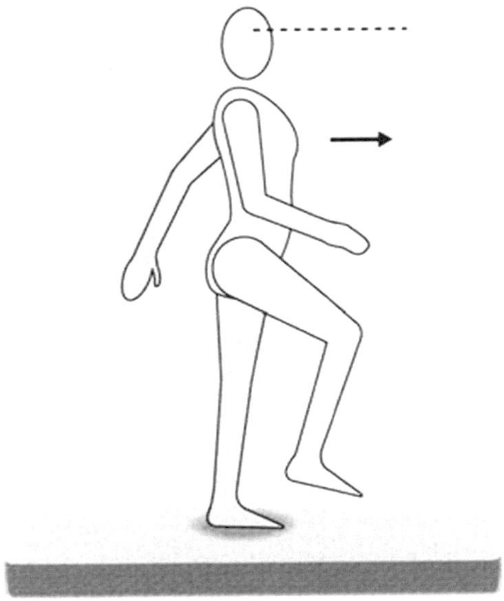

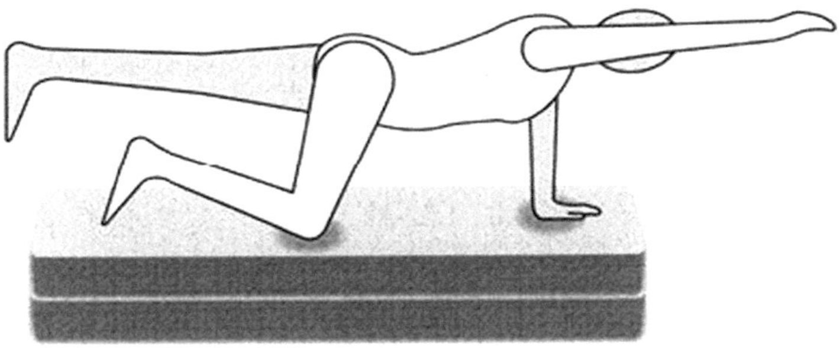

Fig. 12.16 In the quadrupedal position on a double mattress: synchronization exercises (Originally published in Cesarani and Alpini [21] published by Springer © 1999)

16. On the balance board:
    (a) The patient steps on the board with the feet centrally positioned and concentrates on a proper posture using a mirror to see her/his reflection. The therapist destabilizes the patient by means of sagittal or lateral pushes, and the patient has to maintain equilibrium using the mirror as a feedback.
    (b) The patient steps on the board with the feet centrally positioned and concentrates on a proper posture using a mirror. A laser pointer is fixated on the patient's head. A white paper square (approximately 5 cm × 5 cm) is positioned on the mirror at the level of the patient's eyes. The patient is required to maintain the laser spot into the square.

(c) The same exercise is performed while the therapist destabilizes the patient by means of sagittal or lateral pushes.
(d) The patient steps on the board with the feet centrally positioned and concentrates on a proper posture using a mirror to see her/his reflection. With eyes open, she/he transfers her/his weight from one foot to the other with a smooth flowing motion maintaining the laser spot into the square.

12.1.3 Third Week

17. The patient extends her/his right arm and lifts her/his thumb. Then she/he slowly moves the arm to and fro first in a horizontal direction and then in a vertical direction. She/he follows her/his thumb with her/his eyes only, first slowly and then increasing progressively the velocity of thumb displacement.
18. Repeat as above but simultaneously moving also the head trying to maintain the eyes still.
19. The patient opens a book in front of her/him. Then she/he moves it away from her/him extending the arms while reading it at the same time. She/he then moves it closer to her/him slowly, trying to read it, and then moves it away again, and she/he repeats the exercise several times.
20. On the soft mattress:
    (a) The patient stands on the mattress, and then she/he steps up and down, moving her/his head to and fro, during fixation of a target placed on a mirror, according to the following sequence:

Right foot up	Left foot up	Right foot down
Left foot down	Left foot up	Right foot up
Left foot down	Right foot down	

    (b) A laser pointer is fixated on the patient's head. A white paper square (approximately 5 cm×5 cm) is positioned on the mirror at the level of the patient's eyes. The patient is required to maintain the laser spot into the square while walking in place.
    (c) The patient opens a book in front of her/him and reads it, simultaneously moving it to and fro and right and left.
    (d) The patient opens a book in front of her/him, and then she/he moves it away from her/him, extending the arms while reading it. Then she/he moves it closer to her/him slowly, trying to read it. She/he then repeats the exercise several times.
21. On the balance board:
    (a) The patient steps on the board with the feet centrally positioned and concentrates on a proper posture using a mirror. With her/his index finger and limbs extended, she/he tries to touch some visual targets (different coloured paper squares) placed in different positions on a front mirror according to the commands of the therapist.

(b) The patient steps on the board on one leg with the flexed knee. A laser pointer is fixed on the patient's head. A white paper square (approximately 5 cm × 5 cm) is positioned on the mirror at the level of the patient's eyes. The patient is required to maintain the laser spot into the square.
(c) Repeat the exercise with the other leg.
(d) Repeat the exercise with the extended leg.
(e) The b–c–d exercises are performed while wearing pinhole glasses.

12.2 Home Protocol

The aim of home protocol is to maintain the results obtained with the therapist. Exercises have been subdivided according to the sequence of equilibrium. Only the most effective exercises have been comprehended into this protocol because the patient has to repeat them twice or three times a day.

Supine

1. Hold and take both your knees to the chest simultaneously, gently with the help of your hands.
2. Put a pillow under your leg. Bind a 2 kg weight on your ankle with the flexed knee; then extend it alternating the right and left legs.
3. With the legs flexed and the feet on the bed, rotate your pelvis rightward and leftward, keeping your knees flexed and your legs together.
4. Lift your pelvis simultaneously extending your arms over your head. Then reposition your arms along the body lowering your pelvis.
5. Fixate a target on the ceiling and slowly move your head rightward and leftward.
6. Look for two equidistant targets on the ceiling and then fixate them alternately first moving only the eyes and then moving only the head.
7. In the quadrupedal position, inhale and arch your back (hyperkyphosis) taking your head between your arms. Then exhale bending your head and rotating the pelvis in hyperlordosis.
8. From the supine position, shift to sitting position fixating a target straight in front of you.
9. In quadrupedal position, simultaneously extend the right arm and the left leg. Then repeat with the left arm and the right leg.
10. In prone position, lift your left arm and the right leg simultaneously also lifting the head. Then repeat with the right arm and the left leg.

Sitting

11. Extend your right arm and lift your thumb. Move slowly your arm to and fro first in a horizontal direction and then in a vertical direction. Follow your thumb with your eyes only, first slowly and then increasing progressively the velocity of thumb displacement.
12. Repeat as above but simultaneously moving also the head while trying to maintain the eyes still.

13. Move your head first slowly and then faster in all directions, fixating a target straight in front of you.
14. Inhale. Exhaling, bend forward holding your head on the right knee. Wait for 10 s. Inhaling, return to sitting position. Exhaling, bend forward holding your head on the left knee. Wait for 10 s and then inhale and return to sitting position.
15. Inhale. Exhaling, bend forward to pick an object on the floor. Inhale and take it over your head and then fixate it for 10 s. Inhale. Exhaling, bend forward and place the object on the floor.
16. Open a book in front of you. Read it while at the same time moving the book right and left and then to and fro.

Standing

17. Fixate yourself in a mirror. Align your position correctly. Maintain equilibrium for 1 min and then close your eyes visualizing your correct position and remain in this position for at least 1 min.
18. Repeat the same, standing on a soft mattress.
19. Fixate yourself in a mirror; then, keeping your feet still, bend your trunk to and fro and right and left with eyes closed standing on a soft mattress.
20. Hold a small object and lift it over your head. Fixate it. Inhale. Then exhale and bend yourself forward placing the object on the floor. Wait for 10 s, and then inhaling again, lift the object over your head.
21. Standing on soft mattress, hold a small object and lift it over your head. Fixate it. Lift it over your head, and then, with your arms straight, move the object in circles of increasing width, and simultaneously bending your trunk and your knees, take it on the floor.

Moving

22. Walk with eyes closed, moving the head to and fro.
23. Walk while reading a book.
24. Walk on a soft mattress, reading a book.
25. Step up and down, moving to and fro your head, according to the following sequence:

Right foot up	Left foot up	Right foot down
Left foot down	Left foot up	Right foot up
Left foot down	Right foot down	

12.2.1 Counselling

Collar use has to be restricted to the first 3–4 days after the accident [18].

In WABD QTF grades I and II act as usual [19, 20], and, furthermore:

Maintain regular and constant aerobic physical activity, e.g. rapid walking (not running neither jogging) 30′/day three times/week

Sleep using two pillows in order to maintain the head lifted about 20°

Avoid maintaining the same position of the head/neck for more than 30 min
Change position every 30 min and mobilize your head and shoulders
Maintain proper position of the head/neck in particular and check proper position when watching television and working on PC

- Maintain adequate water intake (at least 1.5 l for females and 2 l for males)
- Restrict alcohol intake (less than 120 ml for women and 240 ml for men)
- Restrict smoking and, obviously, avoid drug abuse

Note. The contents of this chapter are partially based on *Dizziness and Vertigo Following Whiplash Injuries* (A. Cesarani, D. Alpini) in A. Cesarani, D. Alpini (1999) Vertigo and Dizziness Rehabilitation – The MCS Method. Springer, Milan, p 168.

References

1. Foreman SM, Croft AC (1988) Whiplash injuries. The cervical acceleration/deceleration syndrome. Williams & Wilkins, Baltimore
2. Spitzer WO, Skovron ML, Salmi LR, Cassidy JD, Duranceau J, Suissa S, Zeiss E (1995) Scientific monograph of the Quebec Task Force on Whiplash-Associated Disorders: redefining "whiplash" and its management. Spine (Phila Pa 1976) 20(8 Suppl):1S–73S
3. Ikeda K, Kobayashi T (1967) Mechanisms and origin of so-called whiplash injury. Clin Surg 22:1655–1660
4. Ommaya AK et al (1968) Whiplash and brain damage. JAMA 204:75–79
5. Pedler A, Sterling M (2013) Patients with chronic whiplash can be subgrouped on the basis of symptoms of sensory hypersensitivity and posttraumatic stress. Pain 154(9):1640–1648
6. Epley J (1992) The canalith reposition procedure: for the treatment of benign paroxysmal vertigo. Otolaryngol Head Neck Surg 107:399–404
7. Semont A, Sterkers JM (1980) Reeducation vestibulaires. Les Cahiers D' Orl 15:305
8. Shih CP, Wang CH (2013) Supine to prolonged lateral position: a novel therapeutic maneuver for posterior canal benign paroxysmal positional vertigo. J Neurol 260(5):1375–1381
9. Sugita-Kitajima A, Sato S, Mikami K, Mukaide M, Koizuka I (2010) Does vertigo disappear only by rolling over? Rehabilitation for benign paroxysmal positional vertigo. Acta Otolaryngol 130(1):84–88
10. Jenkins A et al (1986) Brain lesions detected by magnetic resonance imaging in mild and severe head injuries. Lancet 23:445–446
11. McKenzie JA, Williarns JF (1975) The effect of collision severity on the motion of the head and neck during "whiplash". J Biomech 8:257–259
12. Drukker J, van der Wal JC (1990) Centrai verbindingen van het vestibulaire apparaat. In: Fischer AJEM, Oosterveld WJ (eds) Duizeligheid en Evenwichtsstoomissen. Data Medica, Utrecht, pp 29–45
13. Drukker J, Jansen JC (1975) Compendium anatomie. De Tijdstroom, Lochem
14. Gluckman PD, Beedle AS, Hanson MA, Low FM (2013) Human growth: evolutionary and life history perspectives. Nestle Nutr Inst Workshop Ser 71:89–102
15. Tardieu C, Bonneau N, Hecquet J, Boulay C, Marty C, Legaye J, Duval-Beaupère G (2013) How is sagittal balance acquired during bipedal gait acquisition? Comparison of neonatal and adult pelves in three dimensions. Evolutionary implications. J Hum Evol 65(2): 209–222
16. Bramble DM, Lieberman DE (2004) Endurance running and the evolution of Homo. Nature 432(7015):345–352
17. Ivanenko YP, Wright WG, St George RJ, Gurfinkel VS (2013) Trunk orientation, stability, and quadrupedalism. Front Neurol 4:20

18. Kongsted A, Qerama E, Kasch H, Bendix T, Bach FW, Korsholm L, Jensen TS (2007) Neck collar, "act-as-usual" or active mobilization for whiplash injury? A randomized parallel-group trial. Spine (Phila Pa 1976) 32(17):1933
19. Dehner C, Kraus M, Schöll H, Schneider F, Richter P, Kramer M (2012) Therapy recommendation "act as usual" in patients with whiplash injuries QTF I°. Glob J Health Sci 4(6):36–42
20. Dehner C, Elbel M, Strobel P, Scheich M, Schneider F, Krischak G, Kramer M (2009) Grade II whiplash injuries to the neck: what is the benefit for patients treated by different physical therapy modalities? Patient Saf Surg 3(1):2
21. Cesarani A, Alpini D) (1999) Vertigo and dizziness rehabilitation – the MCS method. Springer, Milan/Heidelberg

13 Phobic Postural Vertigo

The syndrome of phobic postural vertigo (PPV) was described by Brandt [1], and it is characterized by subjective dizziness and a disturbance of balance while standing and walking, despite normal values in clinical balance tests.

PPV is sometimes considered as one of the primary and secondary somatoform dizziness syndromes [2–4] or a visual vertigo [5] or a chronic subjective dizziness [6]. Anyway, it is one of the most frequent causes of chronic dizziness. PPV sometimes represents an impaired compensation of a vestibular neuritis with a consequent high impact on quality of life [7].

Instrumented analysis of postural sway in PPV reveals subtle abnormalities such as increased muscular energy expenditure and high-frequency body sway during quiet standing [8, 9].

The *key lesion* is a shift in the coordination of open- and closed-loop mechanisms of postural control: patients with PPV use sensory feedback inadequately during undisturbed stance, and this impairs postural performance, while equilibrium control is normal when a difficult balance task, such as tandem stance on foam rubber with eyes closed, is required just like to that of healthy persons in the same stance conditions [10].

In other words, in PPV patients, subjective imbalance is caused by inappropriate balance strategies with higher levels of antigravity muscle activity and co-contraction during the conscious concentration on control of postural stability.

In fact, in normal subjects, maintenance of balance is achieved unconsciously and conscious control is required only in unusual and therefore unadapted balance tasks, e.g. on slippery ground or when walking on a beam. The performance of the postural control system in PPV is changed in two ways:

- The steady-state behaviour of the open-loop control mechanisms is significantly altered.
- The effective range of the open-loop regime is shortened and the feedback threshold of the closed-loop regime is reduced.

Thereby the open- and closed-loop control system as a whole is not optimally tuned. The control systems are working but in an inadequate way, so that they are not as smoothly and efficiently functioning as in healthy subject.

D.C. Alpini et al., *Vertigo Rehabilitation Protocols*,
DOI 10.1007/978-3-319-05482-7_13,

The consequent *key impairment* is postural fear and the *key disability* is a decreased motor and social autonomy due to a phobic behaviour.

Patients with PPV use sensory feedback inadequately during undisturbed stance, and this impairs postural performance and the subjective imbalance further increases conscious control of posture. This condition is sustained by a mismatch between general proprioception (from muscle, ligaments and joints) and the special proprioception (from maculae and cristae) during postural control. The integration and elaboration of general and special proprioception by cerebellum has been proposed by Drukker [11, 12]. He described the connections of the vestibular system to the spino-cerebello-vestibulospinal circuitry (Fig.13.1): proprioceptive inputs from muscles, ligaments and joints are integrated and elaborated in the cerebellum together with information from maculae and cristae and then from cerebellum efferent pathways return to spinal motoneurons through another elaboration in the vestibular nuclei (with special regard to the lateral Deiter's nucleus).

13.1 Treatment

Treatment is aimed to obtain the unconsciousness of postural control reducing energy expending. Thus, rehab has to be pointed to restore correct integration between special and general proprioception and the correct internal representation of posture in order to recover appropriate balance strategies.

13.1.1 First Week

1. The patient, with the legs flexed and the feet on the bed, rotates her/his pelvis rightward and leftward keeping her/his knees flexed and the legs together (Fig. 13.2).
2. The patient lifts her/his pelvis taking simultaneously extending the arms extended over her/his head. She/he then repositions the arms along the body, lowering the pelvis.
3. In the quadrupedal position, the patient inhales and arches her/his back (hyperkyphosis), holding the head between the arms. She/he then exhales, flexing the head and rotating the pelvis in hyperlordosis (Fig. 13.3).
4. In the prone position, the patient lifts her/his left arm and the right leg while holding her/his forehead over the bed. She/he repeats with the right arm and the left leg (Fig. 13.4).
5. She/He repeats the procedure as above but also simultaneously lifting the head.
6. In the sitting position, the patient first inhales. Then, exhaling, she/he bends forward holding the head on the right knee. She/he waits 10 s and then, inhaling, she/he returns to the sitting position. Then, exhaling, she/he bends forward holding the head on the left knee. She/he waits 10 s and then, inhaling, she/he returns in the sitting position (Fig. 13.5).

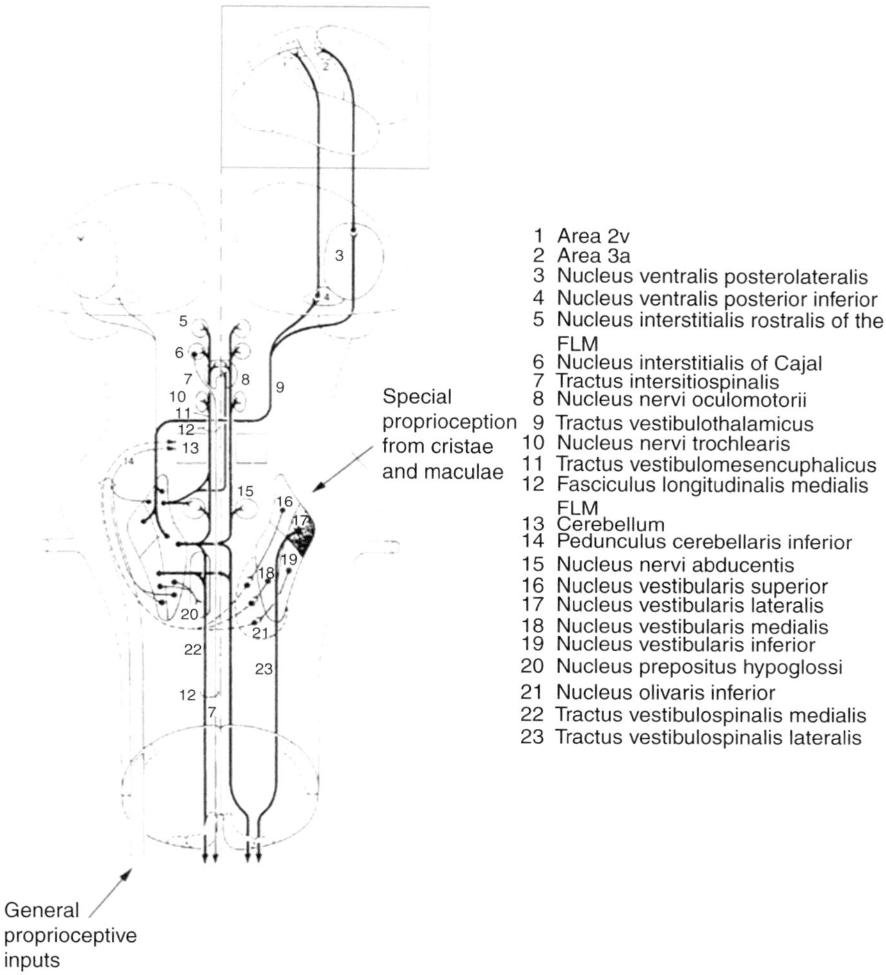

Fig. 13.1 The connections of the vestibular system: efferent connections of the vestibular nuclei and the spino-cerebello-vestibulospinal circuitry: the so-called spino-cerebello-vestibulospinal circuitry is shown. General proprioception information (from muscles, ligaments and joints) is integrated and elaborated in the cerebellum together with special proprioception information from maculae and cristae. From the cerebellum, efferent pathways return to spinal motoneurons through another elaboration in the vestibular nuclei (with special regard to the lateral Deiter's nucleus) (Originally published in Cesarani et al. [14] published by Springer ©1996)

7. In the sitting position, the patient grasps a stick with her/his hands. Then, she/he holds it against the upper part of the sternum at the level of sternoclavicular joint. Then, rhythmically, she/he performs backward displacements of the shoulders in order to mobilize the cervicothoracic junction.

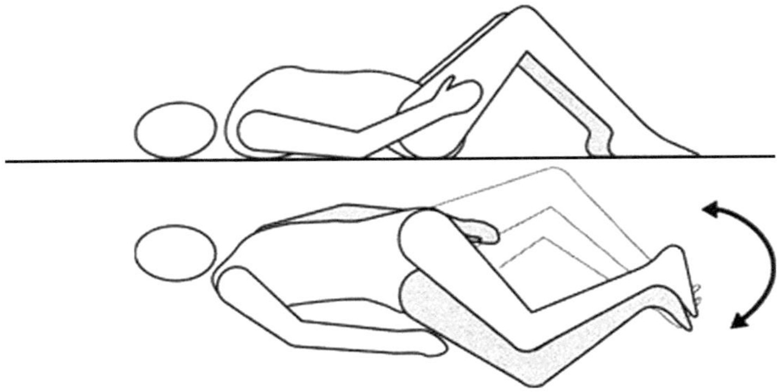

Fig. 13.2 Rotation of the pelvis (Originally published in Cesarani and Alpini [15] published by Springer © 1999)

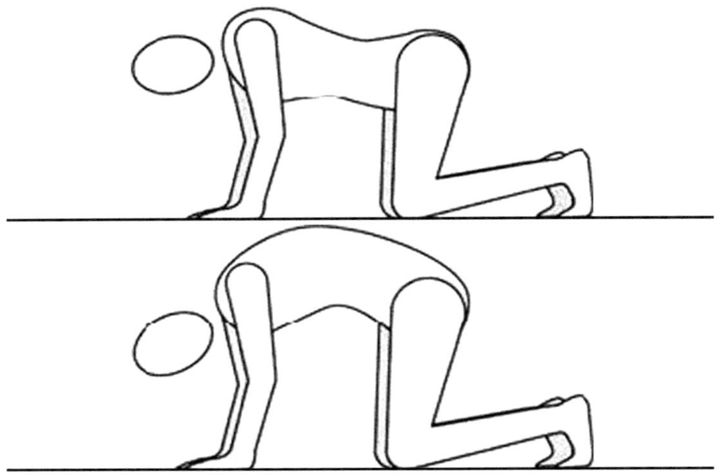

Fig. 13.3 Movements of the pelvis in the quadrupedal position (Originally published in Cesarani and Alpini [15] published by Springer © 1999)

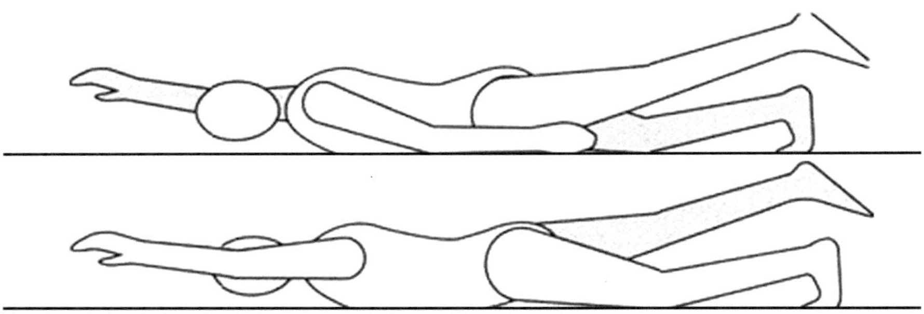

Fig. 13.4 In the prone position, simultaneous extension of one arm and the opposite leg (Originally published in Cesarani and Alpini [15] published by Springer © 1999)

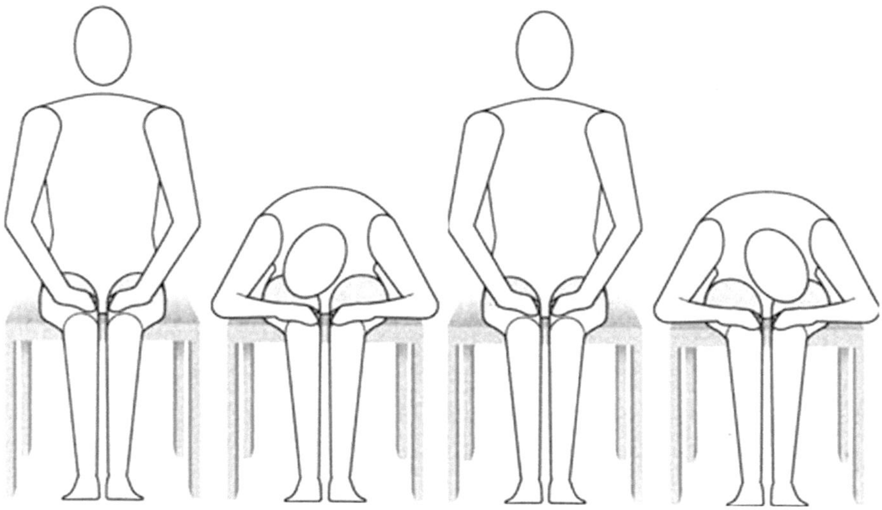

Fig. 13.5 Bending the trunk and holding the forehead on a knee (Originally published in Cesarani and Alpini [15] published by Springer © 1999)

13.1.2 Second Week

8. In the recumbent position, the patient rotates the head rightward and fixates a target on the lateral wall. Then she/he straightens her/his head maintaining the visual fixation. She/he counts until ten and then rotates the head.
9. The patient rotates her/his head leftward and fixates a target on the lateral wall. Then she/he straightens the head, maintaining the visual fixation. She/he counts until 10 and then rotates the head.
10. From the supine position, the patient moves to the sitting position fixating a point on her/his right (Fig. 13.6a).
11. From the supine position, the patient moves to the sitting position fixating a point on her/his left (Fig. 13.6b).
12. In the supine position, the patient moves the head first slowly and then more rapidly in all directions fixating a target straight in front of her/him.
13. Sitting, the patient looks for three targets sited, respectively, in front of her/him, at her/his left and at her/his right. She/he fixates the front target, then moves rapidly the head, fixating the right-hand target. Now she/he turns leftward the head, maintaining the fixation of the right-hand target. She/He fixates the front target. Now, she/he rapidly moves her/his head leftward and fixates the left-hand target. Then she/he turns rightward the head, maintaining the fixation of the left-hand target.
14. Standing, the patient holds a small object and lift it over her/his head and she/he fixate it. She/he inhales. Then exhaling she/he bends forward, picking up the object on the floor. She/he waits 10 s, and then inhaling she/he lifts again the object over the head.

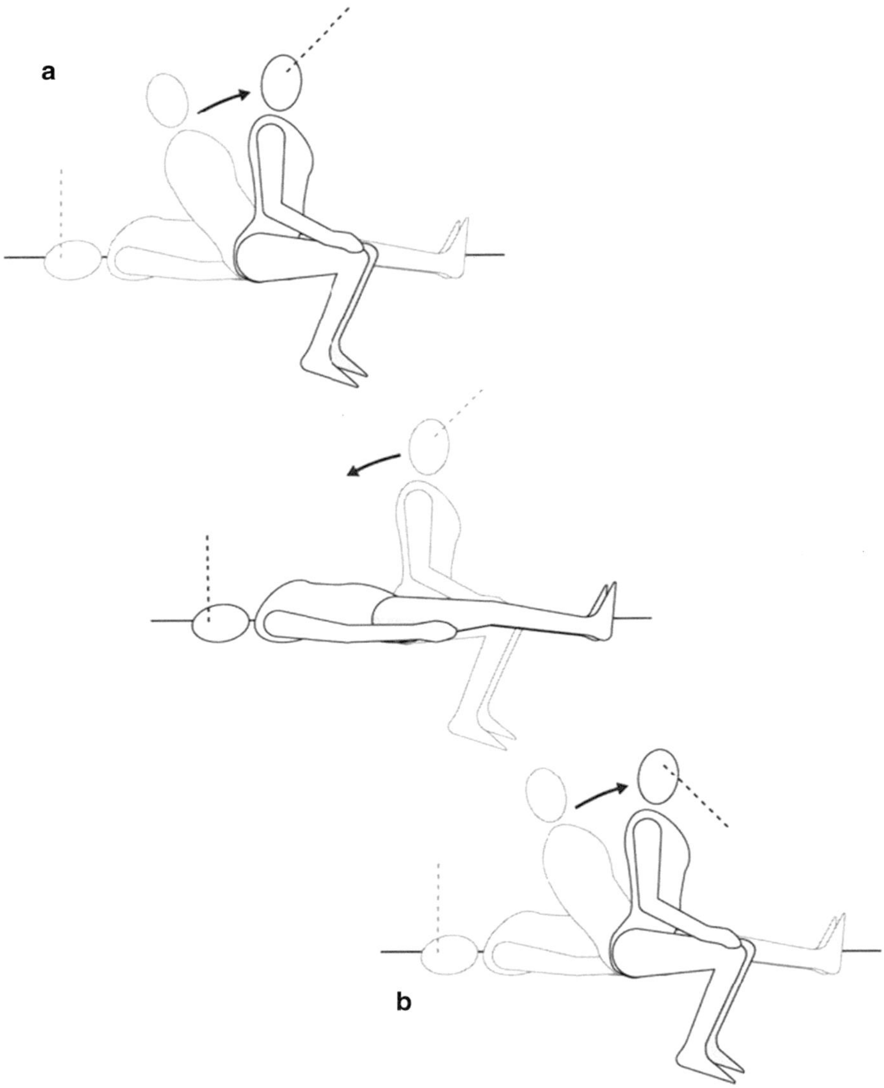

Fig. 13.6 (**a**, **b**) From the supine to the sitting position with simultaneous fixation of a target (Originally published in Cesarani and Alpini [15] published by Springer © 1999)

15. The patient holds a little object and lifts it over the head, fixating it. She/he lifts it over her/his head and then, with straight arms, she/he moves the object in circles of increasing width and, simultaneously bending her/his trunk and knees, she/he picks up from the floor.
16. She/he repeats the exercise on a soft mattress.

17. On a balance board.
    (a) The patient steps on the board with the feet centrally positioned and concentrates on a proper posture using a mirror to see her/his reflection. With eyes open she/he transfers her/his weight from one foot to the other with a smooth flowing motion maintaining a correct postural alignment of the head and the trunk. In this case, feedback is visual, provided by the mirror.
    (b) The patient repeats the exercise but with eyes closed. The therapist controls the patient's movements in order to avoid falls. The therapist is on the back of the patient, helping her/him to maintain correct postural alignment of the trunk. In this case, feedback is somatosensorial, provided by the hands of the therapist.

13.1.3 Third Week

The patient performs the exercises of the cybernertics phase n. 8–9, 13, 15–16, 17 during contemporary TENS stimulation, placing the electrodes on the paravertebral muscles of the both sides [13].

13.2 Home Protocol

Exercises have been subdivided according to different phases of equilibrium, from supine to standing to moving. In each phase, there is a progression from mechanic to synergetics exercises. They are not based on habituation mechanisms, but on sensorimotor learning phenomena.

Home exercises can never substitute the therapeutic programmes shown in the previous section performed with the therapist. Home exercises complete the therapy and maintain the results obtained.

Supine

1. With the legs flexed and the feet on the bed, rotate your pelvis rightward and leftward, keeping your knees flexed and your legs together.
2. Lift your pelvis simultaneously, extending your arms over your head. Then reposition your arms along the body, lowering your pelvis.
3. Grasp a stick. Take your extended arms over your head and then return in the original position.
4. Rotate your head rightward and fixate a target on the lateral wall. Then straighten your head straight, maintaining the visual fixation. Count until ten and then rotate your head.
5. Rotate your head leftward and fix a target on the lateral wall. Then straighten your head, maintaining the visual fixation. Count up to ten and then rotate your head.
6. From the supine position, shift to sitting position, fixating a point straight in front of you.

7. From the supine position, shift to sitting position, fixating a point sited on your right.
8. From the supine position, shift to sitting position, fixating a point sited on your left.

Sitting

9. Move your head first slowly and then more rapidly in all directions, fixating a target straight in front of you.
10. Look for three targets sited, respectively, in front of you, on your left and at your right. Fixate the front target, then move your head rapidly, fixating the right-sited target. Now rotate your head leftward, maintaining the fixation of the right-hand target. Fixate the frontal target. Now, suddenly, move your head leftward and fixate the left-hand target. Then rotate your head rightward, maintaining the fixation of the left-hand target.
11. Inhale. Exhaling, bend forward holding your head on the right knee. Wait 10 s. Inhaling, return to the sitting position. Exhaling, bend forward holding your head on the left knee. Wait 10 s and then, inhaling, return to the sitting position.
12. Inhale. Exhaling, bend forward to pick up an object on the floor. Inhale and take it up over your head and then fixate it for 10 s. Inhale. Exhaling, bend forward and place the object on the floor.

Standing

13. Hold a small object and then lift it over your head and fixate it. With your extended arms, move in circles of increasing width, maintaining the fixation of the object.
14. Repeat with eyes closed.
15. Repeat the exercise again, standing on a soft mattress.
16. Hold a small object and lift it over your head. Fixate it. Inhale. Then exhale and bend yourself forward, placing the object on the floor. Wait 10 s and then, inhaling, lift the object over your head.
17. Hold a small object and lift it over your head. Fixate it. Lift it over your head and then, with your arms straight, move the object in circles of increasing width and, simultaneously bending your trunk and knees, place it on the floor.
18. Repeat the exercise on a soft mattress.

13.2.1 Counselling

It is important to pay attention to lifestyle and to maintain usual daily activities.

The main suggestions are:

- To control own Body Mass Index (BMI)
- BMI is correlated to body fatness and it is calculated as body weight (in Kilos) divided by square height (in metres); e.g. a subject weighed 70 kg and 1.74 m height has a BMI as follows: $70/(1.74 \times 1.74) = 23.1$. Normal values are between 18,5 and 24,9 (World Health Organization, WHO).

- To avoid to remain too much hours in own home sitting on a chair watching television
- To walk alone at least 30 min twice a day
- To perform regular and constant aerobic physical activity: e.g. rapid walking (not running neither jogging) 30′/day three times/week
- To maintain a diet rich of fruit and vegetables (five servings/day) especially in autumn and spring
- To maintain adequate water intake (at least 1.5 l for females and 2 l for males)
- To avoid industrial food
- To restrict alcohol intake (less than 120 ml for women and 240 ml for men)
- To restrict smoke and, obviously, to avoid drug abuse
- To maintain regular sleep/awake cycles, sleeping at least 8 h/night starting before midnight
- To sleep using two pillows in order to maintain the head lifted about 20°

References

1. Brandt T (1996) Phobic postural vertigo. Neurology 46(6):1515–1519
2. Furman JM, Jacob RG (1997) Psychiatric dizziness. Neurology 48(5):1161–1166
3. Eckhardt-Henn A, Breuer P, Thomalske C, Hoffmann SO, Hopf HC (2003) Anxiety disorders and other psychiatric subgroups in patients complaining of dizziness. J Anxiety Disord 17(4):369–388
4. Best C, Eckhardt-Henn A, Diener G, Bense S, Breuer P, Dieterich M (2006) Interaction of somatoform and vestibular disorders. J Neurol Neurosurg Psychiatry 77(5):658–664
5. Bronstein AM (1995) Visual vertigo syndrome: clinical and posturography findings. J Neurol Neurosurg Psychiatry 59(5):472–476
6. Staab JP, Ruckenstein MJ (2007) Expanding the differential diagnosis of chronic dizziness. Arch Otolaryngol Head Neck Surg 133(2):170–176
7. Brandt T, Strupp M, Novozhilov S, Krafczyk S (2012) Artificial neural network posturography detects the transition of vestibular neuritis to phobic postural vertigo. J Neurol 259: 182–184
8. Krafczyk S, Schlamp V, Dieterich M, Haberhauer P, Brandt T (1999) Increased body sway at 3.5–8 Hz in patients with phobic postural vertigo. Neurosci Lett 259(3):149–152
9. Holmberg J, Karlberg M, Fransson PA, Magnusson M (2003) Phobic postural vertigo: body sway during vibratory proprioceptive stimulation. Neuroreport 14(7):1007–1011
10. Wuehr M, Pradhan C, Novozhilov S, Krafczyk S, Brandt T, Jahn K, Schniepp R (2013) Inadequate interaction between open- and closed-loop postural control in phobic postural vertigo. J Neurol 260:1314–1323
11. Drukker J, van der Wal JC (1990) Centrai verbindingen van het vestibulaire apparaat. In: Fischer AJEM, Oosterveld WJ (eds) Duizeligheid en Evenwichtsstoomissen. Data Medica, Utrecht, pp 29–45
12. Drukker J, Jansen JC (1975) Compendium anatomie. De Tijdstroom, Lochem
13. Chu H, Li MH, Juan SH, Chiou WY (2012) Effects of transcutaneous electrical nerve stimulation on motion sickness induced by rotary chair: a crossover study. J Altern Complement Med 18(5):494–500
14. Cesarani A et al (1996) Whiplash injuries – diagnosis and treatment, 1st edn. Springer, Milan/Heidelberg
15. Cesarani A, Alpini D) (1999) Vertigo and dizziness rehabilitation – the MCS method. Springer, Milan/Heidelberg

Autonomic Vertigo 14

In 2003 Pappas [1] showed a subgroup of patients with spontaneous vertigo who also demonstrated symptoms and findings consistent with poor autonomic regulation, that is to say, vestibular symptomatology can occur in relation to autonomic dysfunction. He defined this clinical entity as autonomic vertigo (AV).

Patients affected with AV describe symptoms consistent with spontaneous, rotational vertigo or postural vertigo and distinct lightheadedness. In some cases, vertigo failed to improve or worsened with prior treatment of low-sodium diet or diuretics.

Autonomic symptoms include palpitations, chronic fatigue, cold extremities and previous fainting. A history of mitral valve prolapse is frequent.

More recently Kim and Lee [2] showed that in patients with benign paroxysmal positional vertigo (BPPV), residual dizziness after successful treatment may be associated with sympathoneural autonomic dysfunction.

The *key lesion* of AV is dysregulation of autonomic vestibular responses. Although the neural signals generated from the hair cells of the otolith organs and semicircular canals are important in the maintenance of equilibrium and orientation, they influence also autonomic control, and thus, the third group of vestibular reflexes are the vestibulosympathetic or vestibulo-autonomic reflexes (VAR), provided by the labyrinth, through vestibular nuclei, besides the vestibulo-ocular (VOR) and the vestibulospinal (VSR) reflexes [3, 4].

Evidence suggests that the vestibular system plays a role in postural-related adjustments in blood pressure. Much like equilibrium, blood pressure regulation involves multiple feedback systems. The most recognized feedback system for blood pressure regulation is the baroreflex that senses mechanical changes in the blood vessels of the aortic arch and carotid bodies. However, Carter and Ray [5] provided direct evidence that the vestibulosympathetic reflex is a robust vascular reflex in humans and that the vestibular system is important in postural blood pressure regulation. Aging, through aging processes involving hair cells, attenuates the vestibulosympathetic reflex in humans and, in this way, it may contribute to the increased prevalence of orthostatic hypotension with age [6].

D.C. Alpini et al., *Vertigo Rehabilitation Protocols*,
DOI 10.1007/978-3-319-05482-7_14,

The vestibular autonomic reflexes influence also muscle sympathetic nerve activity (MSNA) which responses are specific to activation of the otolith organs and not the semicircular canals [7]. Sauder et al. [8] showed that the sensitivity of the vestibulosympathetic reflex is greater in the upright compared with the prone position supporting and further expanding the concept that the vestibulosympathetic reflex is a robust autonomic reflex.

Yates [9] showed that considerable evidence exists to suggest that both sympathetic and respiratory outflow from the central nervous system are influenced by the vestibular system and otolith organs that respond to pitch rotations seem to play a predominant role in producing vestibulosympathetic and vestibulo-respiratory responses.

Carter et al. [10] showed the additive neural interaction between mental stress and the vestibulosympathetic reflex: this interaction may induce post-traumatic stress disorders with vertigo and dizziness [11].

The autonomic nervous system, the hormonal systems and the postural control are strictly interconnected as assessed, for example, in adolescent idiopathic scoliosis in which the pathogenesis of developmental disharmony between somatic and autonomic nervous systems is postulated [12]. In fact, normal mechanisms involved in trunk growth, acquired in evolution and unique to humans, are driven hormonally and supplemented by the sympathetic nervous system acting symmetrically. Hormonal abnormalities, e.g. insulin resistance and hyperinsulinemia, are frequently observed in AV patients.

Pappas proposed as management of AV fluid loading, dietary changes, exercise and patient education.

Rehab is aimed to improve postural control and to re-coordinate visuo-vestibular balance control with respiration.

14.1 Exercises in the Gymnasium

14.1.1 First Week

1. The patient lifts her/his left leg, extending the knee; she/he maintains this position for 10 s and then she/he extends the right knee (Fig. 14.1).
2. The patient extends the left arm over her/his head and simultaneously she/he moves the flexed right leg to the chest, with the help of her/his hands. She/he maintains this position for 10 s and then repeats with the opposite arm and leg (Fig. 14.2).
3. The patient holds her/his left leg against the chest with the knee flexed, maintaining this position for 10 s and then repeats the exercise with the right leg. She/he then holds both knees against her/his chest (Fig. 14.3).
4. In the quadrupedal position, she/he extends her/his right arm and left leg and then repeats with the opposite arm and leg. She/he repeats this exercise in prone position (Fig. 14.4).

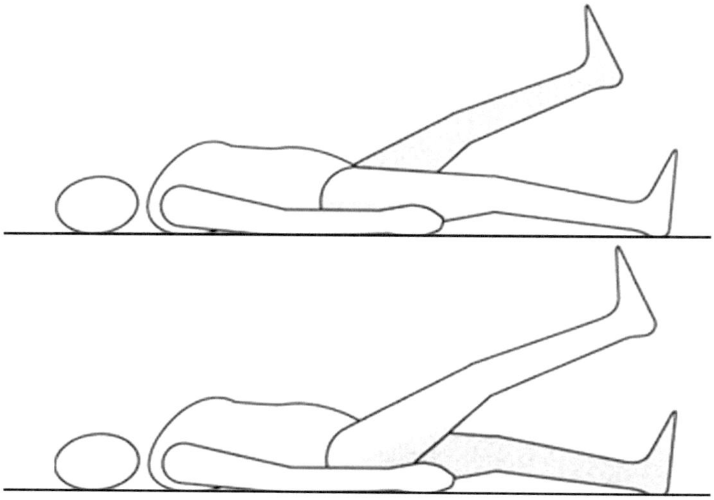

Fig. 14.1 Extension of the knees (Originally published in Cesarani and Alpini [14] published by Springer © 1999)

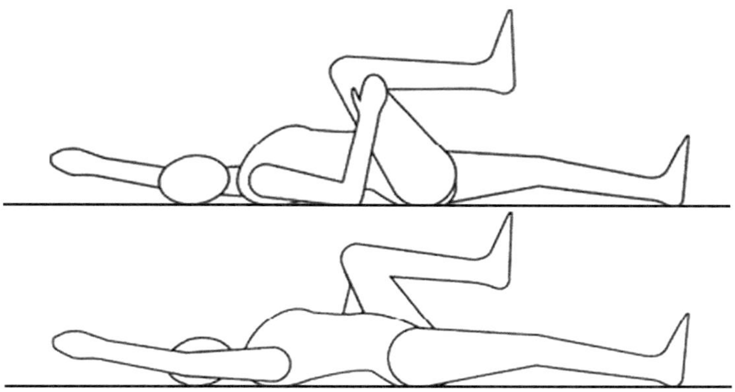

Fig. 14.2 Flexion of the knee with simultaneous extension of the opposite arm (Originally published in Cesarani and Alpini [14] published by Springer © 1999)

5. The patient, with the hands on a chair, lifts her-/himself on tiptoes, maintaining this position for 30 s (Fig. 14.5a).
6. The patient, with her/his hands on a chair, lifts her-/himself on her/his heels, maintaining this position for 30 s (Fig. 14.5b).
7. The patient walks (Fig. 14.6a) with the arms still.
8. The patients oscillates her/his arms rhythmically as during gait (Fig. 14.6b).

a

b

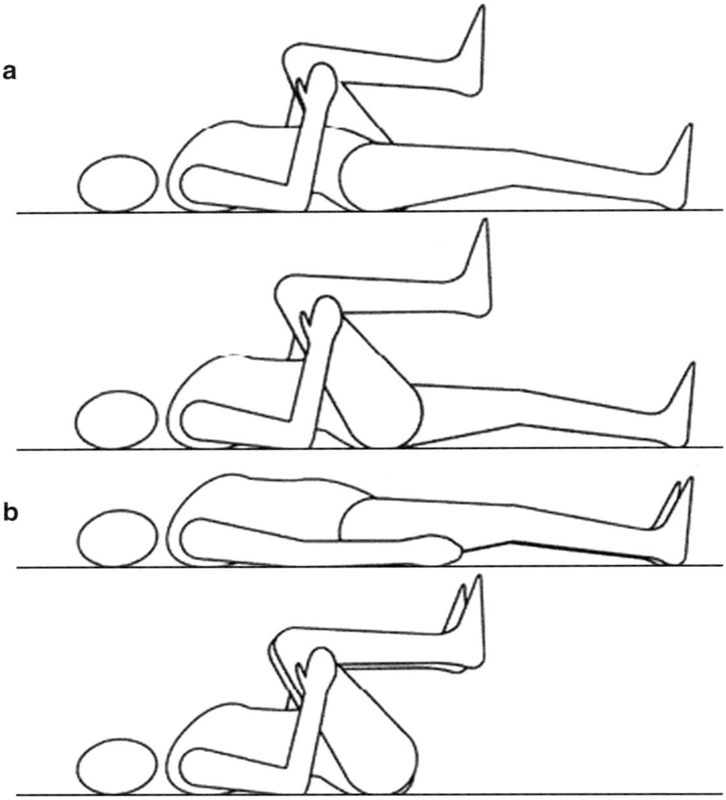

Fig. 14.3 (**a**, **b**) Exercises of the knees for the pelvis (Originally published in Cesarani and Alpini [14] published by Springer © 1999)

9. She/he repeats the stepping movement, oscillating the arms at the same time (Fig. 14.6c).
10. Standing on a balance board:
    (a) The patient oscillates to and fro, maintaining equilibrium with the arms.
    (b) The patient oscillates from side to side, maintaining equilibrium with the arms.

14.1.2 Second Week

1. The patient stands quietly in an upright position standing on tiptoes and fixating a target on a mirror. In this case, she/he receives from two planes of fixation: the target and her/his image. She/he needs to be able to extract the correct fixation information from visual inputs (Fig. 14.7a).
2. The patient repeats the same exercise standing on heels (Fig. 14.7b).

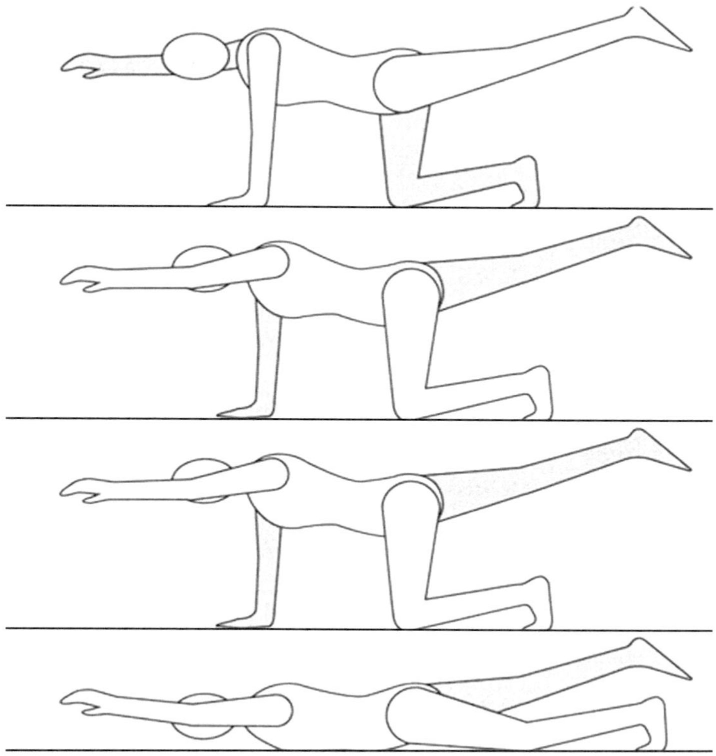

Fig. 14.4 Arm–leg synchronization (Originally published in Cesarani and Alpini [14] published by Springer © 1999)

3. The patient rides a cylinder, fixating a target on a mirror and the therapist destabilizes her/him (Fig. 14.8).
4. Standing on a soft mattress:
   (a) The patient swings around her/his ankles, maintaining fixation of a target on a mirror (Fig. 14.9a).
   (b) The patient repeats oscillations but now using the hip (Fig. 14.9b).
   (c) The patient holds a small object over the head. Fixating it, she/he moves the object in small circles. Then, maintaining circular movements of the object and its fixation, she/he bends her-/himself, placing the object to the floor, paying attention to breathing (Fig. 14.10).
   (d) The patient maintains equilibrium in different conditions, fixating a target on a mirror (Fig. 14.11): in quiet standing (A), crossing her/his legs (B), resisting to therapist's destabilization and (C) standing on one leg (D).
   (e) The patient synchronizes her/his arm and leg (Fig. 14.12): in quadrupedal position (A) and standing on the mattress during stepping (B): It is better if two mattresses have been overlapped.

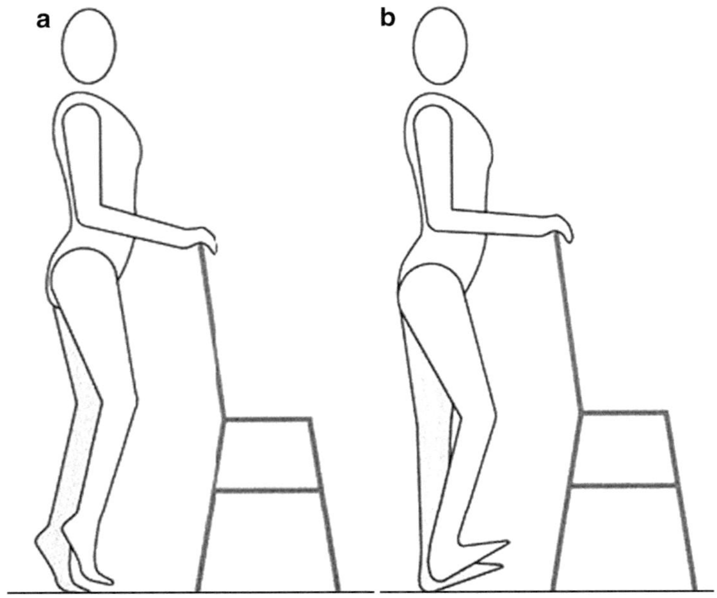

Fig. 14.5 (**a**, **b**) Equilibrium on tiptoes and heels (Originally published in Cesarani and Alpini [14] published by Springer © 1999)

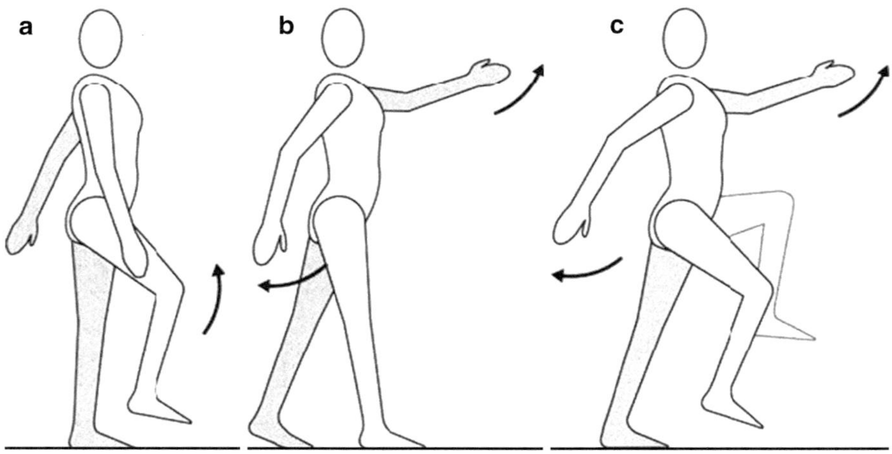

Fig. 14.6 (**a**) Stepping; (**b**) oscillations of the arms; (**c**) stepping with simultaneous oscillations of the arms (Originally published in Cesarani and Alpini [14] published by Springer © 1999)

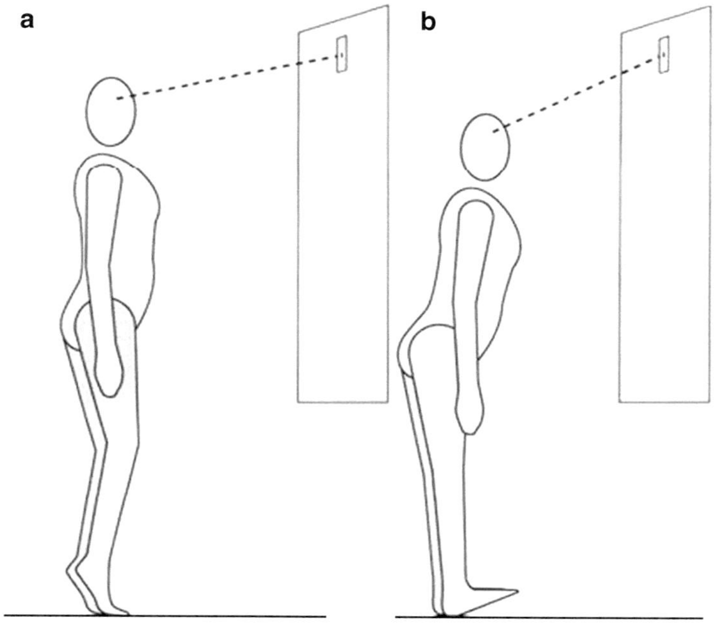

Fig. 14.7 Exercises on tiptoes (**a**) and heels (**b**) fixating a target on a mirror (Originally published in Cesarani and Alpini [14] published by Springer © 1999)

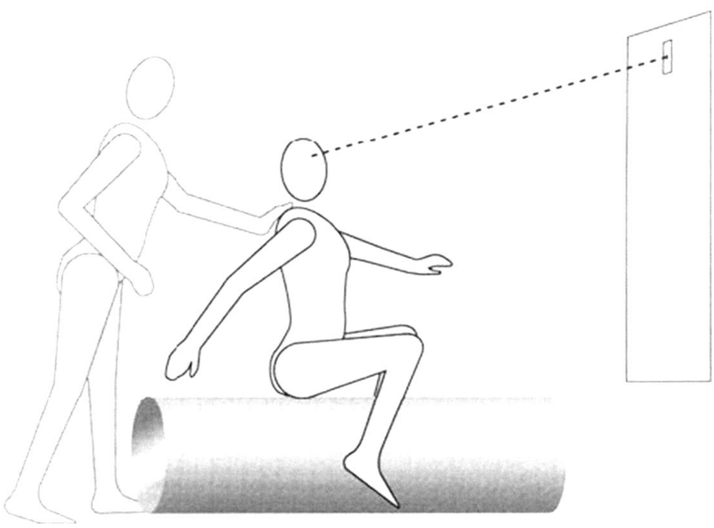

Fig. 14.8 Equilibrium riding a cylinder fixating a target on a mirror (Originally published in Cesarani and Alpini [14] published by Springer © 1999)

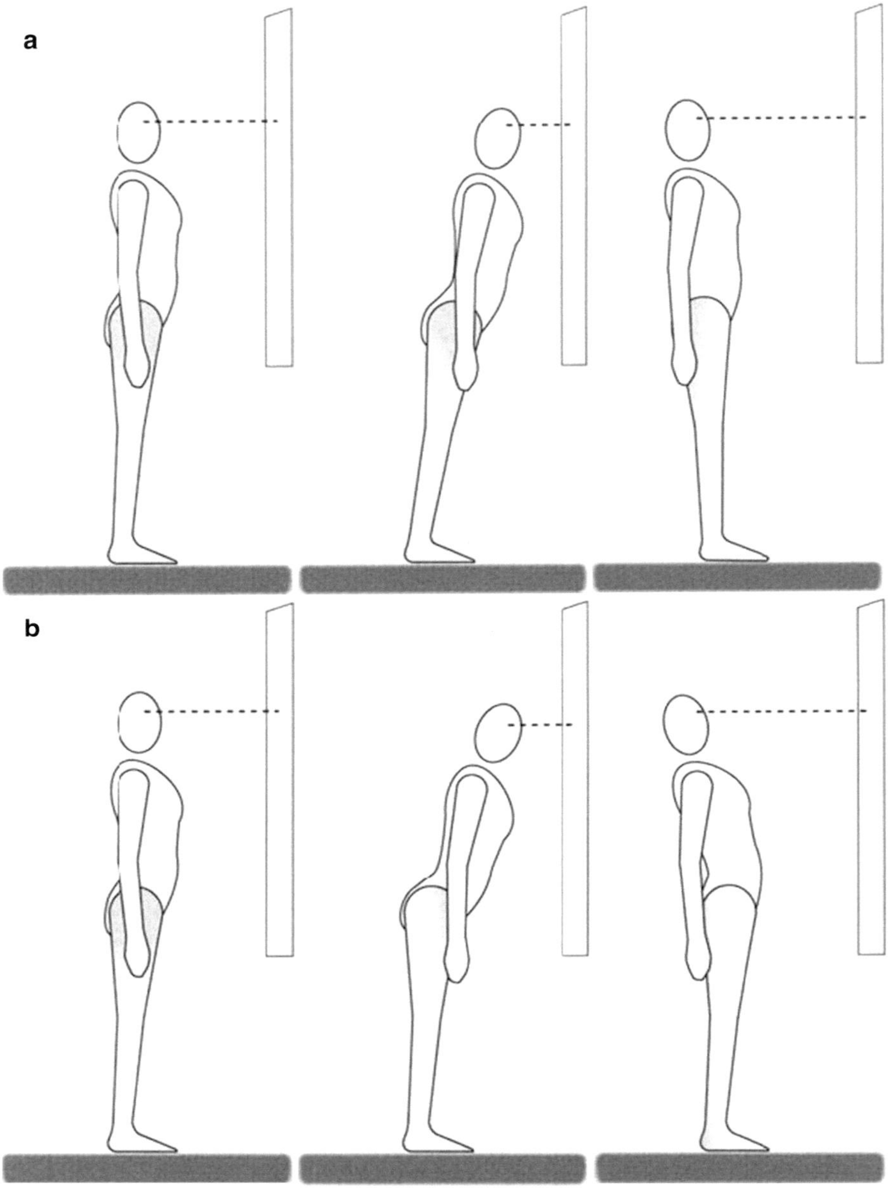

Fig. 14.9 Ankle (**a**) and hip (**b**) oscillations standing on a mattress (Originally published in Cesarani and Alpini [14] published by Springer © 1999)

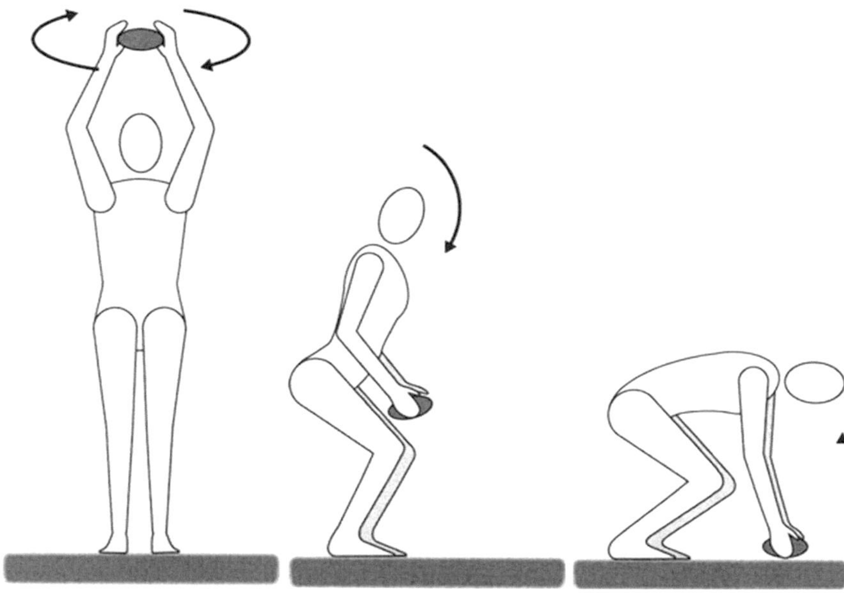

Fig. 14.10 Lifting over the head an object and turning it during fixation. The patient then places it on the floor (Originally published in Cesarani and Alpini [14] published by Springer © 1999)

5. Standing on a balance board:
   (a) The patient stands quietly on the platform and rhythmically she/he oscillates the arms, maintaining equilibrium.
   (b) The patients repeats the same exercise while fixating a target on a mirror

   In both exercises, the therapist helps the patient to pay attention to breathing.

14.1.3 Third Week

1. The patient stands quietly on a soft mattress:
   (a) In front of her/him, there is a mirror with several targets placed in different positions (paper squares of different colours or marked with different numbers). According to the therapist's orders, he has to point one target as fast and as precisely as possible (Fig. 14.13).
   (b) The patient tries to maintain equilibrium during hyperventilation.
   (c) The patient repeats the same exercise while fixating a target on a mirror.
2. The patients stands on a balance board trying to maintain equilibrium during hyperventilation.
   (a) The patient repeats the same exercise while oscillating the arms.
   (b) The patients repeats the same exercise while fixating a target on a mirror.

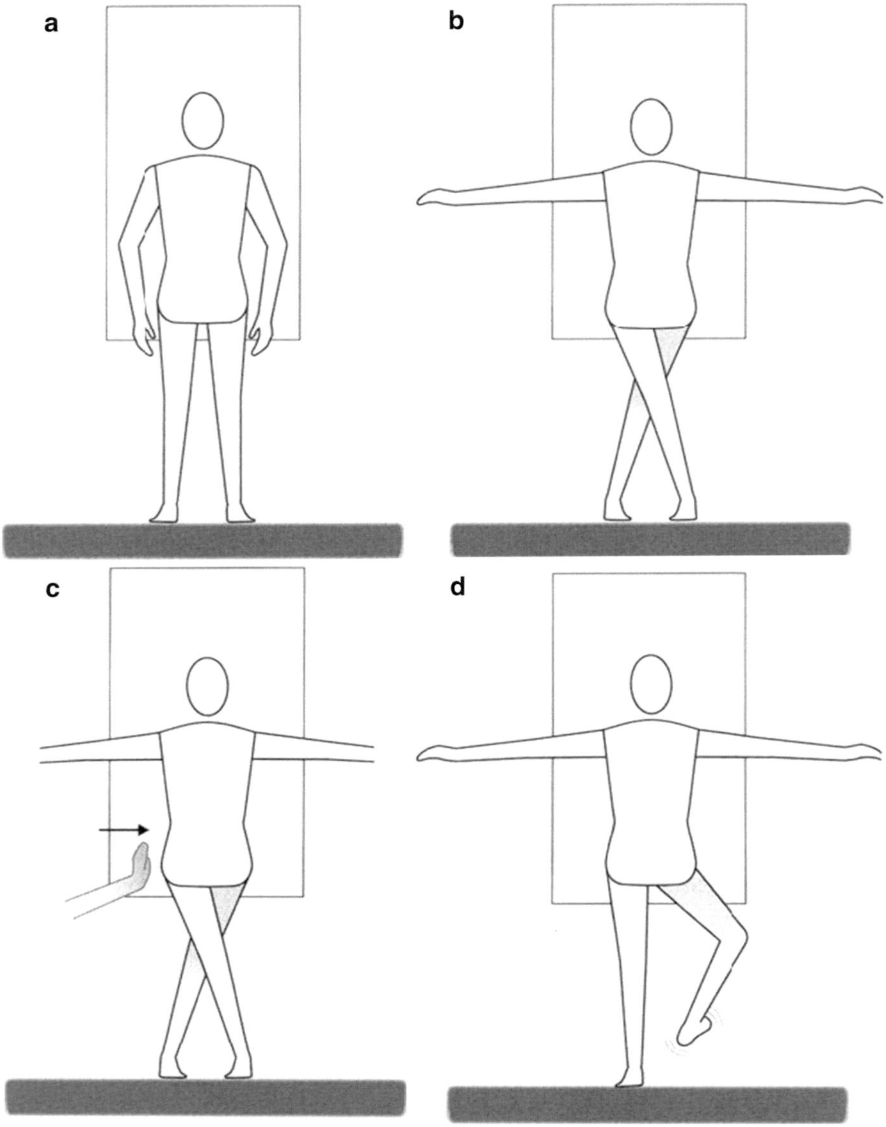

Fig. 14.11 (**a–d**) Equilibrium exercises on the mattress (Originally published in Cesarani and Alpini [14] published by Springer © 1999)

3. By visual feedback devices. The patient is stable on the stabilometric platform, without shoes, wearing pinhole glasses.
   (a) The patients moves her/his centre of gravity toward the targets (Fig. 14.14a, b).
   (b) The patient fixates a central target trying to maintain the CoG control during hyperventilation.

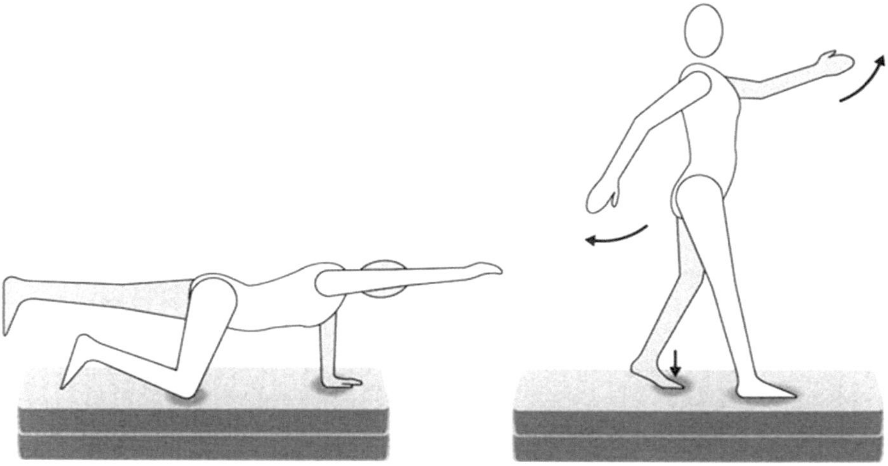

Fig. 14.12 Arm–leg synchronization on the mattress (Originally published in Cesarani and Alpini [14] published by Springer © 1999)

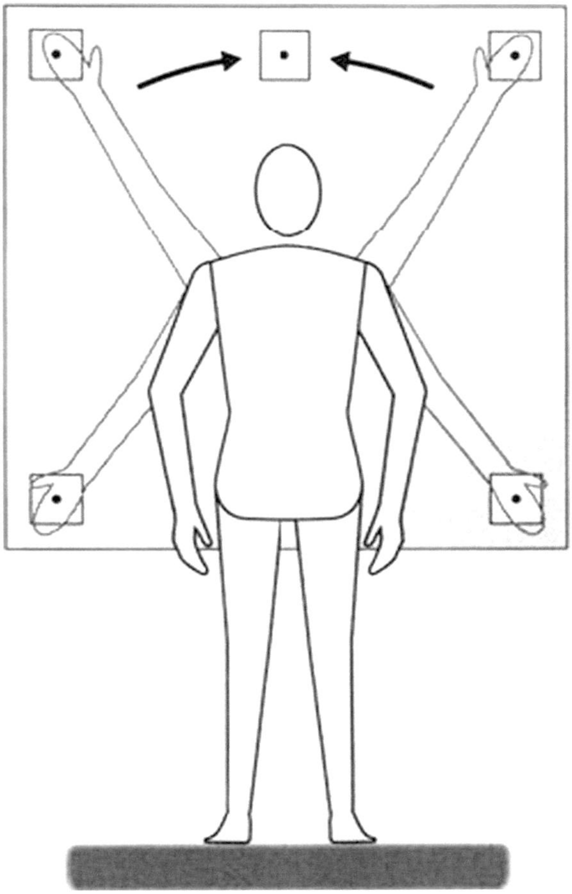

Fig. 14.13 Pointing to different targets on a mirror, standing on the mattress (Originally published in Cesarani and Alpini [14] published by Springer © 1999)

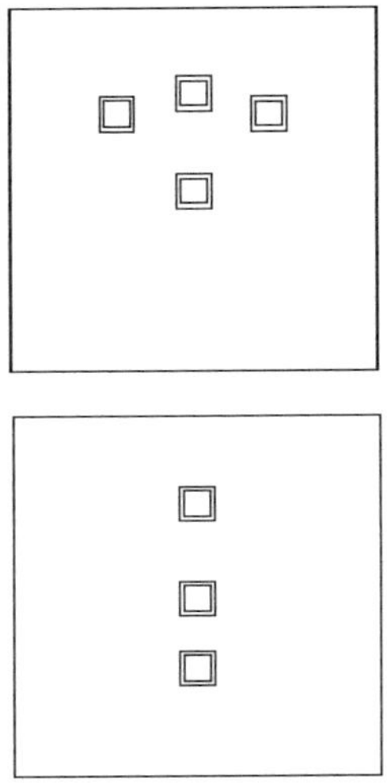

Fig. 14.14 Stabilometric visual feedback exercise performed wearing pinhole glasses. In (**a**) the exercise improves the latero-lateral control; in (**b**) it improves the anteroposterior control (Balance Master, reproduced with courtesy of NeuroCom International, Inc, Clackamas, Oregon, USA) (Originally published in Cesarani and Alpini [14] published by Springer © 1999)

14.2 Home Protocol

The exercises are subdivided according to different phases of equilibrium, passing from supine to standing to moving. In each phase, there is a progression from mechanic to synergetic exercises. Home exercises can never substitute for the therapeutic programmes shown in the previous section, performed with the therapist. Home exercises complete the therapeutic programme and maintain the results obtained.

Supine

1. Extend your left arm over your head and at the same time hold the flexed right leg to the chest, with the help of your hand. Maintain this position for 10 s and then repeat alternating the arm and leg.
2. Lift your left leg with the knee extended.
3. Lift your right leg with the knee extended.
4. Repeat with the tip of the foot outward.
5. Repeat with the tip of the foot inward.
6. Fixate a target on the ceiling and slowly move your head rightward and leftward.
7. Look for two equidistant targets on the ceiling and then fixate them alternately first moving only the eyes and then moving only the head.
8. From the supine position, shift to sitting position fixating a point sited on your left.
9. From the supine position, shift to sitting position fixating a point sited on your right.

Sitting

10. Extend your arms and lift your thumbs. Move your arms along a horizontal plane at about 50 cm from your eyes and then fixate your thumbs alternately. Begin slowly and then increase progressively the velocity of alternating the fixation.

11. Extend your arms and lift your thumbs. Move your arms along a vertical plane at about 50 cm from your eyes and then fixate your thumbs alternately. Begin slowly and then increase progressively the velocity of alternating the fixation.
12. Extend your right arm and lift your thumb. Move your arm slowly to and fro first in a horizontal direction and then in a vertical direction. Follow your thumb with your eyes only, first slowly and then increasing progressively the velocity of thumb displacement.
13. Repeat as above but at the same time also moving the head trying to keep the eyes still.
14. Move your head first slowly and then more rapidly in all directions fixating a target straight in front of you placed on a mirror.
15. Open a book in front of you. Read it while moving simultaneously right and left and then to and fro
16. Open a book in front of you. Move it away from you extending your arms. Read it. Then move it closer to you, slowly, trying to read it. Then move it away. Repeat several times to and fro.

Standing

17. Fixate a target placed on a mirror. Align your position correctly. Maintain equilibrium for 1 min and then close your eyes visualizing your correct position and remain in this position for at least 1 min.
18. Repeat the same exercise standing on a soft mattress.
19. Fixate a target placed on a mirror. Then oscillate to and fro and right and left, around your ankles keeping your pelvis still.
20. Fixate a target placed on a mirror; keeping your feet still, bend your trunk to and fro and right and left.
21. Repeat 19 and 20 standing on a soft mattress.
22. Open a book in front of you. Read it while moving simultaneously to and fro and right and left.
23. Repeat this exercise on a soft mattress.
24. Open a book in front of you. Move it away from you extending your arms. Read it. Then move it closer to you, slowly, trying to read it. Then move it away. Repeat several times to and fro.
25. Repeat on a soft mattress.

Moving

26. Walking, fixate a target placed on a mirror in front of you.
27. Walking, read a book.
28. Walking on a soft mattress, read a book.
29. Walk for five steps along a corridor forward and backward while fixating a target.
30. Walk for five steps along a corridor forward and backward moving your head to and fro, maintaining your fixation of a target.
31. Walk for five steps along a corridor forward and backward while reading a book.

After the first week of home treatment, the protocol will be reduced to the following exercises to be performed at least once a day: 12–15, 16–18, 19–20, 21–25 and 28–30

14.2.1 Counselling

It is important to pay attention to lifestyle and to usual daily activities.

The main suggestions are:

- To control own body mass index (BMI). BMI is correlated to body fat, and it is calculated as body weight (in kilos) divided by the square of the height (in metres); e.g. a subject weighing 70 kg and 1.74 m height has a BMI as follows: $70/(1.74\times1.74)=23.1$. Normal values are between 18.5 and 24.9 (World Health Organization, WHO)
- To maintain a diet rich of fruit and vegetables (five servings/day) especially in autumn and spring.
- To maintain adequate water intake (at least 1.5 l for females and 2 l for males) especially during warm season.
- To maintain adequate salt intake especially in the warm periods.
- To maintain a distributed supply along the day (five times a day).
- To avoid industrial food.
- To avoid white sugar, preferring for brown sugar and honey.
- To avoid alcohol and smoking and, obviously, to avoid drug abuse.
- To perform regular and constant aerobic physical activity: e.g. rapid walking (not running neither jogging) 30′/day three times/week
- To maintain regular sleep/awake cycles, sleeping at least 8 h/night starting before midnight. In some cases, supplementation with melatonin 3 or 5 mg 30 min before sleeping may be useful to maintain regular day/night cycles [13]
- To sleep using one or more pillows placed under the mattress in order to maintain both the head and the legs lifted about 20°.

References

1. Pappas DG Jr (2003) Autonomic related vertigo. Laryngoscope 113(10):1658–1671
2. Kim HA, Lee H (2014) Autonomic dysfunction as a possible cause of residual dizziness after successful treatment in benign paroxysmal positional vertigo. Clin Neurophysiol 125(3): 608–614. doi: 10.1016/j.clinph.2013.08.008
3. Doba N, Reis DJ (1974) Role of the cerebellum and the vestibular apparatus in regulation of orthostatic reflexes in the cat. Circ Res 40:9–18
4. Ray CA, Carter JR (2003) Vestibular activation of sympathetic nerve activity. Acta Physiol Scand 177(3):313–319
5. Carter JR, Ray CA (2008) Sympathetic responses to vestibular activation in humans. Am J Physiol Regul Integr Comp Physiol 294:R681–R688
6. Ray CA, Monahan KD (2002) Aging attenuates the vestibulosympathetic reflex in humans. Circulation 105:956–961

7. Ray CA, Hume KM, Steele SL (1998) Sympathetic nerve activity during natural stimulation of horizontal semicircular canals in humans. Am J Physiol Regul Integr Comp Physiol 275:R1274–R1278
8. Sauder CL, Leonard TO, Ray CA (2008) Greater sensitivity of the vestibulosympathetic reflex in the upright posture in humans. J Appl Physiol 105:65–69
9. Yates BJ (1996) Vestibular influences on the autonomic nervous system. Ann N Y Acad Sci 781:458–473
10. Carter JR, Ray CA, Cooke WH (2002) Vestibulosympathetic reflex during mental stress. JAppl Physiol (1985) 93:1260–1264
11. Fife TD, Giza C (2013) Posttraumatic vertigo and dizziness. Semin Neurol 33(3):238–243
12. Geoffrey Burwell RG, Aujla RK, Grevitt MP, Dangerfield PH, Moulton A, Randell TL, Anderson SI (2009) Pathogenesis of adolescent idiopathic scoliosis in girls – a double neuro-osseous theory involving disharmony between two nervous systems, somatic and autonomic expressed in the spine and trunk: possible dependency on sympathetic nervous system and hormones with implications for medical therapy. Scoliosis 4:24
13. Macchi MM, Bruce JN (2004) Human pineal physiology and functional significance of melatonin. Front Neuroendocrinol 25(3–4):177–195
14. Cesarani A, Alpini D) (1999) Vertigo and dizziness rehabilitation – the MCS method. Springer, Milan, Heidelberg

The Quantification of Rehabilitation Outcome

15

15.1 Introduction

Quantification of rehabilitation outcome is particularly important to evaluate efficacy and efficiency of rehab protocols. We have many times underlined the importance of distinguishing between lesion, impairment and disability and that human balance is mainly a behaviour rather than a complex function. Thus, it is possible that the adopted protocol is able to solve the impairment of that specific patient but not her/his specific disability nor her/his handicap. Sometimes it is not possible to completely solve the disability; thus in this case it is important to teach to the patient how to cope and how to manage her/his balance handicap.

On the basis of these considerations, also rehab outcome has to be planned in order to collect information about lesion–impairment–disability and the level of coping and/or management of the residual handicap. Furthermore, the outcome planning we propose is inspired by the same concept of efficacy and efficiency, that is to say, to collect the most useful information in the simplest way.

15.2 The Overall Impact of Balance Disturbances

The overall impact of balance disturbances, vertigo and/or dizziness and/or unsteadiness (VDU), can be quantified using questionnaires about activities of daily living (ADL) [1–5]. As with functional scales, there is a tendency to use different standards, depending on the type of lesion one aims to study. However, the usefulness of ADLQ estimations should not be underestimated. The clinician may well use this expertise to enhance the objective assessment of the patients. Basic activities of daily living (ADL) consist of activities that are performed daily, habitually and universally, such as dressing, bathing and eating (Table 15.1). In contrast, instrumental ADL require organization and planning and include such tasks as shopping, using transportation, preparing meals, handling finances, keeping the house and using a telephone. However, such estimations may be biased

D.C. Alpini et al., *Vertigo Rehabilitation Protocols*,

DOI 10.1007/978-3-319-05482-7_15, © Springer International Publishing Switzerland 2014

Table 15.1 Activities of daily living questionnaire (ADLQ)

Instructions: circle one number for each item
1. *Self-care activities*
A. Eating 0 = No problem 1 = Independent, but slow or some spills 2 = Needs help to cut or pour; spills often 3 = Must be fed most foods 9 = Doesn't know
B. Dressing 0 = No problem 1 = Independent, but slow or clumsy 2 = Wrong sequence; forgets items 3 = Needs help with dressing 9 = Doesn't know
C. Bathing 0 = No problem 1 = Bathes self, but needs to be reminded 2 = Bathes self with assistance 3 = Must be bathed by others 9 = Doesn't know
D. Elimination 0 = Goes to the bathroom independently 1 = Goes to the bathroom when reminded; some accidents 2 = Needs assistance for elimination 3 = Has no control over either bowel or bladder 9 = Doesn't know
E. Taking pills or medicine 0 = Remembers without help 1 = Remembers if dose is kept in a special place 2 = Needs spoken or written reminders 3 = Must be given medicine by others 9 = Does not take regular pills or medicine *OR* doesn't know
F. Interest in personal appearance 0 = Same as always 1 = Interested if going out, but not at home 2 = Allows self to be groomed or does so on request only 3 = Resists efforts of caretaker to clean and groom 9 = Doesn't know
2. *Household care*
A. Preparing meals, cooking 0 = Plans and prepares meals without difficulty 1 = Some cooking, but less than usual or less variety 2 = Gets food only if it has already been prepared 3 = Does nothing to prepare meals 9 = Never did this activity *OR* doesn't know B. Setting the table 0 = No problem

Table 15.1 (continued)

- 1 = Independent, but slow or clumsy
- 2 = Forgets items or puts them in the wrong place
- 3 = No longer does this activity
- 9 = Never did this activity *OR* doesn't know

C. Housekeeping
- 0 = Keeps house as usual
- 1 = Does at least half of his/her job
- 2 = Occasional dusting or small jobs
- 3 = No longer keeps house
- 9 = Never did this activity *OR* doesn't know

D. Home maintenance
- 0 = Does all tasks usual for him/her
- 1 = Does at least half of usual tasks
- 2 = Occasionally rakes or some other minor job
- 3 = No longer does any maintenance
- 9 = Never did this activity *OR* doesn't know

E. Home repairs
- 0 = Does all the usual repairs
- 1 = Does at least half of usual repairs
- 2 = Occasionally does minor repairs
- 3 = No longer does any repairs
- 9 = Never did this activity *OR* doesn't know

F. Laundry
- 0 = Does laundry as usual (same schedule, routine)
- 1 = Does laundry less frequently
- 2 = Does laundry only if reminded; leaves out detergent, steps
- 3 = No longer does laundry
- 9 = Never did this activity *OR* doesn't know

3. *Employment and recreation*

A. Employment
- 0 = Continues to work as usual
- 1 = Some mild problems with routine responsibilities
- 2 = Works at an easier job or part time; threatened with loss of job
- 3 = No longer works
- 9 = Never worked *OR* retired before illness *OR* doesn't know

B. Recreation
- 0 = Same as usual
- 1 = Engages in recreational activities less frequently
- 2 = Has lost some skills necessary for recreational activities (e.g. bridge, golfing); needs coaxing to participate
- 3 = No longer pursues recreational activities
- 9 = Never engaged in recreational activities *OR* doesn't know

C. Organizations
- 0 = Attends meetings; takes responsibilities as usual
- 1 = Attends less frequently
- 2 = Attends occasionally; has no major responsibilities
- 3 = No longer attends
- 9 = Never participated in organizations *OR* doesn't know

(continued)

Table 15.1 (continued)

D. Travel 0 = Same as usual 1 = Gets out if someone else drives 2 = Gets out in wheelchair 3 = Home or hospital bound 9 = Doesn't know
4. *Shopping and money*
A. Food shopping 0 = No problem 1 = Forgets items or buys unnecessary items 2 = Needs to be accompanied while shopping 3 = No longer does the shopping 9 = Never had responsibility in this activity *OR* doesn't know
B. Handling cash 0 = No problem 1 = Has difficulty paying proper amount, counting 2 = Loses or misplaces money 3 = No longer handles money 9 = Never had responsibility for this activity *OR* doesn't know
C. Managing finances 0 = No problem paying bills, banking 1 = Pays bills late; some trouble writing checks 2 = Forgets to pay bills; has trouble balancing checkbook; needs help from others 3 = No longer manages finances 9 = Never had responsibility in this activity *OR* doesn't know
5. *Travel*
A. Public transportation 0 = Uses public transportation as usual 1 = Uses public transportation less frequently 2 = Has gotten lost using public transportation 3 = No longer uses public transportation 9 = Never used public transportation regularly *OR* doesn't know
B. Driving 0 = Drives as usual 1 = Drives more cautiously 2 = Drives less carefully; has gotten lost while driving 3 = No longer drives 9 = Never drove *OR* doesn't know
C. Mobility around the neighbourhood 0 = Same as usual 1 = Goes out less frequently 2 = Has gotten lost in the immediate neighbourhood 3 = No longer goes out unaccompanied 9 = This activity has been restricted in the past *OR* Don't know
D. Travel outside familiar environment 0 = Same as usual 1 = Occasionally gets disoriented in strange surroundings 2 = Gets very disoriented but is able to manage if accompanied 3 = No longer able to travel 9 = Never did this activity *OR* doesn't know

Table 15.1 (continued)

6. *Communication*
A. Using the telephone 0 = Same as usual 1 = Calls a few familiar numbers 2 = Will only answer telephone (won't make calls) 3 = Does not use the telephone at all 9 = Never had a telephone *OR* doesn't know
B. Talking 0 = Same as usual 1 = Less talkative; has trouble thinking of words or names 2 = Makes occasional errors in speech 3 = Speech is almost unintelligible 9 = Doesn't know
C. Understanding 0 = Understands everything that is said as usual 1 = Asks for repetition 2 = Has trouble understanding conversations or specific words occasionally 3 = Does not understand what people are saying most of the time 9 = Doesn't know
D. Reading 0 = Same as usual 1 = Reads less frequently 2 = Has trouble understanding or remembering what he/she has read 3 = Has given up reading 9 = Never read much *OR* doesn't know
E. Writing 0 = Same as usual 1 = Writes less often; makes occasional spelling errors 2 = Signs name but no other writing 3 = Never writes 9 = Never wrote much *OR* doesn't know

Scoring:
For each section (e.g. self-care, household care, etc.), count the total number of questions answered (i.e. questions that are NOT rated as "9", doesn't know). Multiply the total number of questions answered by 3. This equals the total points possible for that section
Add up the total score (i.e. the sum of the responses) for that section and divide by the total points possible. Multiply by 100 to get the per cent impairment

and they cannot easily be quantified or documented for studies or evaluation of the effect of treatment.

ADLQ is as complete as time-expending for the requirements of balance control rehab outcome. *Visual Analogue Scale* (VAS) is the easiest way to quantify, on a decimal scale, the global impression of the patient about his/her global disturbance, that is to say, the overall impact of symptoms on patient's life [6–10].

15.3 The Quantification of Human Balance Control Lesion

Lesion may be quantified by means of a semi-subjective scale, the vestibular index, developed by Haid and Wigand [11] to quantify the impact of eighth nerve schwannoma on vestibular function (Table 15.2). All the main vestibular signs are represented. The examiner assigns a score ranging from 0 (normal or absent) to 4 (severely impaired) to each item. In this way the scale is semi-objective, and it allows quantification, but it is, obviously, examiner dependent. No inter-examiner validations have been performed. Anyway, vestibular index is still the unique published scale which specifically regards vestibular lesion. The original vestibular index has been slightly modified by the authors of this book in order to be better used for the scope of balance control rehab.

15.4 The Quantification of Human Balance Control Impairment

To get better objective estimations, several functional scales have been developed, generally designed for the study of a certain group of patients, thereby lacking the quality of general applicability.

Table 15.2 Vestibular index by Haid and Wigand [11]

Instructions: the examiner assigns a score ranging from 0 (normal or absent) to 4 (severely impaired) to each item	
Signs/symptoms	**Scoring**
Spontaneous vertigo or dizziness or unsteadiness	0 absent, 4 disabling vertigo
Positional or positioning vertigo/dizziness	0 absent, 1 one-side Hallpike or McClure manoeuvres, 2 Hallpike or McClure manoeuvre both sides, 3 Hallpike AND McClure manoeuvres, 4 head-hanging position
Gait unsteadiness	0 normal, 3 possible only with aid, 4 gait impossible
Spontaneous nystagmus	0 absent, 1 I degree¸ 2 II degree or gaze ny, 3 vertical ny, 4 multiple ny
Head shaking Ny	0 absent, 1 brief horizontal HS ny, 2 long-lasting horizontal or vertical HS ny, 3 horizontal AND vertical HS ny, 4 horizontal or vertical long-lasting and very symptomatic ny
Positional/positioning Ny Positional symptoms may be present with or without nystagmus	0 absent, 1 one-side Hallpike or McClure manoeuvre, 2 Hallpike or McClure manoeuvre both sides, 3 Hallpike AND McClure manoeuvres, 4 head-hanging position
Eye movements – saccades	0 normal, 1 hyper- or hypometric, 2 increased latency, 3 dissociated, 4 gaze palsy
Eye movements – smooth pursuit	0 normal, 1 irregular, 2 clearly impaired in the vertical plane but only irregular in the horizontal plane, 3 impaired in both planes, 4 horizontal cogwheel pursuit
Romberg test	0 normal, 1 slight deviation, 2 clear side deviation, 3 backward deviation, 4 stance impossible
Stepping test	0 normal, 1 lateral translation, 2 rotation until 45°, 3 rotation <45°, 4 ataxic gait
Total	

The *Timed Up and Go test* (*TUG*) may be considered a test which regards the patient's ability to manage position changing and thus acceleration managing. It is a simple test to assess a person's mobility because it uses the time that a person takes to rise from a chair, walk 3 m, turn around, walk back to the chair and sit down. During the test, the person is expected to wear their regular footwear and use any mobility aids that they would normally require The TUG is used frequently in the elderly population, as it is easy to administer and can generally be completed by most older adults. Scores of 10 s or less indicate normal mobility, 11–20 s are within normal limits for frail elderly and disabled patients and greater than 20 s means the person needs assistance outside and indicates further examination and intervention. A score of 14 s or more suggests that the person may be prone to falls. Alternatively, a recommended practical cut-off value for the TUG to indicate normal versus below normal performance is 12 s [12, 13].

TUG is well correlated to Berg Balance Scale Score. The *Berg Balance Scale* (*BBS*) is a widely used clinical test of a person's static and dynamic balance abilities. For functional balance tests, the BBS is generally considered to be the gold standard [14, 15]. The test takes 15–20 min and comprises a set of 14 simple balance related tasks, ranging from standing up from a sitting position to standing on one foot. The degree of success in achieving each task is given a score of zero (unable) to four (independent), and the final measure is the sum of all of the scores. The BBS has been shown to have excellent inter-rater (ICC = 0.98) and intra-rater reliability (ICC = 0.98) and is internally consistent (0.96). The BBS correlates satisfactorily with laboratory measures, including postural sway, and has good concurrent criterion, predictive criterion and construct validity. Considerable evidence indicates that the BBS is also a valid measure of standing balance in post-stroke patients, but only for those who ambulate independently, due to the tasks that are required of the patient.

Another well-known scale is the Tinetti scale. The *Tinetti test* (*TT*), or *Performance Oriented Mobility Assessment* (*POMA*), is a common clinical test for assessing a person's static and dynamic balance abilities. It is named after one of the inventors, Mary Tinetti et al. [16]. The test is in two short sections, one examining static balance abilities in a chair and then standing and the other examining the gait. The two sections are sometimes used as separate tests.

Some TUG aspects and Berg and Tinetti scale item measures the same functions. Thus, in 1997 Tesio et al. [17] validated a simplified combination of Berg and Tinetti scales in order to reduce time necessary to quantify static and dynamic balance. A preliminary 10-item version encompassed sit/stand manoeuvres, standing with eyes open and closed, standing with eyes closed and head extended, leaning forward while standing, picking up an object from floor, resisting nudges on the sternum, turning around and tandem stance. The Rasch analysis was adopted to explore the psychometric validity of the scale. Two items (stand-to-sit and standing with eyes open) were deleted, as they were too easy and thus uninformative. The remaining 8 items made up a scale (called *Equi-Scale*, Table 15.3) complying with the requirements of unidimensionality and reliability.

Table 15.3 Equi-Scale by Tesio et al. [17]

For each situation a different score is assigned on the basis of patient's balance abilities
I – from sitting to standing
2. patient is able to stand up without using the hands
1. patient is able to stand up, with difficulties, using her/his hands
0. patient needs examiner's help to stand up
II – standing with eyes closed and arms folded
2. patient is able to maintain stance for at least 20″
1. patient is able to maintain stance for at least 5″
0. patient maintains stance for less than 5″
III – standing with eyes closed, head backward and feet together
2. patient is able to maintain stance for at least 30″
1. patient is able to maintain stance for at least 10″
0. patient maintains stance for less than 10″
IV – pushing forward with the arms for 25 cm
Patient has to try to push forward with the arms extended to reach a target at 25 cm distance (the wall, the examiner's fingers, etc.) without moving the feet
2. patient is able to push forward for at least 25 cm
1. patient is able to push forward for at least 10 cm
0. patient is able to push forward for less than 25 cm
V – collecting an object from the ground
The object (e.g. a pen) is on the ground, about 30 cm from patient's feet
2. patient is able to collect the object at the first attempt
1. patient is able to collect the object after 1–2 attempts
0. patient is not able to collect the object
VI – thrusts
Patient has to maintain stance with feet together when the examiner pushes her/his sternum (3 times in 15′)
2. patient maintains stance without moving the feet
1. patient maintains stance but moving the feet
0. patient falls
VII – 360° rotation
Patient has to rotate completely, first rightward and then leftward
2. patient is able to rotate in both directions in less than 4″ each
1. patient is able to rotate in 4″ only in one direction or in both directions but in more than 4″
0. patient is not able to rotate
VIII – standing with feet in tandem position
Test is performed first with right foot forward and then with left foot forward
2. patient is able to maintain position for at least 15″ in both trials
1. patient is able to maintain position for at least 15″ in only one trial
1. patient is able to maintain position for at least 5″ in both trials
0. patient maintains position for less than 5″

15.5 The Quantification of Human Balance Control Disability

It is a fact that vertigo, dizziness and/or unsteadiness seriously impact on patient's quality of life. Thus the SF-36 could be the adequate instrument of measure. The SF-36 is a standardized questionnaire derived from a larger set of questions used in the US Medical Outcomes Study in the mid-1980s [18]. The SF-36 was designed for use in clinical practice and research, health policy evaluations and general population surveys. The SF-36 includes one multi-item scale that assesses eight health concepts: (1) limitations in physical activities because of health problems, (2) limitations in social activities because of physical or emotional problems, (3) limitations in usual role activities because of physical health problems, (4) bodily pain, (5) general mental health (psychological distress and well-being), (6) limitations in usual role activities because of emotional problems, (7) vitality (energy and fatigue) and (8) general health perceptions. The survey was constructed for self-administration by persons 14 years of age and older and for administration by a trained interviewer in person or by telephone. The history of the development of the SF-36, the origin of specific items and the logic underlying their selection are summarized. The content and features of the SF-36 are compared with the 20-item Medical Outcomes Study short form.

Self-reported health measures introduce an element of subjectivity into health status measurement. This is useful in providing a more "consumer-centred" view of health and places the measurement emphasis on quality of life or well-being. The SF-36 is a widely used questionnaire for measuring self-reported physical and mental health status but still little used in balance disturbances and vestibular rehab outcome measurements [19].

The SF-36® Health Survey requires an administration time of 5–10 min. The SF-36 also includes a single-item measure of health transition or change. The SF-36 can also be divided into two aggregate summary measures, the Physical Component Summary (PCS) and the Mental Component Summary (MCS). In the standard version of the SF-36, all scale questions refer to a 4-week time period. Answers to each question are scored. These scores are then summed to produce raw scale scores for each health concept which are then transformed to a 0–100 scale. Scoring algorithms can then be applied to produce the PCS and MCS scores.

In the field of balance disturbances and vestibular rehab, disability may be quantified in the easiest way by means of the Dizziness Handicap Inventory proposed by Jacobson and Newman [20] (Table 15.4). The 25-item Dizziness Handicap Inventory (DHI) was developed to evaluate the self-perceived handicapping effects imposed by vestibular system disease. The preliminary version included 37 items while the final versions 25 items. The items are subgrouped into three content domains representing functional, emotional and physical aspects of dizziness and unsteadiness. Cronbach's alpha coefficient was employed to measure reliability based on consistency of the preliminary version. The final version demonstrated good internal consistency reliability. Test–retest reliability is high. A DHI short form (13 items) has been developed by Tesio et al. [21] (Table 15.5) which measures the severity of self-reported balance deficits. The scale was constructed and validated by Rasch analysis. Rasch analysis was applied to rescore or remove any items that are misfitting, redundant or off-target, until an optimal instrument is obtained. The 25-item, 3-level Dizziness Handicap Inventory was, thus, reduced to the 13-item, 2-level DHIsf. The retained items explore the domains of eye–head movements, full body activities and mood alterations. The Rasch statistics showed that the 13 items evenly fitted a hierarchy of

Table 15.4 Dizziness Handicap Inventory, by Jacobson and Newman [20]

Instructions: the purpose of this scale is to identify difficulties that you may be experiencing *because of* your dizziness or unsteadiness. Please answer "yes", "no" or "sometimes" to each question. Answer each question as it pertains to your dizziness or unsteadiness problem only. Score is calculated as 2 (yes), 1 (sometimes) and 0 (no)
Does looking up increase your problem?
Because of your problem, do you feel frustrated?
Because of your problem, do you restrict your travel for business or recreation?
Does walking down the aisle of a supermarket increase your problem?
Because of your problem, do you have difficulty getting into or out of bed?
Does your problem significantly restrict your participation in social activities such as going out to dinner, going to movies, going dancing or going to parties?
Because of your problem, do you have difficulties in reading?
Does performing more ambitious activities like sports, dancing and household chores such as sweeping or putting dishes away increase your problem?
Because of your problem, are you afraid to leave your home without having someone accompany you?
Because of your problem, have you been embarrassed in front of others?
Do quick movements of your head increase your problem?
Because of your problem, do you avoid heights?
Does turning over in bed increase your problem?
Because of your problem, is it difficult for you to do strenuous housework or yardwork?
Because of your problem, are you afraid people may think you are intoxicated?
Because of your problem, is it difficult for you to go for a walk by yourself?
Does walking down a sidewalk increase your problem?
Because of your problem, is it difficult to concentrate?
Because of your problem, is it difficult for you to walk around your house in the dark?
Because of your problem, are you afraid to stay at home alone?
Because of your problem, do you feel handicapped?
Has your problem placed stress on your relationships with members of your family or friends?
Because of your problem, are you depressed?
Does your problem interfere with your job or household responsibilities?
Does bending over increase your problem?

Table 15.5 Dizziness Handicap Inventory short form By Tesio et al. [21]

Instructions: the purpose of this scale is to identify difficulties that you may be experiencing that can cause your dizziness or unsteadiness. Please answer "yes" or "no" to each question *even if* disturbances are caused by problems different from vertigo, dizziness and unsteadiness. Score is calculated as 1 (yes) or 0 (no)
Does looking up increase your symptoms?
Do you restrict your travel for business or recreation?
Do you have difficulty getting into or out of bed?
Do you have difficulties in reading?
Do quick movements of your head increase your problem?
Do you avoid heights?
Does turning over in bed increase your problem?
Is it difficult for you to go for a walk by yourself?
Does walking down a sidewalk increase your problem?
Is it difficult for you to walk around your house in the dark?
Are you afraid to stay at home alone?
Are you depressed?
Does bending over increase your problem?

difficulty within a homogeneous construct. The DHIsf compares favourably with the original Dizziness Handicap Inventory, shows some consistency with the instrumental findings and provides original information on the severity of imbalance syndromes, as it is seen from the patient's perspective (Table 15.4). The questions are not restricted to the patient's problem (vertigo and dizziness), but they investigate the patient as an entire person. For example it is possible that vertigo and dizziness don't cause difficulties in reading (answer "no" in DHI) but the patient may have a vision impaired for ophthalmological problems. In this way the correct answer in the DHIsf will be "yes" because, in every way, reading is difficult and impaired vision, for any cause, may impair balance.

15.6 Minimal Approach to Rehab Outcome

Despite the numerous available questionnaires and scales, in our experience, an effective and efficient approach to outcome measurement is based on:

- *VAS* as measurement of overall subjective impact of VDU
- *Vestibular index* as measurement of vestibular lesion
- *Equi-Scale* as measurement of balance impairment
- *DHIsf* as measurement of balance disturbances handicap

References

1. Dai CY, Huang YH, Chou LW, Wu SC, Wang RY, Lin LC (2013) Effects of primary caregiver participation in vestibular rehabilitation for unilateral neglect patients with right hemispheric stroke: a randomized controlled trial. Neuropsychiatr Dis Treat 9:477–484
2. Aratani MC, Perracini MR, Caovilla HH, Gazzola JM, Ganança MM, Ganança FF (2011) Disability rank in vestibular older adults. Geriatr Gerontol Int 11(1):50–54
3. Lee HJ, Choi-Kwon S (2009) Quality of life and the related factors in patients with dizziness. J Korean Acad Nurs 39(5):751–758
4. Kaya BK, Krebs DE, Riley PO (1998) Dynamic stability in elders: momentum control in locomotor ADL. J Gerontol A Biol Sci Med Sci 53(2):M126–M134
5. Cook CE, Richardson JK, Pietrobon R, Braga L, Silva HM, Turner D (2006) Validation of the NHANES ADL scale in a sample of patients with report of cervical pain: factor analysis, item response theory analysis, and line item validity. Disabil Rehabil 28(15): 929–935
6. Scholtz AW, Steindl R, Burchardi N, Bognar-Steinberg I, Baumann W (2012) Comparison of the therapeutic efficacy of a fixed low-dose combination of cinnarizine and dimenhydrinate with betahistine in vestibular neuritis: a randomized, double-blind, non-inferiority study. Clin Drug Investig 32(6):387–399
7. Morozetti PG, Ganança CF, Chiari BM (2011) Comparison of different protocols for vestibular rehabilitation in patients with peripheral vestibular disorders. J Soc Bras Fonoaudiol 23(1):44–50
8. Ricci NA, Aratani MC, Doná F, Macedo C, Caovilla HH, Ganança FF (2010) A systematic review about the effects of the vestibular rehabilitation in middle-age and older adults. Rev Bras Fisioter 14(5):361–371
9. Giray M, Kirazli Y, Karapolat H, Celebisoy N, Bilgen C, Kirazli T (2009) Short-term effects of vestibular rehabilitation in patients with chronic unilateral vestibular dysfunction: a randomized controlled study. Arch Phys Med Rehabil 90(8):1325–1331

10. Hansson EE, Månsson NO, Håkansson A (2004) Effects of specific rehabilitation for dizziness among patients in primary health care. A randomized controlled trial. Clin Rehabil 18(5): 558–565
11. Haid T, Wigand ME (1984) The vestibular index of patients with cochleo-vestibular insufficiency after neurolysis of the eighth cranial nerve. Acta Otolaryngol Suppl 406:275–277
12. Podsiadlo D, Richardson S (1991) The timed 'Up & Go': a test of basic functional mobility for frail elderly persons. J Am Geriatr Soc 39(2):142–148
13. Bischoff HA, Stähelin HB, Monsch AU, Iversen MD, Weyh A, von Dechend M, Akos R, Conzelmann M et al (2003) Identifying a cut-off point for normal mobility: a comparison of the timed 'up and go' test in community-dwelling and institutionalised elderly women. Age Ageing 32(3):315–320
14. Berg KO, Maki BE, Williams n, Holliday PI, Wood-Dauphinee SL (1992) Clinical and laboratory measures of postural balance in an elderly population. Arch Phys Med Rehabil 73:1073–1080
15. Downs S, Marquez J, Chiarelli P (2013) The Berg Balance Scale has high intra- and inter-rater reliability but absolute reliability varies across the scale: a systematic review. J Physiother 59(2):93
16. Tinetti ME, Williams TF, Mayewski R (1986) Fall risk index for elderly patients based on number of chronic disabilities. Am J Med 80(3):429–434
17. Tesio L, Perucca L, Franchignoni FP, Battaglia MA (1997) A short measure of balance in multiple sclerosis: validation through Rasch analysis. Funct Neurol 12(5):255–265
18. Ware JE Jr, Sherbourne CD (1992) The MOS 36-item short-form health survey (SF-36). I. Conceptual framework and item selection. Med Care 30(6):473–483
19. Lorin P, Manceau C, Foubert F (2010) Effect of vestibular neuritis on postural control using wavelets and fractal analysis. Rev Laryngol Otol Rhinol (Bord) 131(4–5):235–241
20. Jacobson GP, Newman CW (1990) The development of the Dizziness Handicap Inventory. Arch Otolaryngol Head Neck Surg 116(4):424–427
21. Tesio L, Alpini D, Cesarani A, Perucca L (1999) Short form of the Dizziness Handicap Inventory: construction and validation through Rasch analysis. Am J Phys Med Rehabil 78(3):233–241

Index

D.C. Alpini et al., *Vertigo Rehabilitation Protocols*,
DOI 10.1007/978-3-319-05482-7, © Springer International Publishing Switzerland 2014

T

U

V

MIX
Papier aus verantwortungsvollen Quellen
Paper from responsible sources
FSC® C105338

If you have any concerns about our products,
you can contact us on
ProductSafety@springernature.com

In case Publisher is established outside the EU,
the EU authorized representative is:
Springer Nature Customer Service Center GmbH
Europaplatz 3, 69115 Heidelberg, Germany

Printed by Libri Plureos GmbH
in Hamburg, Germany